The Conscious Anatomy

Healing the Real You

By Case Adams, Ph.D.

The Conscious Anatomy: Healing the Real You

LOGICAL BOOKS
http://www.logicalbooks.org

Printed in USA
Front cover art by Sebastian Kaulitzki
Back cover "Vitruvian Man" with notes, by Leonardo da Vinci, est. 1487

Publishers Cataloging in Publication Data
Adams, Case
The Conscious Anatomy: Healing the Real You
First Edition
1. Health. 2. Medicine
   Bibliography and References; Index

Library of Congress Control Number: 2009904971

Paperback ISBN 978-0-9816045-7-2
Ebook ISBN 978-1-936251-03-2

OTHER BOOKS BY THE AUTHOR:

ARTHRITIS SOLVED NATURALLY: The Real Causes and Natural Strategies for Rheumatoid Arthritis, Osteoarthritis, Gout and Other Forms of Arthritis

ASTHMA SOLVED NATURALLY: The Surprising Underlying Causes and Hundreds of Natural Strategies to Beat Asthma

BOOSTING THE IMMUNE SYSTEM: Natural Strategies to Supercharge our Body's Immunity

BREATHING TO HEAL: The Science of Healthy Respiration

DEPRESSION AND ANXIETY SOLVED NATURALLY: The Science for Relief of Mood Disorders with Dozens of Proven Natural Strategies

DIABETES SOLVED NATURALLY: Discovering the Causes, and the Foods, Herbs and Natural Strategies for Type 1 and Type 2 Diabetes

ELECTROMAGNETIC HEALTH: Making Sense of the Research and Practical Solutions for Electromagnetic Fields (EMF) and Radio Frequencies (RF)

HAY FEVER AND ALLERGIES: Discovering the Real Culprits and Natural Solutions for Reversing Allergic Rhinitis

HEALING WITH LIGHT: The Science of Natural Light Therapy

HEALING WITH SOUND: The Science of Sound Therapy

HEALTHY SUN: Healing with Sunshine and the Myths about Skin Cancer

HEARTBURN SOLVED: The Real Causes and How to Reverse Acid Reflux and GERD Naturally

HOLISTIC REMEDIES FOR ALZHEIMER'S: Natural Strategies to Avoid or Combat Dementia

MUCOSAL MEMBRANE HEALTH: The Key to Preventing Inflammatory Conditions, Infections, Toxicity and Degeneration

NATURAL CANCER SCIENCE: The Evidence for Diets, Herbs, Superfoods, and Other Natural Strategies that Fight Cancer

NATURAL SLEEP SOLUTIONS FOR INSOMNIA: The Science of Sleep, Dreaming, and Nature's Sleep Remedies

NATURAL SOLUTIONS FOR FOOD ALLERGIES AND FOOD INTOLERANCES: Scientifically Proven Remedies for Food Sensitivities

ORAL PROBIOTICS: Fighting Tooth Decay, Periodontal Disease and Airway Infections Using Nature's Friendly Bacteria

PROBIOTICS: Protection Against Infection

PROBIOTICS SIMPLIFIED: How Nature's Tiny Warriors Keep Us Healthy

PROVING HOMEOPATHY: Why Homeopathy Works, Sometimes

PURE WATER: The Science of Water, Waves, Water Pollution, Water Treatment, Water Therapy and Water Ecology

THE ANCESTORS DIET: Living and Cultured Foods to Extend Life, Prevent Disease and Lose Weight

THE GLUTEN CURE: Scientifically Proven Natural Solutions to Celiac Disease and Gluten Sensitivities

THE HEALTHY BACK: Strategies for Low Back Pain (Course)

THE LIVING CLEANSE: Detoxification and Cleansing Using Living Foods and Safe Natural Strategies

THE MEANING OF DREAMS: The Science of Why We Dream, How to Interpret Them and How to Steer Them

THE SCIENCE OF LEAKY GUT SYNDROME: Intestinal Permeability and Digestive Health

TOTAL HARMONIC: The Healing Power of Nature's Elements

YOUR PLAN FOR LIFE: Personal Strategic Planning for Humans

Table of Contents

Introduction

We humans walk the earth with extravagant certainty and ownership. We assume we are the most advanced race. We assume we are the most intelligent. We assume our eyes are equipped to see everything, and if we do not see it, it must not exist.

We seem oblivious to the relationship between our biochemistry and life itself. We should know that chemicals are not conscious. This can be empirically proven simply by extracting functional biochemicals from a conscious living organism. Once extracted and isolated, there is no life left in those chemicals. They will lie purposeless in the Petri dish.

We must therefore begin the journey of not only distinguishing between matter and life, but also understanding how life is animating and moving within matter. Once we can see the role of consciousness and how it intertwines with matter, we can purposefully determine how to pursue a healthy relationship between our consciousness and the physical world that exists around us.

In recent history, humankind has invested significant time, money and other precious resources into probing the body's anatomy to find what makes the body "tick." Humankind's relatively impressive technologies have still offered only shadowy surface views of a technology vastly superior to any we have yet been able to imagine, let alone devise. The synchronization between genes and cells; the immaculate yet flexible timing of the body's clockworks; and the amazing scanning identification systems resident within the body's immune system are engineering feats beyond comprehension.

Even with our technologies, humans are still debating what drives the body's technologies. Within a mechanical view, its cellular, genetic, tissue, probiotic and organ systems have been disconnected from the goals and aspirations evident from consciousness. Science has instead proposed an accidental process of chaotic evolution from molecule to humankind.

Yet the responses and activities of living systems do not indicate chaotic behavior. Consciousness implies goal-oriented behavior, and goal-orientation contradicts chaos. Quite simply, consciousness and chaos are contradictory terms. This fact has been illustrated by thirty years of random event generator research performed and confirmed by scientists with impeccable credentials and methodologies. REG research showed that conscious intention can be transmitted through events previously considered random. These studies also revealed that element western science has conveniently chosen to ignore over the past few centuries of research: The element of consciousness.

The conscious element has been complicated by the plethora of alternative health literature of recent years. A lot of vague jargon has been thrown about regarding "body, mind and spirit." As are many words utilized in the "new age" lexicon, the practical elements behind these words lie undefined, undisclosed, and quite frankly, nebulous. Loose terms such as *"vibration," "energy-healing,"* and *"channeling"* come to mind among others. These have inherited a new context and vernacular, along with a mass rejection by the modern scientific world as being *"pseudoscience."*

This rejection is probably not ostentatious. Still, in reality modern science and western medicine provide little if any explanation or acceptance for the role of consciousness within the body aside from the admittance of the *placebo effect* or the positive role the family has in the healing process. These are obviously the effects of consciousness, yet science has provided no suitable explanation for its existence within the living organism, let alone its effects upon the health of the organism.

The primary view provided by medical schools into the human body comes through the lenses of pharmacology and diagnostic technologies, in principle not unlike the crude instrumentation utilized in Hooke's microscope. This view of the body from a perspective of brute mechanics, Newtonian physics and even quantum physics provides little explanation for the living forces within the body.

We might compare this to the perspective of a car mechanic. The mechanic can get under the car and find the brakes low or the timing off. He would be shortsighted, however, if he did not realize the role the driver played in the causation of the problem. The car certainly did not drive itself. Rather, the car was driven by a conscious person who interacted with the car through its steering wheel, accelerator and brakes. Two cars by the same manufacturer, for example, might appear identical when driven off the lot, but their future failures depend largely upon the decisions and actions of each individual driver as they drove their cars.

The purpose of this book is to reconcile the mechanical elements of the body with the conscious aspects of its driving forces. This will be done by probing the functions of the body together with the science illustrating the effects of individual consciousness. To arrive at some clarity, a combination of the latest scientific research is presented together with the wisdom of the ancients. This should provide us with a revised and clarified view of the design of the energetic human anatomy.

This conscious view of the human anatomy opens to us a new doorway of awareness. By viewing the human anatomy within the 'scope' of consciousness, we become freed of many of the incongruities existing within medical science relating to issues of addiction, pain and death.

I hope the reader will gain from this information as much as I have.

Chapter One

The Intentional Body

The Pulse of Consciousness

The human organism cycles through life with a series of pulsating, resonating and mostly harmonious rhythms—in much the same way multiple musicians might play a song with different instruments playing a variety of melodies: Each instrument might have a different sound, yet together they produce a harmonious song. While our hearts typically beat fifty to eighty times per minute to distribute blood, our lungs pull in oxygen and push out carbon dioxide at roughly fifteen to twenty times per minute. Meanwhile, four cranial ventricles pump cerebral spinal fluid through our brains at eight to fifteen times per minute, while periodic skeletal muscle contractions squeeze lymphatic vessels to pump fluid throughout the lymph system. Larger cycles orchestrate through periodic hormone cycles: Puberty sets in at eleven to twelve years. Ovulation in women cycles in twenty-eight to thirty days. Menopause enters the cycle at about forty-five to fifty years. Men of course have their own cycles revolving around testosterone. Interspersed within these cycles are various metabolic functions marching to synchronized clockworks. For example, the Krebs and other energy cycles are driven by respiration rhythms and glucose levels. Thermoregulation cycles are driven by thyroid hormones in sync with sleep patterns and brainwaves. Blood sugar levels are regulated by insulin and eating cycles. Inflammation pathways are driven by plasmin factors regulated by corticosteroids. Energy and sleep rhythms cycle with alternating melatonin and cortisol secretions. Digestion cycles with peristalsis, the vagus nerve, digestive enzymes and probiotic colonies. Mood rhythms are driven by serotonin and dopamine fluctuations. Nerve pulses cycle with neurotransmitter chemistry. And the cells cycle with hormone stimulation in process with weak electromagnetic pulses.

The physical body is moving in a constant orchestrated rhythm. Here we will illustrate that the body's rhythms not only connect with the larger clockworks of the sun, earth and nature, but they also interact with and rely upon conscious intention.

The research on the human body performed over the past few decades by dedicated scientists has unveiled a physiology precisely tuned and connected to the physical universe through a variety of *waveform conductors*. The waveforms provide information, while the conductors translate and carry the information through the body. The body's primary conductors are the senses and sensory nerves. The sensory system conducts waveforms from the outside world into the body's command centers—effectively bridging the physical world with consciousness.

Information Circuits

On first impression, the functioning of the body uncovers a similarity to an electrical appliance. An electrical appliance serves a practical purpose by converting current into a physical operation. To access the current, the appliance must be connected to an electrical circuit. It must have an electrical cord or other wire channel designed to access the circuit. This usually comes in the form of an outlet plug and wire, which will plug into an outlet of a house circuit. The wire serves as a *channel* into the appliance, connecting the circuit to the appliance.

However, the capacity, resistance and conductance of the appliance must match the amperage and voltage specifications of the circuit from which it draws its electricity. For example, a home circuit in the United States will circulate 110 volts of alternating current (other countries will range—for Australia it is 120 volts). The voltage is the amount of potential power, or power pressure available. An appliance draws current in amps, based upon the wattage potential of the appliance.

A circuit consists of a closed loop of current running from one terminal point to another through appropriate grade wiring, together with the various switches, fuses, resistors and grounding mechanisms. The utility power grid is a network of electrical circuits connecting houses to power generating facilities. This is also a circuit—albeit a larger one. Once power is delivered from the grid to a house, it is led into a number of smaller circuits—each distributing power into the different regions of the house. Each circuit is opened and closed with a circuit breaker wired into a main panel: The current for each circuit travels from the distribution panel through that area of the house and then back to the panel. Outlets and switches are linked in to allow the circuit of electrical current to link to the electrical appliances. Assuming the appliance has the right capacity, resistance and conductance; it will bring in and modulate this incoming electricity into the specific pulses needed to drive its particular equipment.

Now if an appliance set up for 12 volts of direct current were connected to 110-volt circuit of alternating current, it would probably fry from being overwhelmed with power. Conversely, an appliance designed for 240 volts connected to a 110-volt circuit would not even run. The capacity of the appliance must meet the output of the circuit.

For simplicity-sake, scientists explain electricity as the movement of electrons through a conducting mechanism like copper. This Newtonian physics view has been proven limited over the past 150 years. In reality, electricity is an *electromagnetic waveform.* Most currents conduct in a sine-oriented waveform that has both electrical and magnetic characteristics. Furthermore, an alternating current's waveforms have alternating motion—moving in one direction for a time before moving in the opposite direction for the same period of time.

Electricity contains a repeating and consistent pulse because a current is rhythmic. This pulsing rhythm is the increase and decrease of power potential—a consistent series of power surges. As this surging in power potential is graphed against time, a consistent waveform becomes apparent. Prior to the quantum understanding of electricity as a waveform, this pulsing or surging was visualized as tiny little units of matter called electrons. Further physics research gradually made scientists aware that electricity was quite a bit more complex than little balls of current.

The pulse of electricity is complicated by its magnetic field. The magnetic field also pulses, but it pulses in a direction perpendicular to the motion of the electricity pulse, affecting its local environment with magnetism. For this reason, wires that carry electricity are double-stranded and shielded. The double stranding allows the magnetic fields to cancel each other, while the shielding prevents leakage of current. These strategies effectively prevent the alternating current in most home installations and appliance wires from spraying their magnetic fields around the room.

If the waveform current were to surge inconsistently, the appliance may become damaged in some way. Spikes in electrical current often occur during a lightning storm or power interruption. To avoid these surges, circuit breakers and surge protectors are often installed into the house circuit. Without a good surge protector, there is a good chance the circuits of computers and other sensitive appliances will be fried by power surges.

Most appliances also contain their own miniature circuits. Electricity will be filtered through these appliance circuits using a series of resistors, transistors and capacitors. Most of today's appliances use integrated circuits to bring a greater number of resisters and transistors together into a single compact chip. These are designed to modify the waveform qualities of the current, and translate them into the waveform requirements of the appliance. The integrated circuit is thus designed to modulate and translate waveforms from one type to another. Digital appliances convert alternating current into a series of pulsed digital waveforms using integrated circuitry. These digital waveforms contain unique patterns, which create the programming instructions (often called machine code) to operate the appliance. Meanwhile, power will also be channeled directly into the hardware of the appliance, to give it the power to execute the operation physically.

An appliance may also bring other waveforms. A radio or television will use an antenna and a receiver to channel in broadcasted radiowaves moving through the air. For this reason, most radios and televisions have tuners that focus their receivers into particular waveform frequencies. Once received, these waveforms will have to be modulated and converted as they are brought into the appliance. Once the waveforms are crystallized, integrated circuits will convert those waveforms into digital pulses. These digital pulses are converted into informational pulses that drive the speakers and/or screen—giving sight and sound to televisions and radios.

The majority of modern electrical circuits are conducted through copper because copper is a good conductor of electrical potential. Copper is by far the most prevalent metal used in wiring systems also because of its stability under changing electric loads. This stability makes it less likely to cause a fire. Aluminum was popular for wiring in decades past. However because aluminum is not as stable as copper under a load, electrical fires were found to be more prevalent in aluminum-wired households. For good reason, insurance companies now prefer copper wiring.

Other types of substances are considered partial conductors of electrical potential. In other words, they allow for only a muted or partial transmission of electricity: These are called *semiconductors.* Most natural semiconductors have a crystalline structure such as silicone or germanium—whose crystal structure compares to a diamond. Other compounded elements like indium phosphide are also used to provide specific semiconductance. Silicone is probably the most popular semiconductor used today, primarily because of its relatively low cost.

We must not ignore one of the most essential elements of the receiving electronic appliance and circuitry, however: The ultimate observer of the information. For a television, computer or radio, this would be the person listening or watching the information, and ultimately responding to it. Without such a conscious person, the circuitry would be quite meaningless, yes? Once the conscious observer receives the translated information through the circuitry of the appliance, there is a natural response. This response is usually accommodated with particular tuning devices that adjust, compensate or allow a response to the information.

The appliance of the human body also takes in and modulates waveforms in much the same way a computer, radio or television appliance does. While the circuitry is infinitely more complex, the human body indeed utilizes a variety of circuitry and biochemistry to conduct and translate information and intelligence into specific physical operations. The crystals used by early radio receivers and the various semiconductor materials used in today's digital devices provide the same process that particular biochemicals provide in the body. The senses and their specialized cells receive transmitted waveforms much the same way a radio or television antenna and receiver does. Once received, these waveforms are converted and translated from the electromagnetic spectrum into informational waveforms suitable for transmission within the circuitry of the body. These converted waveforms are transmitted through a vast array of cells and biochemicals on their way towards a conscious observer. Once the conscious observer within reviews the transmitted information, the conscious observer responds. The type of response given depends on the particular intentions and desires of the observer.

The response by the observer also utilizes specialized cells to accommodate and/or respond to the information transmitted. These responses of the observer are then transmitted through the circuitry of the body. The hormones, proteins, neurotransmitters, enzymes and DNA all act as crystals or semiconductors to convert and transmit this information, ultimately converting intention to waveform pulses and then physical action.

The connection between electricity and the body was established in 1937. Harold Saxton Burr, Ph.D. and Professor of Anatomy at Yale University's School of Medicine, began his research on what he described as living organisms' *bio-magnetic field.* Later he named these fields *L-fields,* or *fields of life.* Dr. Burr believed the electromagnetic property of living tissue provided its "organizing principle." This, he thought, prevented the cell from descending into chaos. Dr. Burr also established that physical disease in a living organism is preceded by particular electromagnetic changes.

To establish living organisms' electromagnetic properties, Burr developed an instrument and measurement system sensitive to very weak electromagnetic waveforms. Through his observations with his specialized equipment, he concluded that living organisms conducted and resisted electricity in the 10^{-6} volts range—small enough to be called *microvolts.*

In one trial, using his specially designed microvolt meters with transistors, Dr. Burr suspended salamander eggs into a saline solution. To screen out the potential galvanic action of the solution, Dr. Burr inserted minimizing silver nitrate electrodes between the microvolt meter probe and the saline. He also set up a spinning disc with a measurable sinusoidal voltage waveform, which allowed him to establish a net increase in voltage when the egg was added. This design allowed Dr. Burr to accurately measure any subtle changes in electronic potentials. To provide some controls, Dr. Burr also tested and compared electric potentials of salamander unfertilized eggs. The results were compared with the readings of fertilized eggs and salamanders immediately after hatching. Using a control group of about 100 eggs, Dr. Burr's testing provided clear evidence that the salamander eggs possessed electromagnetic circuitry. Furthermore, he established that the eggs exhibited increasing levels of electromagnetic energy as the eggs matured.

Dr. Burr also discovered that a particular point on the equator of the eggs had a higher voltage than anywhere else on the egg. Points 180 degrees from that point on its equator had a significantly lower voltage. As the eggs matured and hatched it became evident the higher voltage points corresponded with the salamander's head and the lowest voltage points corresponded with the salamander's tail. Dr. Burr duplicated these results with frogs' eggs and chick embryos. It became evident that a voltage circuit occurred along the alignment of the body's nervous system, with the greatest voltage differential occurring between the top and the bottom of the spine.

Dr. Burr's studies with the living bioelectrical field expanded into diverse areas in the following decades. He published or contributed to nearly one hundred scientific papers on the subject. One of the more fascinating studies Dr. Burr conducted was on the relationship between disease and the bioelectric field. Here he discovered that within about two weeks of contracting cancer, mice would experience an abnormal spiking of their bioelectric field. Confirmed with over 10,000 measurements, it became obvious that most organisms emit a bioelectric surge in advance of contracting disease (Burr 1938).

Another notable result from Dr. Burr's research on various animals and humans was the observation of abnormal bioelectric voltage changes during episodes of metabolic stress. For example, notable voltage changes were observed during wound healing, ovulation, drug use, and a variety of illnesses (Burr 1936; Burr 1937; Burr 1972).

The nervous system is not the only bio-electromagnetic system of the body. The entire body contains multiple circuits and conducting mechanisms. This has gradually become apparent to mainstream science with the discoveries of a multitude of various types of *ion channels.* These are tiny *gateways* lying within cell membranes, typically consisting primarily of proteins. These primarily protein channels reside within the phospholipid cell membranes. They provide the primary passageways through which the cell's electronic balance is established. The gates themselves are stimulated through voltage potential changes, which can take place through the conductance of minerals such as sodium, calcium, magnesium, potassium and others.

Voltage potentials are negotiated through these ion channel gateways. As a gateway is stimulated with a particular ion waveform, it will open or close, conducting particular information into the cell. The process compares favorably to the opening of an electrical circuit to power an appliance. Just as electrical impulses are transmitted through intelligent (including manual) switching to open the circuits within an electric appliance, ion channel gates within the body are stimulated to open or close by informational signals, spurring the channel to conduct information. This means that particular ion polarities affect the gates to open or close. These polarities are networked to provide pathways or circuits for informational messaging.

The metabolic importance of these channels throughout the body cannot be overstated. Should any of these channels fail to respond or react to a particular voltage parameter, or should they close or open at the wrong times, signaling cells to shut down or perhaps signal the wrong action—the body would begin to breakdown.

Ion channels networks function very similarly to circuit breakers, resistors and capacitors. They are the gateways for the informational currents running through our body. Just as copper conducts electricity through our house wiring systems, the various mineral ions like calcium, sodium, potassium and others conduct information and energy through our bodies. They provide the means through which electromagnetic information is passed from one part of the body to the other. Some circuits are conducted through a network of neuron cells tied together with ion channels. These linked neurons create the pipelines we call nerves. Nerves utilize ion channels to pass a particular piece of information—a particular waveform or waveform collection—from neuron to neuron.

Ions, however, provide only a subsystem of many levels of bio-conductance. Other complex molecules such as enzymes and proteins facilitate a macro-molecular exchange of electromagnetic information throughout the body. Like integrated circuits, each cell, from membrane to cytoplasm to nucleus and organelles—all act to conduct, resist, transist and provide instructional coding for all the body's operations.

The body conducts complex information through the broadcasting mechanisms of hormones and neurotransmitters. Hormones and neurotransmitters both fall within a grouping of specialized proteins called *ligands*. Ligands have molecular structures that transfer unique waveform combinations. These unique waveform combinations provide specific information. Information is transmitted from ligands to specialized gateway channel biomolecules called *receptors*. Within the body are innumerable types of receptors and ligands, equipped to send and receive different sorts of information. Receptors are very similar to ion channels. Like ion channels, they respond to the specific waveform nature of specific ligand messengers. Similar to ion channel gateways, receptors have several optional responses. These depend upon the ligand signal. Ligand signals can switch on an activity within a cell, discontinue an activity, or significantly alter an activity.

For example, on the surface of most cells are insulin receptors. These will respond to the information communicated via the (ligand) hormone insulin. As part of a vast array of mechanisms including glucose reception and surtuin instigation, insulin receptors are stimulated and 'switched on' by insulin. When insulin receptors are switched on, the cell becomes receptive to glucose. This will allow the cell to readily absorb glucose molecules for energy utilization. Should the insulin receptors become altered over time from surging insulin levels, the receptors can become less sensitive to switching on from insulin. This insensitivity can contribute to the condition of adult-onset diabetes—which is now increasingly being seen among children due to glucose sweetener overload. As a strategy to prevent the surging of insulin into the bloodstream, high fiber foods can be eaten with every meal. These high fibers slow the absorption of glucose into the bloodstream—giving the blood somewhat of a timed release of glucose and insulin (as nature intended). This timed release of insulin and glucose will over time increase the sensitivity of insulin and glucose receptors, thereby providing efficient entry and use of glucose.

Innumerable ligand-receptor transmission circuits conduct information throughout the body. These range from thyroid hormones, growth hormones, cortisol, melatonin, dopamine, serotonin, epinephrine, and so many others. Some ligands communicate specific instructions to cells from endocrine command centers, while others facilitate cell-to-cell communication. Neurotransmitters are examples of the latter. Through neurotransmitters, particular waveforms are transmitted from nerve cell to nerve cell. Neurotransmitters and hormones are functionally the same in that they broadcast messages. However, hormones tend to broadcast a tighter range of instructions. Neurotransmitters appear to have a broader range of informational transmission.

Hormones and neurotransmitters are extremely complex biochemical molecules. Most are proteins, consisting of hundreds of amino acids joined with other elements. We might compare them to miniature radio stations because they will broadcast received information, while filtering and even sometimes distorting the information to fit their particular design and situation. Within each hormone or neurotransmitter lie semiconductors and integrated circuits. They also have their own broadcasting beacons—the ligand portion of the molecule. These ligand portions conduct electromagnetic information. Prior to conductance, information is modulated, filtered or regulated as it is processed through the molecule. This translation function gives these molecules tremendous power within the body. Incidentally, these larger biomolecules are often crystalline with helical or spiral shapes. This would compare favorably with some of our semiconductor crystals such as silicon and germanium.

The complexity of these *bio-semiconductors* reflects the programming involved within the various circuits of the body. Digital appliances use a system of 1s and 0s compiled together into bytes, which translate information. The on and off gateway states of ion channels, hormones and neurotransmitters create groups of on-off states. These provide complex instructions in the same way a gathering of computer bytes can provide a machine with complex instructions.

Consider again the pulsing—the rise and fall—of a waveform. An on state would be the equivalent of the peak of the wave, and the off state would be considered to be its trough. As different waveforms *interfere* with each other, they can form a particular pattern, depending upon the waveforms that collided. This collection of combined waveforms provides a type of information unit, comparable to the byte.

As computers have progressed, their byte length systems have increased. Only a couple of decades ago, computer processing programs worked on an 8-bit byte. This meant that a combination of eight 1s or 0s could fit within a particular byte. Certainly there is a limitation in the combinations of 1s and 0s in an 8-bit byte. Today most personal computers communicate on a 32-bit byte, and some run with 64-bit or even 132-bit. This increases the productivity of the computer by requiring fewer bytes to conduct more complex information.

The intersection of multiple waveforms creates a platform for information exchange within their *interference patterns*. This allows for an almost limitless opportunity for possible patterns and complexity. Suffice to say that our bodies are not limited to the 8 or even 132-bit combinations. In the body there are also multifarious gateway switches at different levels, with a multiplex of variances at any level. Comparing the 1s and 0s on-off states of digital processing with the body's gateway states is like comparing checkers with three-dimensional chess—multiplied by a billion-fold.

The electrical nature of the body was illuminated by the controversial work of Russian researcher Semyon Kirlian. In 1917, Kirlian attended a presentation by Nikola Tesla, who at the time was experimenting with a new phenomenon called corona discharge. Working as an electrical equipment technician at the time, Kirlian noticed a light flash between an electrotherapy apparatus and a patient's skin. This gave Kirlian another type of flash. For the next few years, he and his wife Valentina worked to develop an oscillating generator. This allowed an observer to look through an optical filter at the electrical activity arising from the skin's surface. This is dramatically similar to the sun's coronal effect as seen during an eclipse or through telescopic equipment.

The ability to photograph the body's *corona effect* was developed by the Kirlians early in the process. They began to notice several interesting correlations as they compared coronal images between different people in different circumstances: The color and activity of the corona seemed different between healthy people and diseased people. They also noticed inter-relationship between the corona and the Chinese *meridian* points.

Observations of *auras* have also been recorded in ancient texts, some thousands of years old. Halos and illuminations have been described in various circumstances throughout Biblical texts. The ancient Vedic literature of the Indus Valley described the pranic aura field surrounding the body and the instance of certain personalities with greater effulgence thousands of years ago. The outward effects of *chi* as an effulgence around the body was also described in ancient Taoist texts. Pythagoras recorded the notion of an outer human energy field around 500 B.C., and Paracelsus described it in the sixteenth century as the *"vital force"* that *"radiates round him like a luminous sphere…."*

More recently, Romanian physician Dr. Ion Dumitrescu led to a startling discovery in the late 1970s. This illustrated that the living electromagnetic aura also has a homuncular holographic nature. Dr. Dumitrescu utilized an electrographic process with a scanning mechanism. In one study, various leaf images were photographed before and after portions of the leaves were removed. Interestingly, the leaf's corona, despite the removal of a section of leaf, would still be in the shape of the entire leaf as if the leaf were still intact. The phenomenon was even more dramatic when a hole in the center of the leaf was cut out. Through this hole, the electrographic photo revealed a tiny leaf shape, identical to the outer leaf, which also had a hole in it (Gerber 1988).

Western medical science all but dismissed the role of electromagnetics in living organisms for many years. Dr. Robert Becker's early work in the mid-twentieth century illustrated that salamander limb regeneration is accompanied by millivolt potentials (Becker 1985). The perspective of western medicine on the body's electromagnetic nature thus changed.

Continuing studies of *electrotherapy* have confirmed the body's electromagnetic qualities. Electrical stimulation for pain relief is now well established, and today hospitals and pain centers regularly implant *electrostimulators* into the spinal cord region to relieve pain. Current theories regarding the process of pain relief now center around the *gate control theory* first proposed in 1964 by Melzack and Wall. This theory states the closing and opening of a pain-relay gate located in the spine determines the level of electronic transduction of pain signal communication to the brain. Apparent confirmation of this theory has been the successful treatment of lower back neuropathic pain and pain elsewhere. In addition, electrostimulation has proven successful in bone healing. Veterinary surgeons report success rates in the 75% to 80% range for healing fractures and nonunions with electrostimulation (Clark 1987). Healing rates of almost 65% with an 85% effectiveness rate in human patients have also been observed (Heckmann *et al.* 1981).

A number of other studies confirm these. Neurostimulation has been proven successful in a number of other human applications, including urinary and bladder issues (Tanagho 1990, Dalmose 2003, Banyo 2003, Kennedy *et al.* 1995); tachycardia arrhythmias (Volkmann 1991); spinal cord injuries (Beckerman *et al.* 1993, Meinecke 1991); low back pain (Shutov 2007); gastric issues (Deitel 2004); pain (Devulder *et al.* 2002, Siegfried 1988); smoking cessation (White *et al.* 2002); and many other conditions.

The research of Dr. Ronald Melzack and Dr. Patrick Wall eventually led to the famous McGill Pain Questionnaire and other gate control applications. These in turn led to the discoveries of some of the body's feel-good biochemical messengers such as endorphins and enkephalins.

The gate control theories also led to hypotheses regarding the *phantom limb* phenomenon. This curious event—in which an amputee continues to feel pain in an area of an amputated limb—is congruent with Dr. Dumitrescu's *phantom leaf theory* mentioned above.

Observation tells us the body derives energy from food, sunlight, water, and air. However, there is significant evidence to conclude that these are actually different forms of radiative inputs translated from an upstream generating source. A hydroelectric plant generating electricity for millions of homes, for example, is not actually producing that power.

The power is being converted from one type of energy into another. This is also stated in the conservation of energy law of thermodynamics. What is the original source of this power?

The body's energy sources—food, sunlight, water and air—are more appropriately identified as transmitters. Their incoming waveform potentials are received, converted and utilized by the body. The core inputs utilized are smaller units such as ions, amino acids, minerals, vitamins and oxygen. This is illustrative of waveform interference patterns of highly complex molecules and elemental combinations being broken down into their constructive parts. As with nutrition, however, we cannot derive the same benefit from isolated waveforms as we can with their complex combinations. The sum of their power cannot match the individual parts.

The evidence presented here will illustrate the presence of an agent who ultimately directs and organizes waveform energy with an intentional purpose. For example, when a person consciously thinks *I want to get up and go for a walk,* suddenly the body organizes a surge of energy, accompanied by the opening of energy gateways for circuits throughout various cells, creating the metabolic mechanisms for physical activity. Without the original intention, there would be no such activity. Logically, the difference between the body that purposely acts and the body that does not must be conscious intention. If there were no driving force of intention, the body's activity would have no functional purpose or result. There would also be no organization among our society.

Rhythmic Orchestration

Over the centuries, humankind has been observing that our activities and the activities of other organisms within our environment seem to be organized with rhythm. Not one beat or rhythm mind you. Rather, many concurrent rhythms that seem to inter-relate and correlate with each other. The relationships between the various beats or rhythms of the universe have been studied by many prominent scientists over thousands of years. The prevailing conclusion is that the body and its environment are somehow acting within a synchronic relationship.

The appearance of rhythmic behavior within the human physiology is evident from both an external and internal view. Certainly, anatomical characterizations of the physical body present a means to measure and observe the outward structural mapping of the body, just as an architectural drawing of a building allows us to know the dimensions of every room in a building. The weakness of the architectural drawing is that it will not tell us how each of the rooms are being used and who may be living within them. In the same way, our anatomical characterizations of the human body, despite their visual endowment, may present the structural nature of the physiology but hardly the depth of its metabolic functions. The inner workings of the body still primarily confound modern physicians, and thus require a view with a whole other perspective.

As Da Vinci and others have illustrated among nature, should we unfold and measure every living organism's physical development, we observe growth following a unique design. Virtually every occurrence in the natural world follows these same designs. Among these include the *Fibonacci sequence*, which maps out to the *golden rectangle*, the *golden mean* and the *golden spiral* as measured multi-dimensionally.

The Fibonacci sequence, 0, 1, 2, 3, 5, 8, 13, 21, 34, 55.... is observed throughout nature. A *Fibonacci number* is found by adding the two preceding Fibonacci numbers together: 1+2=3, 2+3=5, 3+5=8.... Observed by Italian Leonardo Pisano Fibonacci in the thirteenth century while tracing a family tree of rabbits, the *Fibonacci sequence* is recognized as the fundamental progression throughout nature. Its accounting is observed among every living organism, from shape and growth to genetic heredity. For example, the outward projection of branches and leaves from trees and plant stalks assemble precise Fibonacci fractions: one-half in grasses, lime and elm; one-third in sedges, beech, hazel and blackberry; two-fifths in roses, oak, cherry, apple and holly; three-eighths in bananas, poplar, willow and pear; five-thirteenths in leeks, almond and pussy willow; and eight-twenty-firsts in pine cones and cactus. Some plants are aligned in a related sequence, called the *Lucas sequence,* named after nineteenth century Frenchman Edouard Lucas. Like Fibonacci numbers, Lucas numbers are also assembled by adding two consecutive numbers to get the third. However, the Lucas sequence begins with two and one rather than zero: 1+2=3, 1+3=4, 3+4=7, 7+4=11, and so on, to arrive at 1, 2, 3, 4, 7, 11, 18....

When Fibonacci measurements are arranged into polygons, they form rectangles. One of these rectangles is laid against a square of the next Fibonacci number to become the famous *golden rectangle* or *Phi.* The golden rectangle is made from two adjacent 1x1 squares to become a 1x2 Fibonacci rectangle. This can be laid against a 2x2 square to become a 2x3 Fibonacci rectangle. Laid against a 3x3 square, it becomes a 3x5 Fibonacci rectangle and so on. The Fibonacci rectangle is observed throughout nature, including the outer and inner regions of plant, animal and human organisms and their appendages.

Another pattern observed throughout nature is the spiral. The *golden spiral* is most prominent, determined as an array of concentrically outward *golden sections* with dimensions of 1:1.618. The golden spiral is seen repeatedly throughout the natural world. It is seen in the nautilus shell. It is seen in the sections of tortoise shells and fingerprints. It is seen among the tops of plant florets like cauliflower and broccoli, and among cell and nerve patterns.

The Fibonacci sequence is functionally a *harmonic sequence.* A harmonic sequence repeats a pattern of pacing of either an integer or a ratio of integers. An example of a harmonic sequence would be 5, 10, 15, 20, 25, which has a fundamental integer change of five. This type of sequence produces a wave harmonic. Fibonacci and Lucas sequences are progressive harmonics because the fundamental pace is progressively being updated by the previous two factors of the sequence. We might then refer to the typical music harmonic as a *static harmonic,* and the sequencing in nature as a *living harmonic,* as it engages consciousness.

The harmonic series also provides a specific waveform. A repeating cycle can be broken down and charted over a two dimensional horizontal plane, which converts to the sine wave. Sine waves are the waveforms of light, sound, radiowaves, cosmic rays, gamma rays, the infrared spectrum, the ultraviolet spectrum, and even ocean waves. Over a hundred years ago, French physicist Jean Fourier discovered that almost every physical motion could be broken down into sinusoidal components. This demonstrated his famous mathematic *Fourier series.*

We also see these sinusoidal, helical and spiraling dimensions within all the human body's physiology. From top to bottom, the body illustrates this golden design. Should we look at the top of a human head from above we will see an unmistakable swirling of the hair inward from a location in the area of the occipital fontanel—in the neighborhood as the infant's 'soft spot.' This spiraling appearance is seen throughout the hairs of the body. We can see an inward spiraling of hair growth in key anatomical areas such as the pubis, chin, the back, the belly button and elsewhere. For this reason, shaving typically requires several different angles to accommodate the spiraling nature of hair growth.

A quick review of our fingerprints will display a unique spiraling effect. The osteocytes within our bony structures are also arranged helically, as are many of our nerves and cells. The iris is arranged helically. The ear is arranged in a spiraling fashion, strikingly similar to a dissected wave or weather system. The cochlear inner ear is also spiraled, each bend and curve working to translate air pressure waves into electromagnetic pulses that reflect sound onto the audio cortex. A cross-section of the disks of our spine, if viewed from above, also reveals a noticeable spiraling helix as the vertebra become gradually narrower.

Leonardo Da Vinci exhaustively measured the various appendages of the body. He compared them with other parts and the body as a whole. Da Vinci's famous *Vitruvian Man* illustrates a human body within the context of a circle, with the arms and legs each rotating around the circumference of the circle with the belly button marking its center point. Da Vinci also measured length of hands, feet, arms, fingers, and so on, and found that the length and width of these body parts were all congruent when compared relationally. For example, Da Vinci observed that the arm from the wrist is four times the length of the hand from fingertips to wrist. He also established that at three years old a human male almost precisely half his full-grown height, among many other amazing relativities within the human organism.

Da Vinci also noted the symmetry among movement and metabolism. He once wrote that, *"The same cause which stirs the humours in every species of animal body and by which every injury is repaired, also moves the waters from the utmost depth of the sea to the greatest heights."*

In 1590, Thomas Harriot proposed that the *equiangular spiral,* or *spira mirabilis* could be observed from the side view (with the thumb wrapped under the finger) of the clenched fist. This observation was also described by Descartes and later elaborated on mathematically by Jakob Bernoulli. It was described as the logarithmic spiral. This spiral was noted as strikingly similar to the spiraling nature of the nautilus and the swirling of water, well before many other natural helices and spirals were found among nature by other scientists. For centuries, the medical profession assumed this fist-spiral relationship was correct. The specific measurements between the digits of the fingers and thumb supported the precise measurement of *Phi* (about 1.62—the golden section or golden rectangle). This assumption became the subject of heated debate amongst the medical profession.

The debate has continued to the modern era. A more recent motion analysis by Gupta *et al.* (1998) confirmed experimentally that the fingers' motion path towards fisting follows the equiangular spiral. A later study of the bones of the hand done by Andrew Mark, M.D. and associates in the 2003 *Journal of Hand Surgery* took standardized x-rays from 100 healthy volunteers and found a low correlation to a precise *Phi* measurement within the fisted spiral. At the same time, the authors of this study also concluded that the rotation of the metacarpophalangeal joint to the center of rotation of the interphalangeal joints should still yield the Fibonacci relationship. The center of rotation for each digit pivots though the space between the joints. They concluded that discrepancies could occur between the functional and absolute bone lengths.

In other words, there are unique differences in the development and movement of each body. These are related to individual habits and function. Just as no two fingerprints, ears or retinas are alike between different human bodies; there are subtle individual variances between the various body proportions, depending upon use and medical history. We are not making a case for the body being a machine here. The body has a particular design, but it is also designed to reflect the individual consciousness and history of each individual. This points to the body's metabolism being a flexible yet elegant interplay between nature's design and individual consciousness.

Magnetic Messaging

Advancements in physics during the nineteenth century led to the realization that electricity is not a single waveform. Rather, it is a dual waveform, consisting of an electronic pulse and a magnetic field. Gradually we have also come to the realization that the ionic cellular mechanisms of the body also have this dual waveform nature. Like the electric current, the mechanisms of the body are both electronic and magnetic. As electronic biochemical reactions cascade through our bodies with transport mechanisms, we are also generating magnetic fields. These magnetic fields are dispatched through our local environment with real-time results. Some fields are by-products of electronic processes, while others are specifically magnetic, affecting metabolism directly. The anatomical effects of magnetism are not readily addressed by modern medical science. This is odd, noting the extensive use of diagnosis using magnetic resonance technologies. Magnetic resonance (MRI) utilizes radiative polarity to visual the body's anatomy. Just as electrical currents moving through appliances generate magnetic fields, the various currents running through the body's ionic mechanisms utilize magnetic fields. As physics found over a century ago, magnetism influences electronics and vice-versa.

Scientists have long suspected electromagnetism stimulates response among living organisms. The Greeks, in particular Hippocrates, are thought to have applied the magnetic lodestone as a healing therapy. The lodestone was also apparently used by the ancient Egyptians, as Cleopatra is said to have wore lodestone on her forehead around 2000 B.C. The ancient Ayurvedic medicine of the 2000-3500 B.C. Indus Valley applied *siktavati,* or "instruments of stone" in their therapies, and early Tibetan monks applied bar magnets in their training.

Two thousand years after Hippocrates, William Gilbert, the physician to Queen Elizabeth I, demonstrated a number of logical arguments on magnetism and life in his treatise *De Magnete.* Gilbert believed that the earth was a magnet, and that magnetic forces were somehow tuned to the forces of life. Another great physician to adopt magnetic forces was German physician Franz Mesmer. Mesmer professed that living organisms transmitted a subtle aethereal current crudely translated as "animal magnetism," which could influence biology and provide healing benefit. Due to his being investigated and condemned by a King Louis XVI commission (thought to be encouraged by the jealousy of other physicians for his healing successes); Mesmer's work was abandoned by medicine for many centuries.

The eighteenth and nineteenth centuries brought a renewed focus upon electricity and the living organism. The work of physician Luigi Galvani on electrical nerve conduction eventually led to disappointment when it was found that two dissimilar metals were required for electrical activity ("Volta's pile"). Galvani's nerve "animal electricity" proposal had to be abandoned, and electromagnetism was indelibly dissected from medicine for another century.

The connection between life and magnetism became evident following the publication of the successful research of Finnish scientist Karl Selim Lemström during the late nineteenth and early twentieth centuries. Lemström, an expert on polar and electromagnetic forces, found a connection between tree rings and solar geomagnetic storm activity. He also conducted experiments on plant growth using overhead electrical wires with poles set into the soil. The plants surrounded by electromagnetism grew almost 50% more than similar plants without the electromagnetic wiring environment—which we now know conducts magnetic fields.

Horticultural magnetic research has continued over the past century with consistent results. South Carolinan James Lee Scribner's electromagnetic butterbean trials resulted in twenty-two foot tall plants. Italian Bindo Riccioni treated seeds with capacitors, resulting in 37 percent greater yields. Tests in the Soviet Union during the 1960s also treated seeds with electromagnetic currents. Green mass yields went up to 15 percent higher for corn, up to 15 percent higher for oats and barley, up to 13 percent higher for peas and up to 10 percent higher for buckwheat.

The concept of magnetism within human physiology rose again as a late-nineteenth century Julius Bernstein proposed that nerve impulses transferred through polarization. This *membrane polarization* model became the basis for the later conclusive research of Otto Loewi in the early 1920s, which led to his 1936 Nobel Prize for synaptic transmission. Loewi's experiment—which apparently came to him during a dream—was to extract two frog hearts and retain them in a bath of saline. Some of the solution surrounding the faster heartbeat was extracted and put into the bath of the other heart. This made the other heart beat faster, providing the evidence of the biochemical synaptic transmission.

The polarity exchange between ions and biochemicals is unmistakably magnetic. Magnetism is after all, a polarity issue of ions or atoms aligning in one direction or another. The irrefutable link between magnetism and biological response has been confirmed by study and clinical application during the last half of the twentieth century, as the existence of ion channels has been clarified.

Furthermore, the link between intention and magnetism has become evident. This was illustrated by Dr. Grad's research at Canada's McGill University in the late 1950s and early 1960s, when growth rates of barley sprouts were stimulated by the focused intentions of particularly gifted individuals. Further studies indicated these growth rate effects were similar to the influence magnetism has on plant growth.

The central subject of these investigations was a Hungarian refugee named Oskar Estebany. Mr. Estabany appeared to be able to exert extraordinary intentional effects through his touch. A number of tests confirmed that magnetism was involved in Mr. Estebany's abilities. In one, Dr. Justa Smith at the Rosary Hill College (1973) compared Mr. Estebany's ability to increase enzyme reaction rates with those of magnetic field emissions. After Mr. Estebany affected increased reactivity among enzyme reaction rates, Dr. Smith applied magnetic fields and compared the rates. It turned out that the increased growth caused by Mr. Estebany precisely matched that caused by a 13,000 gauss magnetic field.

Dr. Smith had spent a number of years studying these effects prior to and after her tests with Mr. Estebany. She authored a book on the topic (1969) called *Effect of Magnetic Fields on Enzyme Reactivity*. While this research was considered radical at that time, other scientists soon confirmed her findings. In the 1990s, a flurry of research was published from around the world showing magnetic fields in the 2,500-10,000 gauss range affecting reaction rates of various enzymatic reactions. By 1996, more than fifty different enzyme reactions were found to be influenced by magnetic fields. In two linked studies by University of Utah's Charles Grissom, (1993, 1996), single-beam UV-to-visible spectrum and rapid-scanning spectrophotometers with electromagnets built in were applied to two different cobalamine (B12) enzymes. One enzyme (ethanolamine ammonia lyase) had significantly different reaction rates in response to magnetic fields, while the other enzyme (methylmalonyl CoA mutase) had no apparent response. It could thus be concluded that some biochemical processes are sensitive to magnetic field influence and others are not. This effect is still mysterious, but it has become increasingly evident that within the body lie precise flows of magnetic fields.

There have been a number of controlled studies showing that key body tissues respond to magnetic stimulation. Amassian *et al.* (1989) stimulated the motor cortex with a focal magnetic coil, which rendered movement to paralyzed appendages. Maccabee *et al.* (1991) stimulated almost the entire nervous system with a magnetic coil. This particular stimulation instigated responses from the distal peripheral nerve, the nerve root, the cranial nerve, the motor cortex, the premotor cortex, the frontal motor areas related to speech, and other nerve centers.

Dr. Howard Friedman and Dr. Robert Becker studied human behavior and magnetic fields in the early 1960s. They found *extremely low frequencies* (ELF) such as .1 or .2 Hz affected volunteer reaction times (Becker 1985). This paralleled work by Dr. Norbert Weiner and Dr. James Hamer with low-intensity fields, seen as "driving" waveforms already existing in the body. Spaniard Dr. Jose Delgado's research illustrated that low intensity ELF magnetic fields could influence sleep and manic behavior among monkeys. Furthermore, a substantial amount of evidence demonstrates that magnetic fields generated from powerlines and transformers can modulate physiology, noting these and the effects of electromagnetics on plants. Research linking cancer and powerlines has been controversial. Still, enough evidence enables a conclusion that magnetic fields can alter certain physiological processes.

The magnetic nature of the body is revealed through *nuclear magnetic resonance* (NMR). Its application of *magnetic resonance imaging* (MRI) is now one of the more useful diagnostic machines used in medicine when a true cross-sectional analysis of the body is required. The NMR scan is performed on the human body by surrounding the body with strong magnetic fields. These fields polarize the hydrogen (H+) proton ions in water (as the body is mostly water). As these ions' north poles align, they emit a particular frequency. Radio beams positioned around the body (tuned to this frequency) give detectors a cross-sectional scan of the body via these polarized ions. The body is guided underneath magnetic fields ranging from about 5000 to 20,000 gauss (the earth's magnetic field is about .5 gauss). As the altered polarity of the hydrogen protons become excited with radio signals, a computer calculates the water content differences to form an image of the body. Were it not for the magnetic nature of the body, these three-dimensional images would not be possible.

Over the past few years, researchers are increasingly discovering commercial applications for the tiny ion channels within cell membranes. The magnetic reactivity of these *microchannels* (or *micropores*) has enabled technicians to alter the flow through these channels with certain *nanoparticles* (Wee *et al.* 2005). Exerting magnetic influence on these channels—and even etching new channels onto single-celled living organisms—allows the technician to utilize cell structures as microprocessors, drug testers or tiny manufacturing systems. Various functional nanoparticles are under development, and many are in use today in an attempt to exploit nature's magnetic ion channels. Some ethical concerns have voiced on the use of nanobots. What might these magnetized miniature robots become after several generations of evolved intention?

Biocommunication

In 1966, Clive Backster, a former CIA employee and licensed polygraph examiner, began experimenting with polygraph equipment connected to plants. His first plant was a dracaena cane plant. After connecting the polygraph's electrodes, he immediately began to notice that its *galvanic skin response* readings appeared not so different from human examination charts. What surprised Dr. Backster was that the plant's exam also registered emotional responses of fear. Furthermore, these responses were highest during moments where an intention to harm the plant came to mind. The simple thoughts of considering how the plant would be harmed produced a precise fear response in the plant (Backster, 2003).

The prospect of a plant responding to a threatening intention was certainly incredible to Dr. Backster—then an owner of a polygraph school and research laboratory. Following this incident, Dr. Backster spent the next thirty years carefully conducting controlled experiments to study conscious mechanisms within plants, eggs, and then human cells. Dr. Backster published two scientific papers on the subject, along with a number of popular magazine articles. He also wrote a book on the topic (*Primary Perception,* 2003) and consulted on a number of other titles.

Dr. Backster also appeared on television, radio, and several university lecture series. Dr. Backster carefully conducted hundreds of experiments on emotional intention, devising automated research equipment to remove extraneous influences. Many of these studies were reviewed by well-known scientists, and some even took part in the research. His results were clear, and many were replicated by other scientists—although this also proved to be difficult to the spontaneity required by consciousness research. Dr. Backster discovered that plants were not the only living organism to sense intention. Through exhaustive tests using various subjects and perspectives, he found that human leukocytes separated from their host and kept *in vitro* somehow had the ability to sense and respond to emotions of fear and excitement that occurred within their host *remotely.*

Furthermore and amazingly, he found this effect can occurs at a distance of up to fifty miles.

Anyone who has taken a polygraph will report that the examination is complex and requires some technical training in physiology and psychology. A polygraph examiner is thus typically expert in physical-emotion expression. The equipment utilizes primarily galvanized skin response (GSR) and electrocardiography equipment to monitor the physical reflections of specific emotions. What polygraph examination techniques have taught scientists over the years is that the skin, heart and many other parts of the body will reveal heightened emotions with particular physical responses. One of the most noticeable physical responses results from the emotion of fear. Lie detection has thus become recognized as a verifiable science after over thousands of polygraph examinations and hundreds of studies. Even with the occasional variance in specific results, there is undeniable evidence that the body reflects heightened emotional response. Polygraph research has revealed that some people have the ability to cheat the polygraph, assuming they understand how to control certain emotional and physical responses. Here again, this underscores the connection between intention and physical response. Whether cheating the polygraph or not, intention is being expressed through the various responses of the body.

The human polygraph examination focuses upon our fear of detection. The fear of harm through discovery is the typical emotion being tested. This is also controlled in Dr. Backster's research on plants, eggs and human cells. Because the fear of detection is closely related to the fear of harm, the physiological results of the two emotions are practically identical.

One of the dramatic findings of Dr. Backster's research with plants was that once a person consistently begins caring for a plant, that plant becomes emotionally connected to that person. Dr. Backster discovered that even when the person has traveled miles away from this plant, emotionally charged circumstances occurring in the life of the person would affect the plant. In other words, the plant becomes emotionally tied to the person taking care of them. This sort of emotion is typically referred to as *empathy.*

In vitro cells separated from a human responded very similarly in Dr. Backster's research, but only with their host. Living cells being incubated and electroded with the equipment responded to heightened emotional activity of their former host, even when the host was located rooms or even miles away from the cells. This indicated the separated cells somehow had the ability to receive remote communication transmissions from the host. How is it that cells have this ability? Furthermore, Dr. Backster's research demonstrated that the cells were able to prioritize their responses specifically for their host, even amongst emotional controls set up to distract the response.

Dr. Backster's research controls were thoroughly vetted by a number of scientists. Still, it is regarded as controversial, and has been difficult to duplicate in some cases. Nonetheless, communications between a remote ex-host is not altogether different from the cell's known ability to instantly receive instructions from the brain and other remote locations in the body—located many feet away, amongst trillions of other cells. Medical researchers recognize that the body's nervous systems and various biochemicals such as neurotransmitters and hormones help carry messages from one location of the body to another. This begs the question of how billions of cells can be orchestrated to commit a particular action *instantly* upon the intention of the person? Yes, nerves are certainly high-speed, but every cell in the body is not specifically innervated. So how do all the cells instantly respond to intention?

Every cell making up a living organism is a waveform receiver. Each cell has the ability to receive instructional waveforms just as any radio can receive a local broadcast. In addition, groups of cells can align and organize to receive and respond to specific types of waveforms. Actually, the living organism as a whole is a multi-spectrum waveform sensor. Groups of cells called the senses have organized around receiving specific types of waveforms. We can perceive waves in the visible spectrum with the eyes, infrared radiation with the skin, air pressure waves with the ears, and subtle electromagnetic waveforms with the tongue and nose. These are only a few of the multitude of waveforms that are received and translated throughout the body. This is compounded by the fact that the cells also conduct various waveforms via ion channels and receptors.

The body's cells pick up waveforms beyond our current technologies. This is the only explanation for plants and cells to be able to receive precise information from remote locations. Dr. Backster's research illustrated these waveforms were transmitted through insulated and even metal walls.

Waveform communications outside our range of recognition is not a new paradigm to science. The past few hundred years of research have continuously revealed previously unperceivable waveforms.

The eyes have the ability to perceive a variety of waveforms previously considered outside the visible wavelengths. Wavelengths shorter than violet such as ultraviolet, x-rays, and gamma rays have been observed visually under extraordinary circumstances such as a darkened room penetrated with radiation leakage. Both x-rays and gamma rays have been observed on occasion with the naked eye, as a yellow-green glow. Meanwhile, some have identified nuclear leakage in flashes of blue. As the rods of the eyes sensitize for night vision they also become sensitive to other waveforms. Longer and less damaging radiowaves have also been received by humans in extraordinary circumstances. Hearing radio stations through dental fillings, bridgework, and even bobby pins has been an odd but well-documented occurrence.

The body's cells translate radiowaves into electrical brain impulses just as a radio crystal translates radiowaves into electronic pulses. The senses illustrate this well. Once received through the antenna mechanisms of the eyes, ears, nose, tongue and so on—the crystalline structure of nerve cell molecules convert these waveforms to electronic pulses in the same manner. Individual cells have these same antenna systems. The ability of radiowaves influencing single cells and single-cell living organisms is well documented. In 1958, for example, *The New England Institute for Medical Research* published articles documenting that radiowaves could influence red blood cell movement and bacteria motion. Murchie (1978) observed amebas, euglenas, and paramecia aligning their movement with radiating field lines of five to forty megacycle radiowaves. Many other studies have documented similar effects.

The reception and translation of ultraviolet radiation by skin cells is obvious and well understood. The sun's ultraviolet B waveforms stimulate the production of vitamin D_3 when wavelengths of 270-290 nanometers enter the epidermal layer. The *conrotatory electrocyclic reaction* cycles 7-dehydrocholesterol to pre-vitamin D, and eventually to 1,25 dihydroxyvitamin D, or 25-OHD. During this cycle, melanin production is stimulated to provide a filtering and buffering mechanism for additional rays from the sun. Vitamin D is an essential nutrient to the human body. It is important for immunity, cardiovascular health, nerve health and bones and teeth health. Our primary source is through the sun, although a limited number of foods contain small amounts as well.

For many decades, researchers have been studying the effects of light upon other human cells. We all know about photosynthesis—where plant cells utilize light, water and carbon dioxide to produce starches, sugars and oxygen. The molecular structure of chlorophyll acts as a semiconducting crystal, absorbing some ultraviolet waveforms from the sun while reflecting others. With these absorbed waveforms, the unique biochemical reaction of photosynthesis is stimulated among special chloroplasts—specialized proteins embedded inside chlorophyll.

This process illustrates the intimate connection between waveform conversion and living organisms. The complex transformation of light waveforms to plant nutrition is a conversion related to the intention to survive—a conscious act. This intention creates the impetus for energy transformation. We see a similar transformation process occurring through the human cellular production of energy from oxygen and glucose. Cellular energy production occurs through a waveform transition process called *electron transport* (reminiscent of the characterization of electricity as electron movement). ATP and NADPH are created and water is split, releasing oxygen. Part of this process uses an interesting exchange of phosphorus ions called *phosphorylation.* This process is one of transporting waveform energy through a transport chain to create an NADP+ molecule, after which an additional transformation takes place through a process of *redox* to create an energized NADPH. Some theorized that the continuing process of ATP conversion and glucose takes place without UV. Further research has revealed that light is at least indirectly involved, as it stimulates the production of some of the enzymes used as catalysts.

In the 1920s, a Russian scientist Alexander Gurwitsch picked up a weak photoemission from living tissue. The emissions appeared stronger during mitosis, so he termed these UV-range wavelength rhythms *mitogenetic rays.* The presence of living radiation emitted from dividing cells was confirmed shortly thereafter by some German researchers. Even still, their conclusions were overshadowed by doubts from skeptics. Nonetheless, ongoing biochemical experiments have continued to confirm a link between cellular division and radiation.

The topic did not gain much additional research attention until after World War II. Research teams from Italy, Germany and Britain independently worked on the living photon research. Each confirmed waveform observations from living cells, which they named variously. One name stuck: *low-level luminescence ultraweak chemiluminescence.* The prevailing opinion was that the radiation originated from the oxidation of free radicals.

In the early 1970s German researcher Dr. Fritz-Albert Popp was focusing on cancer cell treatment at the University of Marburg. In one particular trial, he discovered weak emissions coming from both living cells and multiplying tumor cells at wavelengths of 260-800 nanometers. Fascinated, Popp and his associates confirmed this phenomenon over repeated assays over the years. He published many scientific papers and wrote a number of books on the topic. He called these weak emissions *biophotons* because of their resemblance to the waveform properties of light radiation. As for his cancer research, Dr. Popp was able to correlate greater emission levels in expanded cancer cell growth, and lower emissions during slower growth. His tests also indicated anti-carcinogenic therapies had the effect of lowering emission levels, indicating a reduction of tumor growth (Popp 1976, 2003; Chang *et al.* 2002).

Dr. Popp, Dr. Chang and fellow researchers (1976, 1997, 2000) found particular frequencies and waveforms among healthy and diseased cells: Cancerous cells emitted certain frequencies and healthy cells emitted certain frequencies. He also found that cells responded to specific frequencies of light by repairing themselves. Especially productive were responsive emissions from other cells. There appeared to be low-level communications occurring between cells in response to cell damage. Research by Gisler *et al.* in 1983 and Dobrowolski *et al.* in 1987 confirmed this luminescence effect among cancer cells.

Cells each emit unique waveforms, and each living organism emits unique waveforms. Dr. Popp's research confirmed that every living organism emits unique frequencies (Popp and Chang 2000); just as each body has a unique fingerprint. The use of identification methods soon led to the description of *cellular fingerprints*—using signature frequencies and amplitudes to differentiate one from another. This concept correlates with differentiated DNA sequencing among cells as demonstrated by researchers like O'Brien *et al.* (1980) and Thacker *et al.* (1988).

This effect was confirmed variously using different types of cells. Dr. Popp's equipment was also able to distinguish conventionally grown tomatoes from organically grown tomatoes. Their ultraweak emissions were measured using another device he developed called the *photon detector*. In 1991, Dr. Barbara Chwirot and Dr. Popp co-authored a report confirming light-induced luminescence during mitosis among yeast cells. His biophoton device was able to predict the relative germination rate of barley seeds prior to sprouting as well. Apparently, biophoton emissions are connected to cellular communication (Lambing 1992).

Research led by Professor Franco Musumeci at the Institute of Physics of Catania University in the early 1990s confirmed the existence of these weak emissions. Professor Musumeci studied cancer tissue systems and confirmed these ultraweak waveforms among growing tumor lines (Grasso *et al.* 1991). He and his associates (Grasso *et al.* 1992) also compared normal tissues with cancer tissues, confirming consistent variances between the two. In 1994, Professor Musumeci and his associates analyzed food for biophoton emission, finding higher emission levels in freshly picked food. Older, storage-bound food had significantly lower emission levels. While early-picked tomatoes might have had the same red color as ripe-picked tomatoes, they were distinguished by lower biophoton emissions (Triglia *et al.* 1998).

Professor Musumeci's research also focused upon yeast growth and soybean germination: Measuring weak photon emissions during while they grew and sprouted. In his yeast growth studies, he discovered a consistent increase in photon emission levels with increased yeast growth. His soybean germination studies yielded some very interesting results as well. Both active soybeans and devitalized soybeans were tested together, and their photon levels were measured over time and against mass increase (growth). Consistently, the active germinating seeds displayed higher sustained photon emission levels than the devitalized ones. The devitalized soybean seeds had higher initial emission levels however. These decreased over time, while the vital germinating soybeans had increasing emission levels through germination until they leveled off as they matured (Grasso *et al.* 1991).

Cohen and Popp (1997) also conducted human trials, testing 200 subjects for biophoton emissions over a period of several years. These trials showed consistent emission levels among the test subjects. Some tests measured levels of a particular subject daily over an extended period. In one of Cohen and Popp's human trials, human biophoton emission was measured daily for several months. These longer-term measurements demonstrated correlations between biophoton emission and human biowaves. Rhythms estimated at 14 days, one month, three months, and nine months were evidenced by rising and falling emission level rates.

These human biophoton trials also revealed a number of other whole-body trends. These include left-right symmetry among biophoton emissions throughout the body. This symmetry was found to become disturbed in diseased states. Various biophoton channels appeared to be functional within the body, appearing to transfer information between different anatomical regions. They found these corresponded closely with acupuncture meridians.

Cohen and Popp proposed that these biophoton measurements could be useful as non-invasive diagnostic techniques. Emission levels were studied before, during, and after application of skin therapy on psoriasis patients, for example. This confirmed that emissions tend to rise with therapy and an improvement of symptoms.

Other research also correlated biophoton emission with the human immune response. It was determined that during immune activity or wound healing, blood will reflect higher biophoton levels. Biophoton levels increase with greater neutrophil levels, which also happen to be active redox messengers. The blood is naturally extremely sensitive to immune threats, and biophoton levels appear to reflect the rise with immune cell response (Klima *et al.* 1987).

Other studies demonstrated that fibroblasts (cells that participate in injury repair) have greater photon emission levels following mitosis. This provides additional confirmation that the body's healing and immune responses yield greater photon emission levels (Niggli 2003).

Biophoton measurements have also been closely studied by a number of other researchers from other disciplines. Among them, bioluminescence was observed by Edwards *et al.* in 1989 using electrotherapeutics. This research again confirmed a connection between acupuncture meridians and biophoton emissions.

Between 1986 and 1991 Dr. Humio Inaba, a professor at the Research Institute of Electrical Communication at Tohoku University, led a research project focused on these ultraweak photon emissions. Dr. Inaba's work utilized a single-photon counting device with an amplification system to enable photon-counting images with narrow photon ranges approximating single waveforms. His research demonstrated that these biophotons occur coincidentally with biochemical reactions within cells. The possibility that this effect was a response to external light was also eliminated. Although external radiation has been shown to prompt a delayed photon response within the body, these ultraweak biophoton emissions were unique and independent. Using his equipment, Dr. Inaba's research also measured similar biophoton emissions in the germinating seeds of various plants, soybeans, spinach chloroplasts, sea urchin eggs, and mammalian nuclei (Inaba 1991).

In 2003, Dr. Michael Lipkind noted higher photon emissions from cell cultures infected with viruses when compared with healthy cell controls. Virus-infected cells not only had higher but also more peculiar ranges than the more standardized ranges coming from healthy cells. The peculiarity of the virus emissions also closely correlated with the virus replication cycles. These results closely corresponded with the tumor-cell growth studies done by Professor Popp.

In a study by Dr. Chwirot and associates published in 2003, colon lesion cells were measured for biophoton activity after removal with surgery from diseased patients. The biophoton levels significantly differed in colon lesion cells as compared with healthy colon mucosal cells. This has led some to suggest that photon emission testing could be an effective tool in diagnosing colon cancers and lesions.

Further biophoton investigations determined that greater toxic loads in living cells resulted in greater photon emission. As the toxin levels or stressors increased, the emission levels increased. This was confirmed in other studies of plant responses to stressors. Higher lipoxygenase and peroxidase levels in plants correlated with higher emission levels.

Human cell membranes interact intimately with ions such as sodium, potassium and other electron-transporting mechanisms like ATPase. The electro-chemical aspects of ions led to our early discoveries of electricity and its magnetic field qualities. This is because ions are electromagnetic messengers. Ions are activated with pulsed electromagnetic fields. This provides a means to carry and exchange waveform information. As the ionic waveform messaging interacts with other waveform messages from other sources, an interference pattern results, creating a complex information mapping system.

Ion channels have been observed transferring chemical charges and communicating processes such as glucose utilization and immune response between cell membranes and intercellular tissues. These electro-chemical pathways have been correlated with biophoton emissions, illustrating the reality that information-messaging systems exist on more than a chemical basis. Biophoton research indicates that although each cell and each individual appears to emit unique waveforms, a significant level of coherence is observed between photon emissions of various cells. More significantly, coherence is observed as these emissions are broken down into their respective spectra. Coherent waveforms create informational interference patterns—either destructive (reducing) or constructive (expanding). The coherency factor became relevant to Dr. Popp and his fellow researchers as it provided a rational holistic model for information transmission within the body (Popp and Yan 2002; Li 1981; Popp 2003).

In other words, bioemissions are bound together into substantial messages by a common, coherent thread: *Conscious intention.*

Communication messaging systems correlating biophoton activity were demonstrated with *dinoflaggellates* by Chang and Popp in 1994. A dinoflaggellate is a single cell organism that typically lives in the ocean or fresh waters of the world. Many plankton species are dinoflaggellates. Though single-celled, they have tremendous complexity, yielding cellulose armor plates for defense, and the ability to change structural shape to give them tremendous propulsion for escape. They also convert sunlight to nutritional energy. Dinoflaggellates thus provide the foundation for the nutrient content of the marine habitat. They also emit bioluminescence.

Most of us have heard about or experienced the nighttime phosphorescent sparkling of the ocean's surface during plankton blooms. This bioluminescence is a biophoton event, occurring at a wavelength perceivable by human retinal cells. When *lingulodinium polydrum* blooms in red tide events, for example, the billions of dinoflagellates will turn the seashore waters phosphorescent blue. It is quite an awesome scene.

Biologists now reason that dinoflagellates are communicating on a grander level during these bioluminescence events. These communications are referred to as *quorum sensing*. Quorum sensing is created when small organisms communicate a general consciousness to make a mass change when they have significant enough numbers. Pathogenic microorganisms also have this capability within the body. This is why common yeasts like *Candida albicans* can exist in the body without any detriment, but once they grow to certain populations, they can overwhelm other populations of symbiotics or probiotics, and burden the body with various symptoms. Not unlike what is seen among the dinoflagellates, *Candida* microorganisms coordinate with waveform messaging to expand their colonies to take advantage of times of weakened immunity within the host.

Gradually we are learning just how smart other organisms large and small are. Marine researchers have realized for example that sharks actually have keen senses and the ability to 'see' their prey by picking up subtle waveforms. In addition to a keen sense of smell and rather good eyesight, the shark has a series of *electroreceptors* positioned within lateral line channels throughout the shark's head, running down the length of the body into the tail. Many fish and even amphibians also have lateral line organs, allowing the fish to sense various waveforms from the surrounding water environment. In sharks, these lateral line channels are implanted with sensors that allow a shark to pick up subtle electromagnetic pulses of life in its environment. This allows sharks to recognize targets or enemies hiding within the sand or in murky waters. These electroreceptors can also sense motion from extreme distances. The shark can identify the splashing of a seal pup up to two miles away, for example. Through these sensory ampules, a shark can also sense fear or panic among other organisms. What is the shark sensing with these electroreceptors? These are the organism's combined biophoton emissions—waveforms reflecting conscious emotions—given off by the unlucky living organism.

These various waveform processes illustrate the connection between cellular biophoton emissions and message reception. Ion channel transport systems existing within and around each of our cells combine with our DNA's molecular bonding structures to crystallize instructional messaging. Together these systems provide the basis for cellular communication and broadcasting mechanisms. This biophoton messaging system also provides the mechanisms for the holographic display of brain waveforms during vision, hearing and other sense perception, as will be covered in depth later.

Cellular division and replication is the culmination of these biophoton messaging systems. The specific traits of the cell—its genetic blueprint of the body's metabolism—are communicated during this process. The higher levels of photon emissions picked up by researchers during replication illustrate this effect. We can conclude that the basic messaging systems of the body are multi-layered and complex. They provide for a smart mapping network of waveforms, wholly unobservable in cadaver dissection.

As we survey the empirical evidence, we arrive at the reality that along with specialized metabolic functions, each cell is a communication device. Each cell is designed to both receive and transmit information. This exchange of information occurs between cells and the outside environment, between one cell and another, and between each cell and the body's various messaging systems stemming from its master guidance systems.

Ion Pathways

Cells might be compared to smart radio-driven generators with multi-layered reception and transmission communication systems. As physiologists have delved deeper into the activities of the estimated trillion cells in the human body, they have continued to see increasingly deeper levels of biocommunication activity amongst the electrolyte ions within and around the cell. Increasingly, we are finding that ion channels provide a window into this complex network of conscious information messaging.

The ion channel is an informational device because it establishes an on-off state in the form of an open or closed gateway. Actually, the gateway of most ion channels is even a bit more complex. Research has indicated that one of three possible states is produced within the typical ion channel gateway: deactivation, activation or inactivation. Both a deactivated state and an inactivated state are closed, while an activated state is open. The difference between the two closed states is that a deactivated gate is blocked by an opposing open gate, while the inactive gate is simply closed in process after activation. In other words, the latter produces a rhythmic opening and closing adherent to voltage potential changes.

One of the most prominent potential conductors in the body is the sodium ion. Sodium ions negotiate electromagnetic waveforms efficiently. *Sodium channels* thus lie within cell membranes of the most active cells in the body, including muscle and nerve cells. These protein complexes are activated by the voltage potential changes provided by sodium ions as they cycle through their biochemical processes. In response to ionic state changes, many sodium channels will generate a change in electric potential inside the cell by conducting sodium ions through the cell membrane. By changing the cell's electrical potential, the cell's inner polarity and reactive potential with various nutrients and biochemicals will change. This will stimulate particular types of biological processes within the cell. Among sodium channels are various subunit types—specialized for a particular cellular activity, organ or tissue system.

Potassium channels exist in almost every cell in the body. They are involved in regulating the secretion and reception of various types of hormones. Potassium channels also lie primarily within the cell membrane. Much like the sodium channels, they provide voltage gates through which potassium ion charges can travel. Potassium channels are activated by various means with specific response ranges. A newly discovered type of potassium channel system is the double-pore system, quite extraordinary compared to the mostly single pore system of other known ionic channels. This double-pore potassium channel is thought to be a complex regulator in vascular cells—it stimulates tone and flexibility to the artery walls.

Calcium channels provide another type of voltage circuit. Calcium ion channels are found among various specialized cells in brain, organ, and nerve systems. The calcium gateways have been linked with an informational depolarization process. This turns on and off the release of various neurotransmitters and hormones. Like the sodium and potassium channels, calcium channels have various subunit types. These will often produce specific results within specialized cells.

Chloride channels appear to be related to regulating the cell's nutritional contents. No less than thirteen different types of chloride channels have been discovered. Each type regulates different nutrients and informational functions within different types of cells.

These are merely the tip of the iceberg. There are trillions of waveform channels throughout the body. Information flows through each and every one constantly. Other types of voltage potential channels have been isolated by research over recent years. *Cation channels* are activated through a combination of ions. They predominate within sperm cells. Cation-selective double pore channels provide both inward and outward voltage potential changes. *Rhodopsin channels* are activated open through the reception of light. *Transient receptor potential channels*—also called TRPs—have so far been observed among fruit flies. Many scientists suspect these also within humans. TRPs are channels that respond to photoelectric waveforms. There are a number of different types of TRPs with various functions. Another type of voltage channel is the *cyclic nucleotide channel.* These are thought to regulate the entry of various ions and nucleotides, which drive energy use and cellular clockworks activity. The heart's pacemaker neurons function extensively with cyclic nucleotide channels, for example. To the billions of channels of the types mentioned above, we can add the cAMP and IP3 channels, and many others.

There are about 80 known macro and trace minerals in the body. As nutritional research into macro minerals has continued, we have gradually come to understand that every mineral plays an important role. Should the human body be lacking in any of these elements, imbalances in metabolism begin to occur. Some of the more prevalent macro minerals include, among others, calcium, potassium, magnesium, sodium and phosphorus. These are called macro because they exist in larger quantities in the body. These minerals contribute to the ionic informational activities of the vast legions of catalysts, proteins, enzymes, cell walls, artery walls, and so many other structural elements of the body's anatomy. They also facilitate communications between cells by providing gateway messaging mechanisms.

All the trace and macro minerals are vital to metabolism. The balance between both macro and trace elements is one of the key governing factors in maintaining physiological balance. Zinc, for example, was long considered not that critical to health. Some thought that zinc was poisonous. Recent research has found that this trace element is a key factor for at least one hundred enzyme and immune system processes. Zinc is a participant in immune function, growth, wound repair, DNA production and enzyme reaction. Without zinc, the body will function in a depressed immune state. Immunity will drop. Foods will taste bland. Today zinc is considered a critical mineral.

It might be surprising that other important trace elements include fluorine, cadmium, copper, chlorine and even uranium are also utilized by the body, albeit in minute quantities. In larger quantities, these elements can be toxic. They are nonetheless essential for many metabolic functions. They are each involved directly or indirectly in innumerable enzyme functions, protein sequencing, immune cell composition and many other functions. Without a consistent source of trace elements, our body's metabolic operations quickly become handicapped.

Each mineral ion provides a specific polarity and covalence for sub-atomic bonding. Each also provides a unique facility for waveform conductance. Conducting ions provide a bridge for information transmission throughout the body. Mineral-conducting waveforms converge through a variety of ion bridges and channels into interference patterns. From these interference patterns, instructional messages emerge. This might be compared to putting a hand in front of a projector screen. The hand blocks part of the light, allowing the opportunity to communicate through various hand gestures. These hand gestures can communicate an idea or shape. The interference between the hand and the light enable the communication. A mineral might be compared to the hand, with each type of mineral and mineral combination providing a different shape. Just as standard 110 household current can be manipulated by the appliance and transformed into specific functions, minerals provide an ion bridge to energy transfer and biomolecules with mineral combinations provide translating devices.

Interference patterns created from viewing different visual spectrum waveforms through the retina and optic nerve also provide good illustrations. Each light and color reflection waveform seemingly has no meaning alone. When waveforms converge within an interference pattern, however, they create information packages. During cellular reactions, tiny electromagnetic waveforms work to define which reaction will occur when. The specific assembly of minerals provides the basis for the molecular combinations that create the appropriate electromagnetic interference patterns.

The respective interference patterns created by the waveforms transferred through an assembly of minerals and ions form the instructional messages that turn on and off specific biochemical reactions. Without this instructional messaging system, there would be no operational control over the body's reactions. They would simply begin randomly and after beginning, they would run indefinitely, out of control.

This is on-off state is starkly illustrated by the inflammatory pathway. The body responds to an injury with a number of inflammatory repair cells such as plasmin and fibrin to patch up the injury. Blood will usually coalesce around the injury to deliver these and other nutrients required to repair the wound. At some point in the process, signaling molecules will stop the inflammatory process, and initiate a clean out of the area to allow for the next steps of the healing process. Cortisol has been seen as involved as one of the key switching messengers. As cortisol levels increase, inflammation is reduced. Pharmaceutical medicine has discovered this link, prompting today's mass prescription of cortisone-based pharmaceuticals. The switching message communicated by cortisol is transmitted via the electromagnetic molecular structure of cortisol. Without cortisol, the inflammatory process would run out of control.

Cortisol also modulates both sodium and potassium concentrations within the body. It also modulates insulin levels and stimulates gastric juices, and stimulates copper-based enzyme functions such as superoxide dismutase. All of these functions are driven by the messenger functions of the cortisol molecule. Cortisol's molecular structure is made up of a combination of carbon, hydrogen and oxygen, just as are many of the body's molecules. It is the unique combination of electromagnetic bonds between the hydrogen and oxygen ions that facilitate cortisol's multifarious abilities. The commingled arrangement of their electromagnetic waveform interference patterns enables its unique messaging.

In traditional chemistry, acids and bases are defined in hydrogen atoms—or proton proportions. An acid is typically described as a substance with an excess of hydrogen atoms (H+), which acts as a net proton donor. A base, on the other hand, is considered either a hydroxide (OH-) donor or a proton acceptor—a substance often described as having excessive electrons. Net charge is also used to describe these solutions. An acid solution is one with a net positive charge, while a base solution has a net negative charge. An acid is often referred to as *catonic* (with cations) because it has a positive net charge, while a base will have a negative charge and thus is referred to as an *anion.*

We can also describe this in the more suitable context of electromagnetic waveforms. The imbalance between units of positively oriented waveforms and units of negatively oriented waveforms creates the measure of its acidic or basic state. This "orientation" is purported to compose of quantum mechanical elements. We can summarize these as containing multi-dimensional magnetic fields with unique spin directions. As mentioned, every electronic wave is accompanied by a perpendicular magnetic field. This field also relates to the spin orientation and magnetic field direction of the molecule.

A measurement of the level of acidity or alkalinity using a logarithmic scale is called pH. The term pH is derived from the French word for hydrogen power, *pouvoir hydrogene,* which has been abbreviated as simply pH. pH is measured in an inverse log base-10 scale, measuring the proton-donor level by comparing it to a theoretical quantity of hydrogen ions (H+) in a solution. Thus, a pH of 5 would be equivalent to 10^5 H+ *moles* worth of cations in the solution. (A mole is a quantity of substance compared to 12 grams of the six-neutron carbon isotope.) Put another way, a pCl (chlorine) concentration would be the negative log of chlorine ion concentration in a solution, and pK would be the negative log of potassium ions in a solution.

The pH scale is 0 to 14, for 10^{-1} (1) to 10^{-14} (.00000000000001) range. The scale has been set up around the fact that pure water's pH is log-7 or simply pH7. Because pure water forms the basis for so many of life's activities, and because water neutralizes and dilutes so many reactions, water became the standard reference and neutral point between an acid and a base. In other words, a substance having greater hydrogen ion concentration characteristics than water will be considered a base, while a substance containing less H+ concentration characteristics than water is considered an acid.

Of course, a solution concentration may well be lower than log-14 or higher than log-1, but this is the scale set up based upon the typical ranges observed in nature. Using this scale, any substance measuring a pH of 7 would be considered a neutral substance, though it still has a significant number of H+ ions. In humans, a pH level in the range of 6.4 is considered a healthy state because this state is slightly more acidic than water, enabling alkaline ionic current flow through the body. Better put, a 6.4 pH offers the appropriate currency of energy flow because there are enough negatively oriented waveforms present for the passage of positively oriented messaging waveforms. The earthly minerals like potassium, calcium, magnesium and others are typically positively oriented—or alkaline in nature. They thus carry the messaging (and thus nutritional) waveforms transmitted through our living earth.

The proof to these points is provided by conventional science: pH is simplified in conventional chemistry as the level of proton donor capability. Yet we know from emission measurements that the higher the electron orbit, the higher the energy emission. Energy release is measured by waveform emission characteristics such as frequency. If we remove the concept of electron particles from the equation, and replace with this the understanding of wave mechanics, we can then realize that the charge (or message) is *traveling through* a particular medium, and the pH of the substance simply measures the type of messaging able to move through that medium. This is why pH meters are voltage meters.

This concept of current traveling through a medium is understood when we consider how an electric charge can be maintained by a battery. A lead battery is set up to perform two reactions (stated conventionally): One reaction oxidizes lead—in a solution of sulfuric acid—to lead sulfate. During this reaction, energy is given off as electrons are emitted, along with hydrogen protons. The other reaction is a reduction, which converts lead dioxide to lead sulfate. This also releases energy, but this is accomplished as hydrogen protons and electrons are being absorbed to create the lead sulfate. Meanwhile, two types of lead plates attract and adhere to the resulting lead sulfates. The positive plates are filled with lead dioxide to drive the oxidation side, while the negative plates are made of lead to drive the reduction side of the battery. These two processes combine to be called *electrolysis,* which is the utilization of ions to conduct current through a particular medium.

We note in this discussion the obvious: Batteries—between their positive and negative poles—exchange an electrical current. This current is used in an automobile to start the engine, after which a generator will create enough electromagnetic energy to recharge the battery. This event reverses the changes to the lead, lead dioxide and sulfuric acid. We must also note that the initial flow of electricity out of the battery is not a spontaneous reaction, nor is the recharging of the battery. Both of these processes have been designed and assembled by humans with the conscious intention to draw a flow of electricity for a specific purpose: To start our automobile for example. Intent is also needed to keep the battery charged. If our car were not in use for a while, the battery would gradually lose its charge, requiring an intentional charge-up.

As we examine the currency properties of the living body, we recognize the same general features of the battery. The living body performs a number of reactions, some oxidizing and some reducing. In most of these reactions, energy is converted from one type to another—a conversion of electromagnetic bonding energy into different forms of kinetic energy such as movement via muscle cells. The exact utilization of the energy is steered by consciousness, which steers usage. The principal energy conversion of glucose and oxygen into the energies mentioned is a complex oxidative reaction called the Krebs cycle. This Krebs cycle will utilize the waveform bonds of ADP to ATP to generate a transport mechanism, which results in energy and ion release. The body also has similar energy conversion mechanisms such as the NADP transport system. These are only two of the billions of ionic conversion systems working within the human physiology.

All metabolism operates on this waveform conversion process. Our sensory nerves all conduct impulses through waveform ionic exchanges. Taste is driven by the acid or alkaline nature of our foods. Acidic solutions taste sour while alkaline solutions taste bitter. As we taste food, particular waveform orientations set off a chain of ionic messaging through the nervous system. Our taste buds, retinal cells, olfactory bulbs and tactile nerve endings all have similar waveform sensing electrodes with ionic gateways. The different types of waveforms emitted by physical matter simply stimulate these gateways, setting off an ionic charge relay within the body's sensory nervous systems. This relay results in interference patterns within the brain, effectively producing perception.

Biochemical Transmission

Since Loewi's research illustrating the involvement of chemistry in physiological messaging, we have learned a lot about the wave nature of sub-atomic elements, atoms, ions and molecules. Biochemical information pathways have been clearly established. It is evident that within these biochemicals exists a more subtle form of information transmission. This is illustrated by the incredible speed and accuracy of biocommunication within the body. The entire body—all its organs, blood vessels, and other tissue systems—will react instantly to a sensory perception of something potentially harmful. Through an intentionally driven networked biocommunication pathway, the signal of impending danger is broadcast to billions of cells and muscle fibers throughout the body instantaneously— enabling the body to immediately respond to a threat to its survival.

Most researchers are convinced that each hormonal instruction requires that hormone molecules (ligands) must physically touch chemical receptors. This notion was advanced in the early twentieth century by Dr. Morgan Hunt, who discovered a protein existing within the cell membrane—part in and part out. This protein was observed as a switching mechanism, receiving particular ligand instructions, and translating that to the cell's nucleus for activation. This protein was called the *notch gene,* and the notch-transport system of cellular communication has been described as one of the major cell communication pathways that instigated particular metabolic activities and coordination between other cells. Notch information biocommunication was observed among cardiac cells, neurons, bone cells (osteocytes), glandular cells and many others, progressing and stimulating some of their most critical functions. These *transmembrane protein receptors* are purported to require physical contact with a particular ligand, but is often accelerated through a catalyst enzyme process.

It is also assumed that intercellular communication requires physical molecular contact. This is often referred to as *paracrine* activity—messages being translated from one nearby cell to another. In comparison, *intracrines* are considered the cellular messengers within the cell, while *intercrines* are cell-to-cell messengers. Note in this respect that *endocrines* are biochemical messengers produced by specific glands, which are circulated around the body. Each of these messengers is assumed to require a physical chemical interaction between the ligand and its particular receptor.

Two cells are also thought to have what is considered a direct nucleus-to-nucleus interaction. This appears to occur through a type of direct-nucleus receptor called a *connexin protein.* When six of these proteins come together within a group, they form a pore or tube within the membrane called a *gap junction.* This allows cells to exchange genetic instructions, or one cell to inject instructions into another cell.

Many receptors lie on the surface of the cell membrane. Most are connected to ion channels between the cell membrane. These provide a transduction channel for the information to pass from the receptor to within the cell. Many neurotransmitters and hormones utilize this pathway to transmit their information. The assumption is that the ligand (hormone or neurotransmitter) *binds* with the receptor on a chemical basis, creating an electrical signal, which is transmitted through the ion channel.

These assumptions come from observations of ligand biochemicals in the vicinity of physical response. Sometimes new compounds are evident, theoretically indicating a possible binding reaction. It has been justly assumed that these neurochemical molecules must be intimately involved in the dissemination of metabolic messages. However, the notion that physical-chemical touch is required in all cases and among all endocrine transmissions appears unlikely, given the coordinated and instantaneous cell response on a global basis. A physical molecular connection between hormones and receptors on each and every cell membrane—even with some cells communicating with paracrines—would require circulation time for the master hypothalamic hormones, pituitary hormones and endocrine gland hormone pathways to execute simultaneously. It would require enough hormones to be secreted fully into the bloodstream, and physically be pumped from the endocrine glands—sometimes halfway around the body—to chemically and physically touch the appropriate receptor on *every* cell involved in the metabolic change.

Let us consider this scenario carefully. A receptor is a protein with an electromagnetic affinity. This requires either a polarity match, or even a constructive combination of spin or angular momentum between the ligand and receptor. In the human body, it is estimated there is one protein molecule for every 10,000 molecules in and around the cells of the body. Furthermore, there are about 200 trillion cells in the human body, and billions if not trillions of them are activated immediately in fearful or stressful response. Every cell in the toes must be activated immediately to break into an immediate run for example. According to the physical ligand-receptor theory, not only does each hormone molecule have to connect with each and every cell membrane, but each hormone must also locate an open, active receptor on every cell membrane.

Observation and *in vitro* testing has shown receptors to have four basic scenarios: They can be *agonized,* or stimulated. They can be *partially agonized* of partly stimulated. They can be *inversely agonized,* and their response lowered. They can also be *antagonized,* whereby they are blocked by a molecule and thereby not be stimulated. So we ask: How is it these hormones can intelligently weave through every tiny capillary and dense maze of tissue systems to bump into the right receptor without being agonized on every needed cell instantaneously? Now if we perceived parts of our body being activated first and then other parts, corresponding to the circulatory routes these hormones or neurotransmitters take, we might be able to agree with this hypothesis. Consider circulatory restrictions such as atherosclerosis and other artery diseases restricting blood flow. In addition, consider that many tissue cells are reached only through tiny microcapillaries—some barely large enough to be able to allow a single red blood cell through at a time within the diameter of the lumen (the opening). If a response required the blood to deliver a hormone molecule to a receptor on every cell within a particular tissue system before that tissue system could respond, we would really be in trouble if we needed to run from an attacker.

We could only imagine the situation where we were frightened by a tiger in the woods, only to find that our upper hamstrings were ready to take off but our toes were not—leaving us stuck while the tiger pounced. Rather, the toes, hamstrings, knees and every skeletal muscle cell, along with the eyes, lungs, brain, and vocal cords all respond at the same moment as we scream and run instantaneously.

The body's process of stimulating metabolic activity has been a mystery to researchers for thousands of years. In modern research, the process of discovery has been to identify hormone presence using radiography with dye markers to trace the flow of chemicals. This physical 'snap-shot' process is combined with harvesting and analyzing organ chemistry with spectroscopic analysis. Via these two methods, researchers figure that since the hormone/ligands are in the proximity of the response, they must be physically setting off the response of each and every cell. This is often confirmed with the techniques pioneered by Loewi to provide the conclusion. While conferring biochemical presence, finding biochemicals in the region offers no conclusive mechanism. We might compare this to finding a gun near a murder victim. We can assume the gun was involved, but this fact alone does not tell us who shot the murder victim.

For example, we know the thyroid gland is one of the central endocrine drivers of metabolism. Researchers have linked cellular metabolic rates and thermogenesis to the presence of thyroid hormones thyroxine and triiodothyronine. These are also referred to as T4 and T3, respectively. The chemical makeup of these messengers are not that exciting—a combination of the amino acid tyrosine and iodine. However, these rather simple molecular structures T4 and T3 somehow charge trillions of cells throughout the body—increasing the speed and output of their various metabolic processes. Without enough of either T4 or T3 (T3 is considered to be the more active of the two, but T3 is derived from T4) the body begins to cool down. A feeling of fatigue will overwhelm a thyroid hormone-deficient body. Suddenly the most basic tasks become difficult in TSH (thyroid stimulating hormone), T3 or T4 deficiencies. The thyroid also produces calcitonin, which works with parathyroid hormone to balance bone calcium levels.

Once the blood contains enough thyroid hormones it becomes almost suddenly energized. This is evidenced by the oral intake of synthetic and analogous thyroid hormones. How again do all those trillions of cells become energized from a pill or two? Again, the theory of cell reception requires that each cell has a set of little chemical receptor 'locks' on its cell membrane, and these ligand chemicals provide the 'keys.' Thus, each cell receptor must be physically touched and unlocked with those chemical ligands. Are there enough moles of chemicals in one or two pills to circulate through the blood system and basal membrane and reach every cell's receptors to energize them? Or perhaps the paracrine system provides a mechanism for filling the gap for cells the chemicals do not physically bind to?

This problem is complicated by the fact that thyroid hormones are hydrophobic—they are not water-friendly. They are not water-soluble. Since the blood, the cells, and their basal surroundings are mostly water, this makes their journey to every cell difficult. Perhaps thyroid hormones require thyroxine-binding globulins, transthyrein and albumins for adequate circulation. It is thought that these may provide a carrier mechanism to each cell. Somehow, these chemical messengers T3 and T4 manage to instantly and simultaneously make their way around the body to stimulate and energize each cell. In other words, the neck does not warm up first, and then the arms warm up, and so on. All the body parts will become energized simultaneously with some exception for diseased tissue systems.

The cell membrane is composed of a variety of lipids—cholesterol, phospholipids and sphingolipids—specialized proteins and glycoproteins. The lipids making up most cell membranes are structurally double-layered and arranged to prevent unwanted molecules from passing through the membrane. The lipid wall is also hydrophobic—keeping water from penetrating the surface without passing through the cell membrane's complex ion channels.

Some cell membranes—particularly in nerve cells—are *myelin*. Others are *inner mitochondrial* in nature. Mitochondrial inner membranes are made up of electron transport proteins, while a myelin membrane will be composed primarily of plasma with less protein. The lipid cell membrane is negatively charged. This sets up an ionic gradient between the inside and the outside of the cell membrane. Crossing the cell membrane is not a physical experience for most molecules—it is primarily an electromagnetic crossing. Water and nutrients are escorted through the membrane through ionic diffusion. This is complicated by the various proteins that electromagnetically identify substances as they pass. Mineral ions pass through the cell membrane via *ionic transport chains*. Ionic transport chains made from protein are similar to ion channels except they allow entry to key nutrients and minerals needed in the cell—particularly sodium, potassium and calcium but also many trace elements. These ions provide just the right electromagnetic environment to set up channels for ionic instructional messages to pass through the cell membrane into the cytoplasm, where they can stimulate RNA, mitochondria and other organelles into action. Thus, the cell membrane's ionic transport mechanisms escort appropriate nutrients in and out of cell, while receptors receive and transmit the messages of hormones like thyroid hormones, insulin, and acetylcholine through ion channels into the cell.

Some might contend that some biochemical messengers are delivered through tissue spaces and ion channels. Yes, certainly there are basal channels that provide access. Still we must remember the adrenal gland is a very small gland in the abdominal region of the body. The thyroid gland is a tiny gland in the neck. To assume that cortisol, epinephrine, acetylcholine, and thyroid hormones must jettison from these tiny organs to every cell—even in fingers and toes—to stimulate the correct cellular and tissue responses should these appendages come under attack is a stretch. Certainly, a strictly physical chemical delivery system would result in a lot more missing fingers and toes than we generally see.

It is interesting that we can accept that informational messages can travel instantly throughout the body via the nervous system. The nervous system can stimulate a particular skeletal muscle system to activate instantly. The ability of all the support systems to come into play, however, is the result of these biochemical informational messenger systems. A perfect example is vasopressin's ability to concentrate urine in the kidneys and constrict artery walls.

Environmental drivers of hormones include light, temperature, gravity, the changing seasons, and cellular metabolism. Internal drivers, however, stem from emotional consciousness. Hormones are complex body chemicals, made of either glycoproteins or steroids. Among other functions, hormones turn on cellular switches for many metabolic functions. Growth hormones encourage cellular growth. Thyroid hormones regulate cellular metabolism speed and temperature regulation. Follicle stimulating hormones and luteinizing hormones stimulate reproductive mechanisms. Insulin stimulates the clearing and attachment of glucose into cells for energy production. Vasopressin stimulates the decreases urine volume, constricts blood vessel walls and stimulates certain memory functions. Cortisol counteracts insulin, inhibits immune system processes such as inflammation and lymphocyte function, stimulates increased circulation and blood pressure, helps regulate potassium/sodium balance, stimulates stomach acids, increases glucogenesis to name a few.

These are just a few of the hundreds of messaging hormones that make up the complex waveform broadcasting system working within the body. Hormones are directly and indirectly involved guiding all of the physical body's various mechanisms. Hormones turn on and shut off genetic switches in particular cells, typically through stimulating the transmembrane receptors. Hormones work primarily within pathways often referred to as *cascades*. As in the 'domino-effect,' a cascade is the progressive stimulation of one activity, which in turn stimulates another. These cascades fire at tremendous speeds, as ligand-receptor triggers initiate pathways of stimulating mechanisms.

An example of a cascading messaging system is the response stimulated by sensory sensation occurring somewhere in the body and transmitted through the neurons to the brain. The pre-programmed sympathetic response (the reflex arc) is typically accompanied by conscious reception of the sensation via the limbic system. The focal point of this stimulation is the thalamus, which acts as a waveform message translator and decoder. Waveform-transmitting neurons deep within the thalamus are engaged, stimulating waves that combine with others to form an interference pattern—also referred to as a neural mapping. As these waveform interference patterns are decoded, some are reflected back to the cerebral cortex. Here an exchange of waveform patterns takes place. A relay of information is conducted between the cerebral cortex and the thalamus, reflecting the information back onto the prefrontal cortex. Here the information is responded to, followed by a return of pulses that stimulate the hypothalamus gland to secrete biochemicals. These biochemical messengers either stimulate endocrine or cellular function directly, or stimulate the pituitary gland to in turn secrete biochemical messengers that precisely activate endocrine glands and physical response.

The hypothalamus, located at the base of the brain under the thalamus, encapsulates part of the third ventricle. The body's autonomic responses are processed here, some of which in turn stimulate the pituitary gland to release key master hormones. These master hormones signal responses that control the critical phase cycles of metabolism, body core temperature, appetite, thirst and so on.

The hypothalamus responds to waveform inputs from the brain centers and limbic system. These brain centers provide the platforms for conscious interaction with waveform messaging. Waveform interference patterns are created from the various sensory nerve transmissions and response neurotransmitter biochemicals. These interactive interference patterns form the basis for information. This facilitates perspective, and allows a sorting process to prioritize the information within the limbic system. Stresses on the body such as infection and immune response also feed into the limbic system for response. For these waveforms, the hypothalamus activates immediate response cascades using the limbic system's programming.

The hypothalamus and limbic system thus respond to a wide range of stimuli, and construct biochemical responses by activating an orchestrated flow of biochemical messengers to stimulate particular physical responses around the body. Dispatched messengers include dopamine, melatonin, somatostatin and others. The hypothalamus also secretes hypothalamic hormones that stimulate the pituitary to produce a number of master endocrine hormones.

The hypothalamic hormones are sent through the hypophyseal capillary beds before they are delivered to the pituitary gland. Once arriving at the pituitary, these biochemical messengers instruct the pituitary gland to secrete specific 'master' hormones. These in turn stimulate particular endocrine glands and regions around the body to produce yet another level of biochemical messengers. These instructional biochemicals include growth hormones, adrenocorticotropic hormones, luteinizing hormones, follicle-stimulating hormones, prolactins, estrogens, testosterone, thyroid stimulating hormones; as well as neurotransmitters like adrenaline, serotonin, acetylcholine and others.

Amazingly, the subsidiary endocrine glands and tissue centers receive the master hormone messages rather instantly, and react instantly by initiating the release of even more specific informational biochemical messengers. These are hormones and neurotransmitters that precisely and directly affect the body's cellular metabolism, organ function and tissue mechanisms. As we all have experienced, the messages stimulate action almost instantly, at tremendous speeds—perhaps at speeds at or above the speed of light. So not only does the limbic system and master glands respond instantly to sensory stimuli, but the entire cascading system responds instantaneously with biochemical messenger cascades that broadcast precise instructions throughout our body's physiology.

Adrenocorticotropic hormone or ACTH is a good example. ACTH is produced by the anterior pituitary gland. Its function is to stimulate the adrenal cortex to release cortisol, and to a lesser degree androgens such as testosterone. The adrenal cortex also produces aldosterone, which stimulates the retention of urine and heightened blood pressure, involved in the renin and angiotensin cycle. The adrenal medulla is also stimulated by sympathetic nerves into producing epinephrine and norepinephrine. Epinephrine is considered a fight-or-flight hormone because it stimulates glycogen and fat breakdown while increasing the heart rate, dilating the pupils and stimulating a number of cognition mechanisms. Epinephrine also stimulates a cascade that constricts some blood vessels while dilating others—namely those feeding needed muscles. An intelligent gating pathway through the liver using inositol and liver enzymes activates glucose release to coordinate with this. Epinephrine's intelligent combination of constriction in vessels effectively diverts blood and nutrients from unnecessary tissues to those deemed necessary for a well-coordinated fight-or-flight response. How does a chemical—a combination of hydrogen, carbon, oxygen and nitrogen—make this sort of distinction? How does it decide which way to divert circulation? How does it know which muscles will be needed? Can a simple chemical make these sorts of judgments—instantly?

Medical researchers believe this is driven by epinephrine's ability to stimulate multiple receptors, most notably the alpha-1 and beta-2 receptors. The alpha-1 tends to stimulate a liver signaling process affecting insulin, while the beta-2 tends to stimulate the process of converting glycogen to glucose. However, this simplistic version of the process can hardly explain how this hormone can instantly gear the body up for fight or flight mode while concurrently coordinating which tissue groups are fed and which tissue groups are starved.

The pituitary gland also produces follicle-stimulating hormone, which stimulates the ovarian follicle to produce estrogen in women. It also stimulates the testes to produce sperm in men. Estrogens are complex because they will assist in the development of female sex organs and female characteristics like breasts, while they also stimulate the uterine environment by expanding the endometrium at the early part of the menstrual cycle. Indeed, the rhythmic cycles of menstruation and ovulation, and of pre- peri- and post-menopause tell us that estrogens also have complex messaging pathways within various tissue mechanisms—some significantly affecting moods and nerve activity. Testosterone is also complex, as its levels relate not just to prostate health in men, but also to general vitality and overall health among both men and women.

Although modern medical science has assumed a physical proximity particle-molecule receptor binding mechanism for hormone effects within the body, it is a rather academic debate because at the same time, science is thoroughly aware that there is no touching within the subatomic atmosphere of atoms and molecules. Quantum mechanics and the law of uncertainty tell us that subatomic units are particle-waves, which rotate around the nucleus at dramatic relative distances. As atoms merge to become molecules, a sharing of particle-wave orbitals takes place. These orbitals do not have the ability to come into physical contact with each other within the molecule. So even in the paradigm of a ligand bonding with physical proximity to a receptor to create a new molecule, there is only a sharing of electromagnetic orbitals involved, which are of course waveform in nature.

Logically, while we can say that close proximity orbital binding can and does occur with some messaging, the nature of the electromagnetic exchange of information logically should not require physical proximity to transfer the message. We might compare this with two people standing next to each other exchanging information. They conduct this exchange through speaking. The nature of speaking is such that the two people could easily stand further away from each other and still exchange the information through speaking. They may have to speak a little louder, but the passing of the information would suffer no deficiency between standing next to each other and standing several feet apart.

The biochemical signaling process comes without the merit of observation, albeit indirect. Scientists cannot open up a human intercellular process and analyze the process to determine the exact mode of biocommunication. However, lab researchers can isolate a complex metabolic process requiring a signaling event, and run a chemical analysis on the whole region to see what chemical changes occurred. Before and after chemical analyses (typically via centrifuge followed by mass spectrometry, or possibly electron microscope) will illustrate a chemical change within the region. A change in the composition would infer that the biocommunication coincided with the ligand-receptor exchange.

However, this does require an initial assumption that the biocommunication process is indeed biochemical-driven.

With confirmed research results, we cannot deny there was a chemical reaction that coincided with the biocommunication. The question that arises, however, is whether the chemical reaction caused the biocommunication event or whether the biocommunication event caused the chemical reaction. It is altogether possible that one of the byproducts of the biocommunication transmission was a chemical reaction. Chemical changes often coincide with waveform transmissions. The microwaving of food will likely create a chemical change in the food, for example. The sun's rays often spark composition reactions in soil and water as well. In fact, most electromagnetic waveform transmissions result in chemical reactions of some sort, because the waveforms interfere with the electromagnetic bonds within molecules of the substance being struck, creating a chemical response.

This basic question of which comes first might be compared to seeing some blood in a hungry shark's tank and assuming the blood made the shark hungry. It is quite possible (and probably more likely) that the shark was hungry before the water was bloody. It is more likely that the shark's hunger drove him to eat, making the tank bloody from the fish he ate. This is also logical, noting shark behavior.

This is not such a fantastic supposition. Every type of communication signal we receive externally is transmitted via waveforms. The most basic signaling event, vision, is signaled via visible electromagnetic radiation. When we look at a star billions of light years away, we are seeing waveform transmissions that may have traveled for several days or even years before reaching our eyes. Hearing is also a waveform-stimulated process, as our inner ears convert air pressure waves to electromagnetic pulses. If the body conducts its most basic communication events via waveform signaling, why should we assume cells should not share those capabilities? Do we feel our cells are any less technical than the rest of our bodies?

This does not necessitate us completely abandoning the *lock-and-key* mechanisms theorized between ligands and receptors. Waveform communications can also be compared to a lock-and-key mechanism. The concept of the receptor simply has to be expanded to include waveform communications. It is also altogether possible that ligands can stimulate the biocommunication through the lock-an-key biochemical basis in addition to remote biocommunication signaling.

We might justly compare this mechanism with our ability to turn on and off a television. We can either walk up to the television and turn it off by pressing the on-off button "manually" or we can use the remote control to achieve the same purpose. In the same way, hormones may make biochemical contract or utilize waveform transmissions to stimulate a receptor. Furthermore, just as we can walk around our living room with our remote and control our television volume and channel, hormone-signaling molecules can move around the body and stimulate multiple cells into action simultaneously. Just as we are more assured of accurate channel changing when our remote is within close proximity of the television, the body is assured of more accurate responses among the cells when the signaling hormones are within close proximity of the cells and their receptors. It is for this reason that messengers are dispatched. Information exchange can begin instantly using radio signaling between these ligand messengers and their receptors.

These mechanisms were proven by over two decades of research headed up by Jacques Benveniste, M.D. and several other research teams. Dr. Benveniste was one of the foremost experts in the study of ligand-receptor mechanisms within the immune system for many years. He was the research director for the French National Institute for Health and Medical Research (INSERM) for a number of years. Dr. Benveniste's career was very distinguished. Several years earlier, he was credited with the discovery of the platelet-activating factor.

It was during further immune system research on the action of basophils that Dr. Benveniste and his research technician Elisabeth Davenas accidentally discovered that an allergic response in solution took place even though the tested allergen was effectively diluted out of the solution. Because the allergen was responded to without an apparent molecular basis (as the substance was diluted out), Dr. Benveniste began a search for what actually caused the immune response. This led to a four-year study on immunoglobulin IgE response—research included joint trials and confirmations with five laboratories in four countries. The research concluded that even at dilutions of 10^{120} (one part to ten parts with one hundred and twenty zeros behind it), and no probability of available molecules, the same immunoglobulin immune responses would occur as with significant concentrations. After confirming this variously, Dr. Benveniste and his team proposed that water somehow acts as a carrier for immune messaging. What else was left in the solution to carry the immune response messaging?

After eliminating alternative causes of this phenomenon, Dr. Benveniste and his research associates began to focus on the potential for a radio signaling process of some type. After much experimentation, the right technology and equipment led to the understanding that cells respond to low-frequency electromagnetic waves. Remarkably, certain biochemical messengers like acetylcholine produce unique electromagnetic waveforms. The question was now whether these waveforms played a role in the immunoglobulin communication.

Dr. Benveniste eventually developed sensitive audio equipment to record the frequencies of biochemical messengers. In the early 1990s, using his digital sound equipment with computerized technology, Benveniste and his associates recorded thousands of these low-frequency waves from various biochemicals. Amazingly, by playing back these recordings in the midst of cells and tissues, the recorded frequencies were able to stimulate the exact same responses the biochemicals stimulated. After several years of testing, Benveniste and his associates built up quite a library of biochemical waveform recordings. Frequencies of established biochemical messengers such as heparin, ovalbumin, acetylcholine and dextran were digitized and recorded. Unbelievably, these digital recording files were then be put on CD and mailed—or even emailed—to other labs. The other lab would play back the recordings onto various cell tissues—exciting the same responses the physical biochemicals stimulated.

This proposition more accurately fits with the body's ability to bridge consciousness with external stimuli. An advanced signaling process using low- and extra-low frequency electromagnetic frequencies creates a messaging system to elicit instantaneous responses simultaneously from billions of cells, just as radio broadcasts will bridge radio jockeys with millions of remote listeners simultaneously.

This model also supports the observation of some ligands coming into close proximity with cells in certain regions. These ligands may require close proximity to their receptors in order to elicit a response. Others, however, are designed to elicit responses from further distances. This might again be compared to the radio-to-radio frequencies used for communications. A CB-band, walkie-talkie system, remote telephone, or television remote may have a relatively short range of reception, depending upon the power of the signal. Therefore, remote telephones that transmit with greater power can be used at greater distances. Radio station broadcasting is also based upon the strength of the waveform signals. For this reason, some radio stations can be heard at much greater distances than others can. In contrast, other radio frequencies, such as shortwave or ham radios, can transmit over thousands of miles, even at lower power.

We apply this same variance to the intracellular process. Different hormones or ligands within the body have different purposes. Therefore, they each broadcast with different signal strengths, and at different frequencies. Just as we choose different types of communication systems or devices for different priorities, the type of biochemical messenger and signal strength used would relate to the need and timing required.

As we examine signaling broadcasting and reception, the cell's transmembrane receptors must *resonate* with the particular frequency emitted by the ligand. This follows the logic of any radio broadcast. Radios utilize not only a receiver but also a tuner, so the radio can synchronize with the broadcast's frequency. This is also a form of resonation. As we turn the tuner on a radio to find the right station, we are locating a point where the radio's receiver is resonating with the waveforms of the broadcasting station's signals. This process was developed using the radio crystal to receive and semiconduct particular waveforms into particular electronic pulses, notably a focus of the great early twentieth century inventor, Nicola Tesla.

Within the body, waveform signals and their messengers are programmed for broadcast through the pathways of signaling messengers beginning from the pituitary gland and its master gland the hypothalamus. As we trace this programming process back further, we find the various brain cortices like the prefrontal cortex at the center of these pathways—at the seat of consciousness. We might compare this to a song we hear playing on the radio being traced back to a particular radio station broadcast, and eventually back to the musician who originally wrote and performed the song.

Indeed, when we consider every response and movement within the physical body, we are seeing a relayed broadcasting process. These broadcasting pathways stimulate physical activity through the network of endocrine glands, the bloodstream, the nervous system, the basal membranes, transmembrane receptors and of course an army of signaling hormones and neurotransmitters. Every beat of our heart and every hunger pang or skeletal muscle twitch is the result of such a cascading signal process. Waveform broadcasts relay information from one biochemical type to another. We can thus compare the transmembrane protein receptors to antenna, and the genetic translation sequences as radio semiconductor crystals.

Biochemical messengers are not dumbwaiters. They have their own informational fingerprinting and translation processes as well. They translate messages specific to the particular body and situation. In other words, those messages are unique to that body. A person injected with hormones from a donor might have a physiological response generic to that hormone, but the specific message being carried through the donor's hormones will not be translated specifically through the body of the recipient. The message is the specific information about which muscles need to be stimulated, which arteries should be dilated in one region or another, and so on. We can test this by injecting epinephrine donated from one person into another person. The injected person's tissues might still be stimulated in a non-specific way, depending upon the location of the injection and the physical state of the injected subject. However, the injection will not stimulate the precise emotional response the body it was extracted from was carrying out. This is observable. The injected person simply does not process the same physiological responses.

The injection of vaccines has the same affect. The body receiving the injection will not respond identically with the source from which the antigens were derived. The injection will stimulate the body's own immune system to respond, quite possibly to produce similar immunoglobulins to fight the same antigen. Each body will initiate its own unique immunity messaging system because each body is driven by a unique conscious personality.

Consider for a moment the translation of a United Nations speech given by a foreign diplomat into a number of foreign languages concurrently. The translating technology (and/or live interpreters) works to translate each word and each phrase from the speaker's language into these other languages. This allows each UN representative the opportunity to hear the speech in his or her native language simultaneously. It was simply translated in real-time into their respective languages.

As a particular message is sent via one part of the body to another, the message is also being translated in real-time into the various functions necessary for the body. When the hypothalamus sends its hormonal messages to the pituitary, they are encoded with the needed response for that event, which are accompanied by a nervous signaling to supply additional information. The pituitary translates this combined message into a multitude of responses to each part of the body. These are broadcast out for processing to each endocrine gland through secreted hormones. Each endocrine organ then receives this translated message, and each one of these organs each does the same: They translate the message into specific biochemical signals.

This broadcasting and translation system is specific and intelligent. If the translation system at the United Nations incorrectly translated any of the words spoken by the speaker, the speech could be grossly misinterpreted. This could be dangerous. It could theoretically start a war. Therefore, the speech must be translated using an intelligent and impartial translating system.

The messages sent through the endocrine system must also be intelligent. Imagine our endocrine system sending out the same message regardless of whether we were being chased by a tiger, or say were in danger of a head-on collision driving in a car. We simply could not react to these two situations with an identical physiological response.

Specific and complex messages are being broadcast from the intelligent centers of the neural network, whether on a purely sympathetic process or autonomic bandwidth. These messages travel within waveforms just as our radio and television communications travel within broadcast radiowaves. The body's waveform broadcasts utilize crystallized amplification mechanisms called hormones to set the stage for the response. Each endocrine organ—or relay station—receives the signals and translates them into a more specific waveform broadcast. This more specific broadcast is meant to stimulate activity with increased specificity for a particular organ or tissue system. As the message is translated at the endocrine organ, it is again broadcast throughout the body, using protein crystals to regulate, amplify, boost or even restrict the message in some way. This enables a transmission with the ability to resonate with and appropriately instruct specific cells or tissue systems.

The use of these receptors and ligands are quite analogous to the functions of semiconductors and resisters among electrical circuits. Resistors and semiconductors—depending upon their positioning and makeup—will slow, redirect and in general modulate the flow of electrical pulses while providing an insulation process. This dampening affect allows the semiconductor or resistor to prevent the pulse from overloading the appliance or shocking its user.

The messaging biochemicals of the body—the hormones and neurotransmitters—must damper, modulate and sometimes even reverse the instructional flow in order for the messages to be properly and precisely engaged. We want to *just* outrun the tiger without killing the body with a heart attack, for example.

The broadcast signals of these relayed messages come with unique waveforms and sequences. Proprietary wave sequences will connect on a specifically resonant basis with specialized receptors on the cell membranes. The receptors on the cell membranes then *translate* and *reflect* those signals though the cytoplasm through particular organelles, RNA, DNA, or other proteins—imparting specific instructions to stimulate or modulate certain activities. These instructions serve to coordinate each cell's metabolic activity with the needs of the whole body. In the case of T3, the information is sent to the cell's ribosomes—responsible for increasing the rate of ATP transport chain processing—which directly increases the metabolic processes. In the case of insulin, the signaling initiates the preparation of micropores to absorb glucose for energy use, together with signaling other cells—such as liver cells to convert glycogen and adipose cells to store up fatty acids from glycogen.

The receptors on the cell membranes are the smart receivers for this intelligent messaging system. It might be comparable to having a satellite dish set up on a house. The dish is designed to pick up particular signals from particular satellites, and not others. The size of the dish and its positioning is established to pick up the specific waveforms emitting from that particular satellite. In the same way, particular receptors on the cell membrane are tuned to particular waveform messages sent from specific biochemicals. Whether those biochemicals are in close proximity or at a distance, their reception can be instantaneous.

Brainwaves of Consciousness

Nineteenth century researchers tested animals in an attempt to understand the electrical nature of physiology. The electric quality of the body was hard to deny even in the early days of electricity exploration. Gradually the apparatus for this probing were refined. Though possibly crudely applied earlier, Dr. Hans Berger is credited to be the first researcher to use the *electroencephalogram* (or EEG) to record brainwaves in the early 1920s. These efforts gradually gave brainwave testing credibility in psychological research. Today it is utilized for medical diagnostics, psychological testing, biofeedback testing and polygraph detection.

Several types of brain waves, each with unique frequencies, were discovered using EEG testing. Further testing using the later-discovered *magnetoencephalograph* indicated that a variety of subtle magnetic pulses also pulse through the body. First used by Dr. David Cohen in 1968, the MEG picked up another dimension of magnetic polarity among waveform transmission. MEG technology was further developed using superconductors. This equipment has been referred to as *superconducting quantum interference devices* (or SQUID).

The multitude of EEG and MEG studies over the years has confirmed the existence of several major brainwave pulses, ranging from one to sixty cycles per second. Our brains pulse to waveforms with frequency bandwidths that correspond to particular moods, stress levels, and physiological status. As we focus on the complexities of daily life, our brains reflect and emit shorter-frequency *alpha* or *beta* brainwaves. A relaxing mood tends to accompany the deeper *delta* or even the more meditative *theta* waves. The greater the stress, the higher frequencies tend to get. Just as higher-pitched sounds tend to indicate intensity or urgency, higher frequency waves reflect a mind hustling to keep up with life's details. Because initial EEG and MEG research predominantly focused upon the brain, these waves were tagged as brainwaves. Actually, we find these waves resonating throughout the body. They tend to be more predominant among the central nervous system and the brain because the brain and spinal cord tends to be the main collection foci for these waves. As will be detailed further, the central nervous system provides freeways for high-speed wave transit.

Researchers have divided the millions of possible brainwave combinations into five general ranges. Alpha waves are typically the dominant cycle during dream states and light meditation. The alpha waves are oscillations with between eight and thirteen cycles per second (same as hertz). Beta brainwaves are dominant during normal waking consciousness, and range from fourteen to thirty cycles per second. Theta waves are considered to be four to seven cycles per second and dominate during normal sleep and meditation. On the lower frequency side are the delta waves, which range from less than one cycle per second to about three cycles per second. These slow waves tend to be dominating during the deepest sleep or deepest meditation states. On the other side of the spectrum, some of the fastest rhythms recorded in the brain are the gamma waves. The high-energy gamma waveforms typically dominate during periods of advanced problem solving or critical thinking. They oscillate at between thirty and sixty cycles per second. Over the past decade, researchers have discovered the existence of even shorter-wavelength and faster brainwaves. Ranging from sixty to two hundred cycles per second or more, these high-speed waves are referred to as *high gamma waves*. The high gamma waves are thought to accompany critical thought processes and brain functions. Multiple brainwave types occur simultaneously in our body. One type will often predominate, however. Just as multiple tuning forks will align to one dominate tone, the body will typically tune—harmonically—to the predominant waveform driven from a pervading consciousness.

A recent neuroscience study jointly done by the University of California at Berkeley and the University of California at San Francisco (Sanders *et al.* 2006) has concluded that it is likely these brainwaves are conduits for messaging between the various regions of the brain. Dr. Robert Knight, professor of neuroscience at the University of California at Berkeley, and a director of the research observed that some regions of the brain emitted waves, others reflected waves, and still others modulated waves. Meanwhile a particular confluence of these waves corresponded with particular activities, indicating different brain centers were using brainwaves as a sort of information exchange system.

As these respected researchers correlated the type of wave with the part of the brain involved in a particular process correlated with thought patterns, they began to see longer wavelength theta waves synchronizing or *coupling* with shorter wavelength gamma waves. They considered this coupling as part of a hierarchical signaling process. Regions of coordinated neurons produce resonant coherent wave patterns, which provide the means for one neuron (or a group of neurons) to communicate with another (or group). Synchronizing waveforms between neurons appeared to coordinate firing patterns. The brainwave synchronization then appeared to provide a process of ranking between brain regions in operational order. Theta waves appear to provide an executive control mechanism, which bridge the operations of various groups.

Using epileptic subjects, the researchers found consistent relationships between cognition and the occurrence of coherent theta and gamma waves. These two types of waves provide a locked resonation process. As cognitive processes changed, one wave from one region would first couple with, then transition into the next type of waveform. A type of congruent harmonic becomes apparent between these various brainwaves.

Biofeedback therapy has focused on the relationship between stress and brainwave types for a number of decades. Biofeedback research has confirmed that stress directly influences brainwave activity. Researchers have tested brainwave activity with patients in a number of different circumstances. Stressful conditions are linked to higher beta wave levels and lower alpha and theta wave levels. Consequently, a person who feels more relaxed and less stressed will produce more alpha and theta waveforms.

Many of us are aware that certain sounds influence relaxation. Most of us have experienced greater relaxation as we listen to soothing music or the songs of birds for example. Melinda Maxfield, PhD (2006) determined that slowly beating a drum at 4.5 beats per second readily brings about a state of theta brainwave activity. In 2006, Stanford University's Center for Computer Research in Music and Acoustics held a symposium with a purpose of *"interdisciplinary dialogue on the hypothesis that brainwaves entrain to rhythmic auditory stimuli, a phenomenon known as auditory driving."* This symposium brought together some of the nation's leading sound researchers. Many discussed the implications of auditory driving as it relates to our mental and physical wellbeing. The implications of the research, reflected by the consensus of the symposium, were that we are merely at the tip of the iceberg of this research.

The applications of brainwave entrainment through auditory driving are numerous. Successful auditory driving and brainwave entrainment treatments have contributed to resolving psychological trauma, chronic pain, stress, and weakened immune systems. Research comparing normal subjects with schizophrenic subjects (Vierling-Claasen *et al.* 2008) has illustrated how gamma and beta waves interface and guide cognitive processes. Normal subjects will tune to a 40 Hz wave in response to either 20 or 40 Hz driving frequencies. Schizophrenic subjects will typically respond with 20 Hz waveforms. The study's authors comment that these results illustrate *"how biophysical mechanisms can impact cognitive function."* This research confirms that brainwaves provide a mechanism for messaging specific information throughout the physical anatomy.

Biofeedback testing has further demonstrated that with practice and proper feedback access, human subjects can consciously change their brainwave levels. As a stress-reduction technique for example, a person can decrease their beta wave activity and increase their alpha and theta activity. The procedure entails the subject sitting down in front of a computer screen visually displaying rates from an electroencephalograph, photoplethysmograph (PPG—heart rate and blood flow), and/or possibly an electromyograph (EMG—muscle tension) to read waveform activity feeding back from different body parts connected to a variety of electrodes. Electrodes may be placed around the head, typically either on the scalp or in some cases around the cerebral cortex. Skin electrodes may also be applied to the arm, and PPG electrodes may be connected to the chest. The computer will monitor the waveform output of these different locations—displaying the results in a graphic display for the subject and therapist to see.

Most of us will generate brainwave signals reflecting our mental or emotional state—be it anxious, focused, relaxed, tired, angry or asleep. A good biofeedback machine will register several of these waves and their relative strengths around the body. Using a good biofeedback machine, most people can gradually learn to significantly lower or increase their alpha and theta wave strengths. For a few people, there will be an almost immediate ability to influence their waves as soon as the monitoring begins. For most it will take a bit of practice—a number of sessions usually—to be able to effectively modulate ones brainwaves or another other body pulse. Researchers have found that most everyone is able to modulate their waves at one point or other. Researchers have yet to understand why there is such a variance among people's ability to control their brainwaves.

Nonetheless, once people do learn to change their brainwaves using the biofeedback, they can usually transition successfully into being able to adjust their brainwaves without the biofeedback equipment. Bringing about a relaxed mental state through visualizing relaxing situations or hearing relaxing sounds are probably the most successful techniques used for this result. Auditory driving with rhythmic sounds has been increasingly used in biofeedback therapy.

Biofeedback therapy illustrates that our brainwaves are expressions of the role of consciousness within the body. An alteration of brainwaves from primarily beta to theta waves will almost invariably result in a lower heart rate, a slower, deeper rate of breathing, and a lowering of blood pressure. Conversely, a lower heart rate, and slower breathing—as long as there is no mental disruption—will also tend to induce a theta brainwave state. We thus have an intersection between consciousness and the cascade of brainwaves with physiological states.

Physicians specializing in the central nervous system have observed another wave associated with the circulating spinal fluid: Aptly named *cerebrospinal fluid pulse waves* (or CSF waves). The data have suggested this wave is composed of five different harmonic waves, ranging in pressure from .25-1 mm Hg range, and averaging .72 mm Hg (Nakamura *et al.* 1997). This is a pressure-wave. In comparison, the standard atmospheric pressure at sea level is equal to 760 mm Hg. It has not been completely ascertained as to the exact source of the CSF waves. One theory says that the pulse waves are due to the pressure gradient between arteries supplying the spinal cord and the spinal fluid. Another says they are based upon brain pulses sent through the spine's subarachnoid spaces. Many osteopaths, chiropractors, and cranial practitioners believe the cerebrospinal fluid pulses are due to the tiny movements of the cranial bones during breathing. Some research has linked breathing with these pulse waveforms. Correlations with ventricle pressure have also been made.

An interesting connection is made when CSF pulses are measured for wavelength: Beta-frequency waves seem to dominate the CSF pulse. Further EEG testing in controlled environments has demonstrated an interference relationship between the CSF pulses and the neural waveforms exhibited during memory retrieval and cognition. It seems these CSF waves play an important role in the orchestration of brainwave interference patterns.

From biophoton research, we can understand that each cell produces a unique collection of coherent electromagnetic emissions. Because each type of cell function has been connected with different types of biophoton emissions, it is safe to say coherent biophoton emissions by groups of brain and central nervous system cells should yield resonating patterns through constructive interference. The collection of weaker biophoton emissions should yield larger waveforms, just as thousands of stadium fans may each make unique sounds, but their confluence together creates a single sound of the crowd. Most of us have heard someone mimicking the single sound of a large stadium crowd full of cheering and jeering fans—it is not too difficult to do.

As the various subtle waveforms traveling in from our sense organs interface with internal waveforms feeding back from around the body, they combine to form a compounded perception of our body's inner and outer environment. This is accomplished again because these waveforms create multiple interference patterns as they interact. These interference patterns create collective views as they are intermingled with others and transferred onto our brain's cortices—predominated by the prefrontal cortex. The combined collection of interference patterns provides a form of image mapping system to be viewed from a position of consciousness.

Conscious Clockworks

The human body paces to an array of rhythmic cycles, each ebbing and flowing with a different frequency. A cycle charted against time is simply another waveform. The body's various cycles, encompassing just about every activity including eating, sleeping, defecation, labor and relaxation—along with every biochemical rhythm that supports them—are all cycling each day, driven by various external clockworks. These have loosely been called the body's *biowaves.* Generally, there are four types of human biowaves: *Circadian (circa*=about; *dian*=a day) cycles occur more or less in the range of one day. *Ultradian* cycles occur in less than a day. *Infradian* cycles occur in multiple days. Finally, *circannual* cycles occur annually.

Over the past century, researchers have been vigorously hunting for the source for the body's biological clockworks. In 1929, two Harvard researchers John Fulton and Percival Bailey studied disrupted sleep rhythms among patients with hypothalamus lesions. They concluded a mysterious link between the endocrine system and sleep cycles.

In 1958, Harvard's Dr. Woody Hastings and Dr. Paul Mangelsdorf illustrated how the marine species *G. polyedra* lit up the night's ocean timed to the sun's path. Exposing the tiny plant to various light pulses at different times, Dr. Hastings concluded some internal biological mechanism within the organism must respond to the sun, switching on and off its illuminating appearance. Over the next decade, various other organisms—including humans—were observed maintaining rhythmic biological responses in conjunction with light.

This research began a focused hunt to corner the body's biological connection to light. Researchers assumed that plants and animals possessed cell-switching mechanisms sensitive to light. Controversy took hold in the 1960s when researchers from Germany's Max Planck Institute published a study showing that human biological rhythms were not light-driven as had been suggested. Charles Czeisler, M.D., Ph.D., an eminent Harvard sleep researcher for several decades with over 180 research papers under his belt, questioned that research. Upon visiting the Planck facility, he found that although the subjects' outside lighting was controlled, they were still able to switch on and off indoor lights within their rooms. Apparently, even weak indoor lights could disrupt or entrain the body's clocks. In the years following, numerous light studies done elsewhere confirmed humans' biological clockworks responded to light—many led by Dr. Czeisler.

Most human light research has put subjects into caves or other light-controlled dwellings. These dwellings were removed of any cues as to time and place. Multiple studies indicated that the human circadian rhythm was about 25 hours. In 1985, Max Planck's Dr. Rutger Wever monitored temperature cycles, illustrating daily cycles of 21 and 28 hours instead of this 25-hour daily cycle. Furthermore, he found that body core temperatures quickly adjusted to the new light schedules. These studies indicated that the body's circadian cycles, which include the daily cycling of cortisol, melatonin and other hormones and neurotransmitters through the body, appear to be governed by the sun's path.

In 1972, University of Chicago researcher Dr. Robert Moore dropped radioactive label material in rats' eyes and traced its pathway from retinal neurons to two small clusters of neurons deep within the hypothalamus. This was traced to two centrally located pinhead-sized clusters of about 10,000 nerve cells called the *suprachiasmatic nuclei* (or SCN cells). The SCN cells were heralded as the biological clock researchers had been looking for over so many decades. Over the next few years, Dr. Moore, together with Lenn and Beebe, traced synaptic contacts with retinal afferent dendrites though the metabolism of young rats, eventually confirming that the SCN cells entrained their switching mechanisms to light (Lenn *et al.* 1977).

For the next two decades, Dr. Moore and other researchers, including Dr. Charles Weitz, Dr. David Welsch, and Dr. Eric Herzog, investigated these SCN cells from various aspects. Without synchronized SCN cells, an animal's body rhythms would collapse into chaotic patterns. These SCN cells were observed primarily residing within the hypothalamus. It was assumed that the body's clock was located within the hypothalamus.

These SCN cells appear to connect the hypothalamus with the activities of the pineal gland—a small conical structure lying above the posterior end of the third ventricle. The pineal gland receives impulses directly from the optic nerves. This seemed to confirm that SCN cells were the human body's switching mechanisms for light.

SCN cells are implicated in the secretion of most if not all the major hormones and neurotransmitters within the body. They appear to switch on in response to light pulses as they are received by the pineal gland. The mechanism for this appeared to be a double-neuron oscillation guided by a combination of light and genetic expression (Ilonomov *et al.* 1994, Fukada 2002).

As the research on the genetic connection to SCN cell activity unfolded, it became evident the activities of the thousands of oscillating nerve cells making up the SCN cell region are somehow expressed through a set of clock-oriented genes (Kalsbeek *et al.* 2006). Recent genetic research has identified several clockwork genes. The central CLOCK gene has been identified as 3111T/C; rs1801260 (Benedetti *et al.* 2007) and APRR9 in plants. Other clockwork genes have been identified as BMAL, PER, CRY (cryptochrome-12q23q24.1), and DEC genes (Gomez-Abellan 2007, Kato *et al.* 2006). These genes have been identified through responses to light and measured circadian biowaves.

Early suspicions were raised about the assumption that SCN cells only existed within the hypothalamus. Gradually, *in vitro* and *in vivo* testing demonstrated that other cells throughout the body also contain individual SCN cells. In 1970, Yamaoka reported finding SCN cells in the region of the thyroid gland. Over the next few years, enough dissecting had been done to demonstrate that SCN cells exist throughout the human body. Studies on light inducement have confirmed that these genetically expressed switches around the body respond to light, and exist within the testes, ovaries, kidneys, and most other organs. They have also been found in adipose cells, various nerve cells, and even cartilage cells. Each of the SCN genes is expressed through a unique disposition. The PER expression, for example, is increased by light exposure during the night, yet remains unstimulated by increased light exposure during the day (Shearman *et al.* 1997).

Further research concluded that SCN cells are not only responsive to light. They also respond to selected mRNA and prostaglandin switching molecules. It was found that every cell seems to have its own independent clockworks, but groups of cells synchronize their clocks to a common setting. The genetic structures of the SCN cells have been further investigated, indicating these clockworks have precise genetic switching mechanisms (Buijs *et al.* 2006).

The work of Dr. H. Okamura (2005) from the Kobe University School of Medicine confirmed that SCN clock cell genes are located throughout most of the body's major tissue and organ systems. Apparently, the genetic expressions of SCN cell oscillations are coupled with the independent clockwork genes in these various locations of the body. This coupling (or resonating) of genetic expressions appears to synchronize the pacing of the SCN-stimulated activities within the cell.

This tells us that the body's clockworks create an alignment between consciousness and sensory stimuli from the environment. A variance or misalignment between these two would logically lead to a diseased state. Through a combination of *in vitro* elimination and research on animals, a number of studies have confirmed that damage or mutation to these clockwork genes can result in various disease models. For example, damage to the Per1 and Per2 genes has been linked with a number of human cancer models (Chen-Goodspeed and Cheng 2007).

Clockwork genes have also been undeniably linked to the rhythmic release of hormones and neurotransmitters. Clockwork genes are now considered the key regulators (or mediators) for all metabolic processes. Mutations of human clock genes have been linked to metabolic syndrome (Gomez-Abellan *et al.* 2007), bone marrow CD34 immune cell availability (Tsinkalovsky *et al.* 2007), depression (Benedetti *et al.* 2007), and glutathione function (Igarashi *et al.* 2007). Clock genes are disrupted in mania-like behavior (Roybal *et al.* 2007). The clock genes have also been observed mediating expression of the plasminogen activator inhibitor, yielding a greater risk of heart attack (Chong *et al.* 2006). In 2005, researchers from the University of Pittsburgh's School of Medicine found that bipolar disorder was also linked to a disruption of clock genetic expression (Mansour 2005).

The clock genes correlate information from the SCN cells with various cues from around the body as well. One of the more important synchronizing mechanisms for these genes along with light is feeding schedules. There is an apparent entrainment to feeding cycles and energy metabolism connected with the SCN/CLOCK gene interaction (Mendoza 2007). Alcohol consumption also appears to substantially alter the expression patterns of a large population of clock genes. The PER genes—especially among brain cells—are significantly affected by alcohol consumption (Spanagel *et al.* 2005).

Recent research indicates that the clock genes engage in a feedback loop of genetic transcription and translation. This takes place with protein phosphorylation via kinases that reactivate alternating expression loops of the WC-1 and WC-2 proteins. These sequences become switched on and off through the induction of light to heat (Lakin-Thomas 2006). Cry1 seems to mediate CLOCK/Bmal1 complex repression, which sets up the feedback response (Sato *et al.* 2006). Further research has uncovered the potential of prostaglandin-2 as an activation-switch for resetting these genes, leading researchers to propose a connection between pain and the biological clock. These feedback loops have also been referred to as rhythmic, with a conserved control of gene transcription regulation (Hardin 2004).

It also appears that these SCN neurons are coupled to (or resonate with) other cells. Through a co-signaling process linked to glucocorticoid production, sympathetic nerve activity and other metabolic systems, activation of genetic alterations by SCN are stimulated by light and other waveforms. Organ-based SCN neurons also have their own waveform switching mechanisms, which turn on and off the various functions of that particular organ.

SCN cells participate in the production of critical neurotransmitter-hormones melatonin and serotonin. The major on and off switches for these biochemicals include light along with a biochemical switching (inhibitory) neurotransmitter messenger called GABA (Gamma-aminobutyric acid) (Perreau-Lenz *et al.* 2005). The dense network of serotonergic neurons within the central nervous system connects with networks of SCN cells. Light-driven oscillations of the SCN cells thus stimulate rhythmic serotonin release through these neurons' activity (Moore and Speh 2004).

The photoreceptor signaling process is still somewhat mysterious. It appears, however, that a protein called malanopsin is involved in a photo pigmentation process stimulating SCN cells. The signaling transduction pathway proposed with respect to the gene phosphorylation system is Glu-Ca2+-CaMKII-nNOS-GC-cGMP-cGK—>—>clock genes. This is obviously a waveform transmission and semiconductance pathway. The body's crystalline transmission and reception sequences within DNA translate these waveforms into intelligent instructional signals.

In 2005, Dr. Erik Herzog and Sara Aton discovered a peptide that lies between SCN neurons, polarizing their rhythmic oscillations. The *vasoactive intestinal polypeptide,* so named because it was found in the gut, became noteworthy because it is apparently produced within the SCN cell pathway. Dr. Herzog proposes the VIP lying between SCN neurons *"is like a rubber band between the pendulums of two grandfather clocks, helping to synchronize their timing"* (Aton *et al.* 2005).

Dr. Paolo Sassone-Corsi's 2006 studies at the University of California revealed that the CLOCK genes function in a fashion comparable to enzymes in the switching process. A year later, Dr. Sassone-Corsi's research found that a single amino acid within the BAL1 protein provides the initial switching signal that influences a single modification. This amino acid bonding modification appears to stimulate other body clock switching systems.

Other body clock signaling pathways have been discovered as the research has continued. These involve a myriad of biochemicals and gene sequences. The irony here is that scientists have been looking for a particular single biochemical or gene that is ultimately responsible for the entire body's clock mechanisms. Instead, soon after one biochemical, molecule or gene is located and thought to be the clock mechanism; another seems to emerge to replace it. The apparent weakness seems to be in the theory of one particular clock mechanism. We propose that the real weakness lies within the assumption that the clock is a single biochemical switch.

One of the mysteries illustrating a weakness in this single switch theory is that blind people have functional biological clocks. A blind body's clockworks will tune precisely to the sun's clockworks despite no obvious entry of light to the pineal gland's SCN region. It has been proposed that retinal cells contain another type of neural photoreceptor system—one receiving electromagnetic rhythms outside the visual relay system. Another theory proposes a few photoreceptor cells remain in blind people allowing them to stimulate the pineal/SCN system while not having enough activity to stimulate the LGN and visual cortex.

A larger mystery is how these various clockwork genes and cells communicate and synchronize throughout the body. In 2004, Dr. David Welsh and a team of researchers observed individual fibroblasts under various conditions. Fibroblasts are cells that will differentiate into connective tissue cells, osteoblasts and other cells. It turns out that fibroblasts also contain self-regulating circadian clockwork genes, somehow synchronizing their behavior with the rest of the rhythmic activities of the body.

The missing link is consciousness. Imagine a house full of thousands of clocks, each having different timing mechanisms and different alarms, dials, pace, and functions, all requiring occasional resetting to stay coordinated. Who oversees the process of resetting? Who governs the objectives or purpose of the resetting? Without a purpose, we would find a room of coo-coo clocks, ticking away separately without a governor.

The rhythms of all these clockworks remain harmonious through consciousness. A good example is the cycle between cortisol and melatonin. Each is driven by different cascading pathways. Cortisol—known to increase metabolism—levels tends to increase and peak as melatonin—known to decrease metabolism and induce sleep—levels recede in the morning. Then, as cortisol levels recede in the evening, melatonin levels increase correspondingly, peaking around midnight as the cortisol levels have wound down. Seemingly independent pathways are driven by seemingly independent endocrine systems. Somehow, these cycles synchronize with each other, yet do not overlap. Through some intelligent mechanism, one gradually recedes while the other increases. This single feat, repeated billions of times every second, is orchestrated. What is the orchestrating mechanism? What provides the baseline direction or controlling purpose?

Circadian Rhythms

Circadian rhythms cycle and recur daily. The timing of the human body clock's day, however, will vary to the various rhythmic cues of our environment. As infants, we begin life in the body tied to the rhythms of our mother. As we emerge from the womb, our bodies begin their entrainment to the sun's path. This entrainment process takes a little time. Infants progress from almost all day sleep (with some feeding and crying in between) to periodic sleep. Gradually, the frequency of sleep decreases. Not randomly, mind you. Rather, a baby's sleep cycles decrease in daily frequency at a consistent pattern, influenced by geographical location (with respect to the equator) and the amount of artificial light present in the room. In other words, with each passing sunrise and sunset, our bodies slowly and methodologically entrain their rhythms to nature's cycles. By the time our bodies reach adulthood, our clocks have become quite rigid, exhaustively trained by so many daily cycles of the sun over the years. Still, our cycles are entrained through conscious activity.

Over the past forty years, sleep researchers have been intensely studying our entrained circadian clocks by incubating and isolating people and animals. This has been accomplished variously, using caves and isolated chambers with and without the benefit of light. A host of mechanisms related to the body's circadian clockworks has been proposed. Various studies done with and without interaction with light have shown that melatonin rises with the dimming of lights. Melatonin levels also tend to fall with the body's interaction with even a little light. Body temperature also appears to be a major component of the melatonin surge. As the body cools with the dimming of lights in the evening, melatonin begins to pulse into the bloodstream. In the early evening, cortisol levels peak and then begin to fall off with the core temperature, guiding the body into slumber. As cortisol begins its rise around 3am, body core temperature begins to increase, as our body gradually prepares itself for a new day of activity.

The conscious anatomy thus revolves around the sun's path, influenced by many other factors. The sun's path orchestrates the body's rhythms through the activity of the pineal gland, the SCN cells and various clockwork genes, which all resonate throughout the body. Receiving light through the eyes is critical to the pineal's response. Yet light seems to stimulate the pineal with the eyes closed or blinded. There are other receptors around the body that respond to the sun's cues. Then, of course, there is the conscious component. As depression cases have indicated, an intention to rise each day is a requisite to cycling with nature's rhythms.

Assuming continued intention, the sun's electromagnetic waveform mechanisms also adjust the body's rhythms on a daily basis. These adjustments are expressed through biochemical switching and messenger pathways, which stimulate the secretion and activity of the various hormones and neurotransmitters, and their receptors.

Cave studies like Kleitman (1963), Siffre (1972), and Miles *et al.* (1977) have indicated that the human body's daily revolution without the resetting mechanism of daylight is about 24.9 hours. This exact period has been debated, as researchers have also seen body rhythms cycle variously. In a study done by Folkard in 1996, a woman was isolated for twenty-five days without daily light cues. While her temperature cycle was close to twenty-four hours long, her sleep cycle was closer to thirty hours. This study indicated that over time, the clock tends to stretch out without any sun. It also indicates individuality among responses to a lack of daily sun waves. Without the daily resetting mechanism of the sun, we might be going to bed later and later each night, and after a few days, we might be doing all-nighters and sleeping during the daytime.

Consistently, the studies on the body clock illustrate how predictably the body's clockworks mechanisms reset with sunlight. For example, Dr. Czeisler performed studies (1989) with the Naval Health Research Center on Trident nuclear submarine crewmembers. Sub operation schedules required crew to attempt to maintain an 18-hour body clock. Dr. Czeisler's results found this just was not possible. The onboard lights were simply too weak to entrain their body clocks to that schedule. Dr. Czeisler and others had previously established that bright light from between 7,000 and 13,000 (typical daylight) lux was necessary to produce such a dramatic resetting of the body clock (Boivin *et al.* 1996).

The human body can also respond to lower intensities of light, however. In another study, Dr. Czeisler and Boivin (1998) studied eight healthy men with eight control subjects. They found a mere 180 lux of light (typical office lighting ranges from 200-400 lux) had the ability to shift the circadian body clock, together with an increase in body core temperature. In another test, Dr. Czeisler found that 100 lux of indoor light has about half the alerting response as 9100 lux of outdoor light (Cajochen *et al.* 2000). In a study of twelve adults, Dr. Czeisler and his associates (Gronfier *et al.* 2007) found while 100 lux is sufficient to shift the clock, a 25 lux light was not enough to shift or reset the body's clock.

We each have unique responses to light. In one study (Cajochen *et al.* 2003) done at Harvard's Brigham and Women's Hospital in 2003, 45% of the study population responded to 3.5 lux of light for 16 hours rotated with 0 lux during 8 hours of sleep. This report concluded the body clockworks appear to oscillate at between 23.9 and 24.5 hours—refuting the rigid 25-hour body clock assumption, and introducing another factor.

The opinion held by many regarding the cave and isolation experiments is that indoor lighting prevents an accurate measurement of the body clock's entrainment tolerances. As mentioned, even a little indoor light can initiate a clock cellular change. This does not necessarily mean that all the body's systems change at once. Dr. Czeisler and his associates have observed that some of the body's rhythms are more rigid than others. For example, melatonin cycles appear to be more resistant to phase changes, although melatonin periods can vary when sleep schedules are adjusted (Boivin *et al.* 1996; Cajocken *et al.* 2003).

Sleep and body core temperature, or thermoregulation, appears to be intimately involved with the body's circadian rhythms (St Hilaire *et al.* 2007). Studies of people tested in isolation without light have confirmed that if the body has no access to the light-driven rhythms of the physical world, the body clock will stubbornly continue its thermoregulation cycles, but many of its biochemical cycles will gradually stray off. After a couple of weeks in *temporal isolation* chambers—meaning with only artificial light and no time signals—subjects will sleep highly irregular hours. Some days a subject might sleep up to 19 hours a day, while other days the sleep length might be as few as four hours. Interestingly, on days with as little as four hours sleep, subjects did not recognize that they had too little sleep. They might even remain awake for as many as 30 hours in a row without apparent sleepiness. Furthermore, these subjects' body temperature cycles—together with their melatonin and cortisol cycles—

would remain constant despite drastic swings in sleep and waking hours. It appears thermoregulation cycles are not as closely tied to light as are waking and sleeping patterns.

Nonetheless, we can see a larger pattern among research on the circadian body clock. We see a distinct range in the equation. There are a number of variables to consider. These include the season of the study, the environment of the study (artificial light strength and temperature) and then the study participants themselves. We must consider the total environmental response: The proximity to the equator, the phase of the moon, and the earth's rotation period. The earth's rotation period also varies from 24 hours, and its clockwork is regulated as the sun's position is factored in. The earth's *sidereal* is approximately 23 hours, 56 minutes and 4.091 seconds. However when we consider the earth's rotation with respect to the sun, we arrive at closer to 24 hour cycles from setting sun to setting sun, adjusting for seasonal variance. Other cycles in nature are very similar in their slight variation from a static, atomic clock (we would surmise this also varies, infinitesimally). The rhythms of nature allow just enough variance with a myriad of cycles to create unique conscious responses. These, of course, depend upon unique personality and choice.

Slight variances in cycle periods also provide enough flexibility for conscious choice. If all cycles were unchangeable and exact, we would be discussing simple machinery. Environmental variances allow for optional behavior, which allow the conscious driver to assess and select optional choices. Environmental variances and entrainment allow for the effect of consciousness upon the body's clockworks. A person intending to stay up late to enjoy an evening with friends will certainly affect the overall rhythm of their body's clock, for example. According to *placebo* research, the conscious factor should account for at least 33% of the variances.

Isolation chamber subjects will quickly become disoriented with respect to time once their light cues are taken away. Subjects may perceive that 2-3 weeks went by during a month, for example. Despite this confusion, subjects without sleep cues will typically make sleep adjustments in a cyclic way, eventually falling into a new rhythm. Even then, isolation-chamber subjects illustrate a residual 24-25 hour clock with variances cycling at a 127-day rhythm. Their sleep rhythm cycles still somehow reflect an internal resetting rhythm driver. What is this internal driver?

The suprachiasmatic nuclei or SCN system helps entrain the body's rhythms to the waveforms of the outside world. SCN cells are a part of the pathway that regulates the timing and production of melatonin and cortisol. They also directly or indirectly influence thermo-regulation through thyroid hormones and various neurotransmitters. SCN cells, together with the clock genes, the pineal gland and hypothalamus, act as translation conveyer of sorts: Translating the slightly varying rhythms of the outer world into the appropriate waveforms to be handed off via inner biochemical messengers. The varying environmental components are driven not only by the amount of sunlight received by the body, but also by the external waveforms of temperature, humidity, colors, sounds, odors and taste. Conscious responses interplay within these factors.

The mysterious cyclic hormone expressed with this SCN interaction is melatonin. As the pineal gland reacts to the absence of sun or light waveforms, it produces this pervading hormone transduces various clock-like messages around the body. The chemical synthesis of melatonin begins with a hydroxylation of tryptophan to 5-hydroxytryptophan, which decarboxylates to serotonin. Serotonin is then converted to N-acetylserotonin, which is methylated to melatonin. Melatonin affects the cellular biological clock and metabolism in a myriad of ways. Outside of signaling sleep metabolism through the body's network of cells, melatonin is also involved in the signaling of puberty and its related sex hormone levels; the regulating of core body temperature; the constriction of blood vessels; the modulation and release of various mood hormones like dopamine and serotonin; and numerous other metabolic functions.

Circulating melatonin levels in the blood have been shown to increase into the evening, proportionate to the level of darkness. The alternating melatonin and cortisol release is a rhythmic waveform system in itself. Melatonin is also part of the pathway that escorts the cooling of the core body temperatures by instigating a slower rate of metabolism. This release of melatonin and lowered body core temperature requires a calm and soothing atmosphere met with an unanxious consciousness, however.

A combination of an anxious consciousness and late-night bright lights discourages natural melatonin levels. High lux lights at night have been shown conclusively to lower circulating melatonin levels. By design, our bodies produce less melatonin if the lights are left on because lights signal to the body a need to keep working. Critical thinking also increases circulating levels of cortisol. With heightened cortisol levels, melatonin levels fall and the intended ability to work late and not sleep is supported.

Deficient melatonin levels have been linked to lowered immunity and heightened risk of cancer and other diseases. A number of pro-inflammatory cytokines are produced when the body is not sleeping enough or is operating on an irregular cycle. Pro-inflammatory interleukin-6 is one of these, and its release correlates with irregular sleep patterns. Another pro-inflammatory trigger, *tumor necrosis factor* (or TNF), is observed higher in persons with inadequate or irregular sleep cycles. Heightened levels of these cytokines have been particularly evident during daytime sleepiness episodes (Vgontzas *et al.* 2005).

About 90% of our body's melatonin production is eventually metabolized out of the body via the liver. Since there are a number of other hormones related to core body temperature that fluctuate around the daily melatonin cycle—including thyroid hormones, growth hormones, adrenaline and others—it is safe to conclude that melatonin is merely a cog in a larger messaging process designed to align the body with its environment.

Various other hormones and metabolic cycles rotate with circadian rhythms. Many are indirectly or directly electromagnetically entrained. This is evident in woman's menstruation and estrogen hormonal cycles.

Men also cycle hormones. Research on adult males over the past decade has confirmed the circadian patterns among testosterone, aldosterone, luteinizing hormone and inhibin B. A Russian study by Pronina (1992) on males in five different age groups determined that all of these hormones cycled through the day. Rhythm amplitudes of aldosterone and testosterone peaked highest in seven to eight year old boys, while LH rhythm amplitudes peaked highest among thirteen and fourteen year old adolescent boys. In another study (Carlsen *et al.* 1999), thirteen healthy males were tested every 30 minutes for inhibin B—a glycoprotein thought to be a feedback-inhibiting messenger for FSH secretion. Significant daily cycles were noted, with peak values of inhibin B in the morning, and lower values in the afternoon and evening. Inhibin B levels cycled opposite those of testosterone and estradiol levels.

Morning testosterone levels appear to be associated positively with the amount of sleep an adult male gets the night before (Penev 2007). Other hormones, such as growth hormone, have been shown to be related not only to sleep quantity, but to the quality and type of sleep. There is also a conscious relationship here, as stress seems to affect GH levels.

In a study (Van Cauter *et al.* 2000) of 149 men aged between 16 and 83 years old, growth hormone levels and cortisol levels were studied concurrent with brainwave sleep analysis. Regardless of age, daily growth hormone levels slowed as the amount of slow brainwave sleep decreased. The less slow wave sleep the person had, the lower the amount of growth hormone the person produced. This trend also occurred in an age-related basis: The older the man, the less slow brainwave sleep he had, and thus the lower growth hormone production.

The relationship between daily cortisol levels in the Van Cauter study also related to sleep quality. Rapid eye movement sleep or REM sleep was associated negatively with evening cortisol levels among the subjects. In other words, independent of age, less REM sleep equated to more evening cortisol. However, this trend also did occur with age: The older men had progressively lower REM sleep and thus higher evening cortisol levels. This in turn would also reduce melatonin levels, thereby keeping core body temperatures up and lowering sleep quality. Both higher cortisol levels and lower REM sleep are directly related to stress. This is consistent with other sleep studies confirming that adults get less REM sleep as our bodies get older, and an anxious consciousness affects our hormones.

Many other body rhythms vary to stress. Rhythmic hormone release adjusts to our working hours and occupational stressors. Sleep is often the critical factor. In one study (Persson *et al.* 2006) of 75 workers, those who involuntarily worked over 80 hours in a week experienced dysfunctional levels of cholesterol, cortisol, melatonin, prolactin, and testosterone levels on day seven of the workweek. In fact, both groups (the 40-hour workers and the 80-plus-hour workers) experienced decreased levels at the end of the workweek when compared to the beginning of the workweek. This would suggest these hormones and metabolic messengers are destructively interfered by stress. This would be consistent with the conscious body clock model. Stress arises from the disharmony between existing environmental factors and our intentional preferences.

Ultradian Messaging

All living organisms large and small undergo a multitude of cycles multiple times per day. Ultradian cycles have periods of less than a day. The circadian rhythms and their environmental drivers cross over and influence most of the ultradian rhythms. These intersections influence just about every metabolic function, including cellular metabolism, respiration, hunger, thirst, body core temperature homeostasis, mood regulation and many others.

Ultradian cycles vary to the organism. Metabolic cycles among yeasts range from thirty to ninety minutes long, while transcriptional cell division processes cycle at about forty minutes (Lloyd and Murray 2007). Complex organisms display an even greater number of ultradian cycles each day. Ultradian neurotransmitter cycles in humans are connected not only with changes in metabolism and thermoregulation, but also with our changing moods and habits throughout the day. Some hormone and neurotransmitter cycles are circadian, and some cycle in smaller ultradian rhythms. In one study (Evans *et al.* 2007), fifty active seniors at the

University of Westminster were continuously measured for cortisol levels through a forty-eight hour period in their homes. Before and after exams showed ultradian cortisol cycles significantly correlate with changing impressions of psychological well-being. This was significant during the first 45 minutes after awaking from sleep. Those with lower morning cortisol tended to experience increased feelings of well-being, for example.

For most of us, by around three a.m. our adrenal cortex begins to quietly pump cortisol into the bloodstream. With cortisol comes higher body core temperatures and increased metabolism amongst the cells. This process subtly orchestrates our multiple sleep cycles—which are also ultradian. Our body slowly comes out of its low-activity deep sleep state, gliding into a lighter cycle in anticipation of awaking. Cortisol levels gradually build close to dawn. They tend to peak just after daybreak, assuming a "typical" sleep cycle. Most of us, unfortunately, are atypical.

Should the sunrise not be synchronized with our first cortisol cycle, we will find our last few hours sleep is of lower quality and less restful. Getting quality sleep after dawn is increasingly difficult by design, because light stimulates physiological responses that must be addressed consciously.

After waking in the morning and awareness increases, our body's cortisol levels should increase as our body temperature rises proportionally. This cortisol surge should peak about 30-45 minutes after waking, tapering off towards the late morning, accompanied by a late-morning decline in energy. This cycle of lower energy continues into the early afternoon as our bodies head into 'siesta' mode (researchers call this the *lunch challenge*). Then cortisol levels again tend to rise. Depending upon our conscious drivers, eating habits, stressors and environment, another rise in cortisol—not usually as high as the morning's—will begin sometime in the middle to late afternoon.

Cortisol levels will also rise during a situation of conscious urgency. This spike can occur at any time of day, and it will usually be accompanied by increases in other biochemical messengers. These include epinephrine, acetylcholine, and others, which help orchestrate changes in metabolism to respond to an urgency. These will facilitate increased blood flow and nutrients to the muscles, eyes and brain cells, and a decrease in blood flow and nutrients to organs like the liver, immune system and the digestive system. For this reason, a physiology pushed by constant stress will usually result in digestive issues, liver problems and lowered immunity.

Should a person have an abundance of these stressful or anxious situations over a period of time (called *chronic stress*), the morning spike in cortisol levels may be absent or flattened. This will usually lower energy throughout the day. This condition is often diagnosed as *chronic fatigue syndrome* or *fibromyalgia,* often traced to the adrenal gland being overtaxed as a result of a body chronically stressed by an anxious consciousness.

In the later afternoon and early evening, cortisol levels again rise, giving a healthy person a burst of energy at the end of the day and into the early evening. The extent of ultradian cortisol secretion and the amplitude (or slope) of the cortisol cycle is related to internal and external environmental conditions in addition to conscious factors. These include levels of estrogen, lutein phase, inflammation, physical fitness, weather, sound, color, oxygen, anxiety and the range of possible intentions.

There are a number of other ultradian cycles in humans. Many also interplay (or interfere) with the cortisol cycles. For example, multiple daily temperature fluctuations were illustrated among babies by Bollani *et al.* (1997). In a study on cognition by Klein and Armitage (1979), it was shown that study participants' verbal and spatial skills cycled at about ninety-six minutes. Other studies have confirmed several other body rhythms that rotate at intervals close to 90 minutes each (Carlson 1986). The length of these rhythms correlate closely with the close-to-ninety minute cycles of REM and non-REM stage sleeping pattern, as documented over many years of government-sponsored sleep studies by William Dement, M.D. (1999).

Research has connected brainwaves with the various ultradian rhythms occurring throughout the body. Brainwaves are, in fact, also ultradian. Slower brainwave rhythms have been connected with the neural activity within the thalamus and cerebral cortex. An oscillation of *spindle complexes* among these ganglia pathways drive rhythmic pulses through the brain, reverberating throughout the body (Burikov and Bereshpolova 1999). These complex switching neurons have been called *corticothalamic* neurons, and they transduce slow delta waves (Timofeev and Steriade 1996). They also so happen to be implicated in adrenal hormone release.

Meanwhile, the faster alpha waves reverberating through our bodies are connected to the conscious optic nerve response of visual input through the LGN to the visual cortex. This function has been tested by reading subjects' brainwave responses in the occipital region while they were visual recognizing particular shapes and sizes. With the processing of visual information, alpha waves were generated (Shevelev *et al.* 1996). Alpha waves may thus be regarded as indicative of imagery reflected on the visual cortex' conscious scanning process.

The slower theta rhythms—moving at between four and ten cycles per second—are associated with states of relaxation and sleep. In waking adults, theta waves are crowded out by focused consciousness. Some tests have shown that theta waves will still occur with certain short-term memory tasks; episodic and semantic memory recalls; and spatial navigation tasks (Buzsaki 2005). Relaxation and semantic memory recall reveal thoughts of a more abstract basis. These slower waveforms are thus reflective of deeper, more abstract awareness. Several studies of theta waves have concluded that they appear to reflect activity related to the functions of the hippocampus—a central player in the human limbic system. Theta waves have also been linked with rhythmic movement like dancing, along with auditory processing during both waking and sleeping. In addition, they have been observed being active during attention shifting (Gambini *et al.* 2002).

The mysterious theta brainwaves provide a link to the programming mechanisms of autonomic function. Pedemonte and Velluti (2005) found that theta rhythms substantially affect the heart rate and many reflex movements, including programmed functions related to responsive memory. As illustrated by biofeedback, theta brainwaves provide the link between consciousness and autonomic activities.

The organs have their own ultradian rhythms. Nobel laureate Dr. Alexis Carrel proposed in 1912 that rather than the heart being a pump—as it was thought of for the previous millennia—it is more like a turbine, working conjunctively with blood flow, artery pressure and the various biochemical messengers. Dr. Carrel's groundbreaking research on the heart is what ushered medicine into the era of open-heart surgery many years later. The rhythmic ebb and flow of the body's fluids and the biochemical messengers appear unrelated when we focus on any one. Observed together, however, their relative cycles illustrate an orchestration of physiological coordination tied to a conscious component evident from biochemical feedback and response mechanisms.

Hunger and appetite are examples of physiological rhythms linked to consciousness. Appetite is intimately connected to the workings of the hypothalamus. The hypothalamus is also one of the limbic system components involved in pleasure feedback. The hypothalamus is activated by the interaction between consciousness and the entrainment of eating cycles. These combine with the feedback of taste, together stimulating the vagus nerve and the flow of gastrin.

Our gastric juices are merely one of the biochemical responses connecting consciousness with our olfactory senses. Feedback response stimulates the vagus nerve, accelerating peristalsis and digestive enzyme flow.

The study of America's two prime epidemics—obesity and diabetes—relates specifically to this feedback-response cycle of hunger-appetite-satiation. This has unveiled a number of biochemical feedback-response mechanisms bridging consciousness with the limbic system, the stomach, the pancreas, fat cells and working cells.

Insulin—a hormone produced by the beta cells of the pancreas—stimulates cells to become glucose-sensitive, stimulating their utilization of glucose from the bloodstream. Without a natural supply of this valuable hormone, the cells are starved for glucose, even if the bloodstream and liver is saturated with glucose and derivatives. This in turn opens the door to various cardiovascular, circulatory, cognitive and liver-related health problems. Western society's epidemic of adult-onset diabetes—no longer "adult-onset"—relates to insulin and glucose receptor sensitivity at the cell membrane. Insulin production, it turns out, is only a small part of the biochemical messaging mechanisms using a host of ligands and receptors. These are balanced by various enzymes such as alpha-glucosidase, and of course, what we eat—which is a conscious action. A simple choice of eating at consistent times, along with a high-fiber diet, can prevent many of these cases.

In 1994, another biochemical messenger named leptin was discovered. Leptin appears to be implicated in signaling the limbic system with a feedback response from the adipose (fat) cells that the body has enough energy in the form of fat. Of course, the pharmaceutical industry followed this discovery with a synthetic form, in an attempt to provide us with that next great medical miracle. Produced inside adipose cells, leptin is part of the body's natural glucose processing cycle. Should our bodies get plenty of food, and there is a buildup of fat cells in the body, leptin messengers signal back to the limbic system that enough energy is available and additional food is unnecessary. In a healthy organism, this should decrease appetite. The attempt to synthesize this important endogenous feedback biochemical to control obesity was successful. However, its application was useless. The conscious 'fingerprinting' process of the body's biochemical messengers does not always accommodate synthetic manipulation.

The research found that leptin also plays a critical role within the functions of other metabolic and endocrine processes. Leptin interacts with sexual hormones, adrenal hormones, thyroid hormones, growth hormones, and immune system biochemicals. Leptin also plays a role in hypothalamic regulation, glucose transport, and the inhibition of insulin secretion by pancreatic beta cells. It turns out that leptin's role mediates many of the body's metabolic processes (Wauters *et al.* 2000; Aronne and Thorton-Jones 2007; Morton 2007; Coll *et al.* 2007).

The ongoing search for a chemical solution to obesity yielded the discovery of another hormone. This hormone, named ghrelin, is produced primarily in the stomach. Depending upon the levels of glucose, leptin, and stomach contents, this hormone signals the lateral hypothalamus to inhibit cytokine secretion and stimulate gastric acid secretion in the stomach. Ghrelin also appears to stimulate and regulate gastrointestinal gut motility—allowing the intestinal wall to undulate with the rhythms of peristalsis. Following its discovery, it was thought that ghrelin was the key to controlling hunger and thus obesity. Like leptin and other pharmaceutical analogs, the synthetic single-bullet theory was assumed. Again, this did not prevail. Ghrelin's complex activity is immersed with other metabolic and endocrine messengers relating to the balancing of energy, hunger and gastrointestinal function (Skoczylas and Wiecek 2006). These, of course, are stimulated by conscious appetite feedback-response.

It is now apparent that the medicated alteration of gastrin flow into the stomach has negative effects upon the stomach's mucosal lining. It is likely that ghrelin levels are also affected as well. The mucosal lining of the stomach protects the gastric cells of the stomach from toxins, oxidative stress from radicals, and infectious agents like *Helicobacter pylori* (now thought to cause a majority of ulcers). Ghrelin not only helps stimulate the mucosa, but also is an effective antioxidant: It neutralizes radicals and toxins that would otherwise damage the stomach lining (Dong and Kaunitz 2006).

Other hormones and genetic switches have also been discovered in the years following ghrelin's discovery. Resistin, for example, has been linked to glucose tolerance and hepatic insulin resistance. Resistin levels increase in obese patients and decrease with thiazolidinediones (ligands which bind with DNA-linked peroxisome proliferator-activated receptors or PPAR) (Steppan *et al.* 2001). Adiponectin is still another adipocyte-produced hormone linked to glucose regulation and lipid metabolism. Plasma adiponectin is high in normal insulin-sensitive tissues and low in NIDDM insulin-resistance (Weyer *et al.* 2001). Another recently discovered hormone implicated in both types of diabetes is amylin. Amylin is secreted with insulin, and appears to complement insulin's actions. Amylin also provides a feedback-response mechanism for insulin sensitivity.

Leptin appears to be involved in the front-loading of glucose and insulin while resistin and adiponectin seem to mediate PPAR-gamma: Resistin upgrades and adiponectin downgrades insulin resistance through

PPAR modulation (Chatterjee *et al.* 2001, Steppan *et al.* 2001, Weyer *et al.* 2001). The PPAR-gamma receptors modulate the genetic expression of glucose and insulin sensitivity at the cell membrane.

Biochemical energy pathways also involve genetic messages broadcast from DNA molecules within the cells' nuclei. Core instructions appear to be dispatched through the complex crystalline assembly of structures that make up DNA. For example, an enzyme instrumental to leptin regulation is SIRT1, related to on a PPAR-gamma genetic repression. Sirtuins like SIRT1 have been implicated in diabetes because of their ability to affect genetic expression related to issues of degenerative glucose and insulin metabolism. SIRT1 appears to balance glucose levels by modulating the PGC-1alpha molecule. PGC-1alpha is a transcriptional co-activator. When SIRT1 was inhibited *in vivo,* this increased hypoglycemia, increased glucose and insulin sensitivity, as well as increased free fatty acid and cholesterol in the liver. On the other hand, increased SIRT1 expression reversed these effects, but only in the presence of PGC-1alpha and only during fasting (Rodgers *et al.* 2007; Das *et al.* 2005).

The complexity of fat biochemistry does not stop there. Additional messenger systems include peptides PYY and GLP-1, produced in the intestines, cholecystokinins, and a number of other enzymes researchers have found in between. Have any of these findings lost us any weight so far? Synthetic chemical magic bullets simply cannot match the body's regulatory processes involving intertwined messaging of related feedback and response. Because feeding, hunger and appetite are all events that bridge consciousness with the internal needs of the body, we simply cannot isolate one or even several biochemicals out of context. As was illustrated in the body clock research, as soon as we think we have found the mysterious master biochemical, another mystery simply pops up to take its place.

The process is intertwined with behavior. All of these biochemical pathways are connected to our choices, created by appetite, digestion, defecation, muscular activity, and so on. Appetite and food consumption are conscious affairs because we each have the ability to vary our diets, mealtimes and number of meals per day. Thus, those messengers associated with the digestion and processing of these meals are not only interactive, but have their own mini-interactivity, which all must coordinate with our conscious decisions. We are incentified to eat foods that have a good balance of glucose, insulin and all the other signaling mechanisms related to energy metabolism. Overriding this principle is the conscious choice to obtain that balance.

These relationships are all due to communication processes. DNA molecular arrangements provide a signaling apparatus, which allows a holographic reflection of consciousness throughout the network of DNA broadcasting stations among the body's trillions of cells. What science has missed in our fat research is the guiding mechanism of consciousness—the driving force.

Without conscious effort, the body's autonomic nervous system rhythmically engages the various functions mentioned above. The hypothalamus interacts with the anterior pituitary; pacing its activities with timed *releasing hormones.* These releasing hormones stimulate the pituitary to release specific hormones, which in turn pace the various functions of the endocrine system. For example, from ACTH hormone, the adrenal gland is stimulated to release glucocorticoids. The pituitary will release TSH hormone to stimulate the thyroid to produce secondary hormones T3 and T4, which help balance and maintain metabolic balance.

This hormonal relay process is more than just automatic. It is informational. For example, certain pituitary hormone messages will suppress T3 release while elevating rT3 levels during physical stress. Other hormone messengers will reverse this process. These types of interactive messaging are coordinated through switching and feedback mechanisms—quite similar to the ion channel gateways discussed earlier. As the body's physical exertion is slowed, some hormone releases are shunted by other biochemical messaging (Mastorakos and Pavlatou 2005). The relationship between the cell's utilization of glucose with insulin to the production of thyroid hormone becomes evident in the case of hyperthyroidism. Most hyperthyroidism cases also show increased cellular metabolic activity, causing the conversion of glucose into energy and lactate to speed up (Dimitriadis and Raptis 2001). This illustrates how easily the interruption (or in this case the over stimulation) of the normal thyroid cycle of T3 production can cause a negative domino effect, increasing glucose and insulin needs; increasing appetite; eating; and affecting so many other related body cycles.

The complex interplay between energy utilization and homeostasis is beyond our scope. Thyroid hormones have complex switching components that somehow gauge the availability of energy, feeding that back for response. This feedback process appears to relate to the flow of melatonin. Melatonin levels are regulated through a handshaking between the hypothalamus and the pineal gland as the system responds to light reduction and mental status. Along with this cyclic melatonin release, thyroid hormones T3 and T4 cycle in shifts cooperating with cortisol and other corticosteroids—all cycling alternatively with melatonin, and entrained to the passage of the sun through the sky (Wright 2002).

Likewise, further metabolic messengers intertwine with other ultradian cycles such as the beating of the heart and the pacing of respiration. Most of us have experienced how an increase in heat or physical activity will increase the heart rate and the rate of breathing simultaneously. These two rhythms are intertwined with a deeper set of synchronized biochemical waveform messengers. These messengers relate to the pressure differentials between air-borne oxygen and blood-borne carbon dioxide. They relate to the arterial walls' ability to respond to changing environmental conditions with expansion or contraction (vasodilation and vasoconstriction). They relate to the heart's muscles and valves expanding and contracting in a synchronized manner to pump blood around the body. They also relate to the conversion of glucose, oxygen and minerals to energy within mitochondria, in a complex process we call the *Krebs cycle.*

Body temperature, for example, fluctuates with ultradian cycles. The thermal dynamics of the body cycle in a regulatory process called *homeostasis*. Homeostasis is the process the body undergoes to keep its temperature balanced. Should body core temperature rise or fall below a temperature ranging from about 95 degrees F to about a high of 104, the body's metabolic balance is challenged. If it is too cold, various enzymatic functions will slow. If it is too hot, the cells can become overheated, causing exhaustion and havoc among metabolism. Thermoregulation is a balancing act, keeping the various interactive processes tuned to a particular thermal range. In a healthy body, temperature rhythms synchronize to slightly rise and fall throughout the day with the rise and fall of cortisol and melatonin. These rhythms form a pervasive biofeedback-response loop, together with sweating to result in a relatively balanced body core temperature range whether it is hot or cold in the outside environment. This mechanism connects metabolic temperature needs to the rhythms of environmental change, with enough variance for conscious interaction.

Should we plot temperature, metabolism and levels of most of these biochemical messengers over a day's time, we would find that most cycle with levels that would graph to a sine wave. Furthermore, as the various environmental and physiological cycles are examined together, we find they interact as coherent waves. During coherence, waves with constructive interference provide mechanisms for channel gate opening, while destructive interference provides mechanisms for channel gate closing. Just as the magnetic field of the electromagnetic rhythm pushes outward and perpendicular from the plane of the electric vector, these interlocked body cycles all effect the biological environment of the body with an outward direction, expanding heat and motion on a plane ancillary to the functional metabolic cycles.

The field of interactive messaging throughout the body creates innumerable cascading mechanisms. These cascades typically consist of a series of multiple *if-then* commands not unlike a multiple-core semiconductor system. When these cascading responses are functioning coherently to open or close appropriate channels congruent to the metabolic needs of the body, they offer its conscious operator the ability to execute commands.

Consciousness can be transmitted through either constructive or destructive inference, as long as there is an overall coherence between these biochemical messengers. Without coherence, we have conflict within the body. Conflict may be temporary, as the body's coherency readjusts. In chronic disease pathologies, these balancing mechanisms are overwhelmed. Chronic disease outside of normal aging degeneration indicates a prevailing conflict of interference between the body's different messaging mechanisms and its conscious operator.

An interesting example of this multi-dimensional field of coherence is the *peristalsis* cycle of the gastrointestinal system. Peristalsis is a series of rhythmic contractions of the smooth muscles that govern the size and shape of the digestive tract. This tract includes the esophagus, the stomach, the small intestine, the colon and the anus, along with supporting muscle groups and organs. It we were to examine the frequency of peristaltic contraction of smooth muscle around each component, we would find that each paces with a different rhythm. Because the process of digestion within each component has a different mechanism, the frequency of the waves within each component is different. Around the stomach, these waves occur from three to eight times per minute (or 180 to 480 cycles per second; or 180-480 hertz). Throughout the intestine, peristaltic waves vibrate at a rhythm of ten to twenty times per minute (600 to 1200 hertz). In the colon, peristaltic waves move in the same range as the stomach—from 180 to 480 hertz—yet will typically maintain a different wavelength and amplitude from that of the stomach.

Peristaltic waves are considered "slow waves." These waves are driven by fluctuations in electronic potential. Smooth muscle resting potential ranges from -50 to -60 mV. A partial depolarization of these muscle fibers causes a fluctuation of membrane potential of 5 to 15 mV. This electronic fluctuation of potential causes muscle contraction when the potential spikes.

Peristaltic waves escort food through the esophagus, massaging its entry into the cavity of the stomach. There are two primary functions involved here: The propulsion of the food, and the mixing of food with enzymes and gastrin. The first wave that massages food from the esophagus to the stomach typically lasts from 8-9 seconds. Secondary waves will continue as the *bolus* (partially digested food and digestive juices) mixes in the stomach, accompanied by peristaltic waves of faster frequencies. These faster peristaltic waves liquefy the food mixing in the stomach.

Guiding the propulsion and mixing process are two interneuron reflex systems that release neurotransmitters into the neurons that stimulate the smooth muscles. The first is a group of excitatory motor neurons stimulated above the bolus. These nerves initiate the contraction of the smooth muscles using neurotransmitters acetylcholine and substance P as messengers. The second nerve group is inhibitory. These nerves stimulate the relaxation of the muscles below the bolus, allowing the bolus to pass through. This second group of neurons is driven by released neurotransmitters such as vasoactive intestinal peptide and nitric oxide.

The bolus, now together with chyme, moves through the pyloric valve and into the intestines. Peristaltic waves provide the motion that encourages the bolus downward as nutrients are being absorbed through the intestinal wall. Eventually the insoluble fiber and chyme will be moved into the colon, where it is mixed with other biochemicals and liver byproducts, to be dehydrated and prepared for evacuation. Both longitudinal and circular muscle fibers are engaged alternatively around the intestines and colon. Much of this takes place through a process of *local longitudinal shortening,* which shortens the longitudinal muscles, and increases circular muscle tone (Brasseur *et al.* 2007).

As the bolus stretches each portion of the digestive tract, neurotransmitters are released into the smooth muscle. This sensitizes the muscle with the greater membrane potential. As the cyclic peristaltic wave passes over that area, the muscle fibers contract, followed by relaxation. This alternating contraction and relaxation process cumulatively moves food through the digestive tract, and provides a precision of mixing among bile, probiotics and enzymes. The viability of our probiotic systems—essential to health, depends upon peristaltic wave coherence.

The relationships between these individual rhythms of various frequencies and waveforms through the digestive tract illustrate how the body's rhythms are intertwined with coherence. As is with any harmonic relationship, affecting one aspect will have a reflective effect on those other cyclic activities functioning in conjunction. The interruption of any one of the body's rhythms by the introduction of synthetic hormones, gastric inhibitors, neurotransmitter receptor agonists or antagonists—or practically any other type of synthetic interference with the body's flow of hormones, metabolism, reproduction, digestion, and so on—will create an imbalance elsewhere to be reconciled. The imbalanced pharmaceutical approach of modern medicine creates the unfortunate consequence of having to deal with increasingly new disorders and consequences that we had previously not even imagined let alone predicted. The onslaught of various new pathologies over the past few decades including new allergies, fibromyalgia, food sensitivities, autoimmune disorders and various cancers are all signs that our body's messenger coherences are being stressed. This is not to say pharmaceuticals are the only form of attack on our various messaging mechanisms. Within today's environment are so many synthetic toxins, ranging from plasticizers to toxicity in our air and water. For this reason—as we will examine more precisely later—humankind's understanding of the congruity of these coherent messaging systems is vastly incomplete.

One important aspect of our body's conscious messaging systems is the element of uniqueness. Every body is tuned to relatively the same major external stimuli. Yet every body is uniquely individual, just as every personality within is uniquely individual. One body might thus respond quickly and intensely to a particular stressor. Another body might resist such a response, maintaining its cycles with hardly any alteration. This stems from each body containing an individual conscious personality. We find many baseline metabolic patterns common among healthy people. Feeling hungry and eating multiple times per day, sleeping six to eight hours per night and so on, are common among healthy people. Adaptogenic mechanisms uniquely smooth out any incongruities. For example, should we feel fatigued due to overexertion, a good night's sleep will typically stimulate our body's various repair systems to heal the damage. Should we wake up with the sun the next day, our metabolic processes and hormonal rhythms will likely be readjusted and refreshed. One body might require 7.25 hours to achieve this readjustment. Another might require 8 hours. Still another might require 9 hours to regain strength, and still more the next night.

Many of us assume that our body clocks are permanent. Subsequently we figure we are either "evening people" or "morning people" for the body's duration, for example. What we may not realize is that the conscious choices we make involving our activities and dietary choices greatly influence our body rhythms. The subsequent production of cortisol, melatonin, thyroid hormones, sex hormones, growth hormones and the other daily cyclic biochemical flows all tune into and respond to the activities intended by a conscious driver.

This 'consciousness effect' was illustrated in a study of 1572 children from fourth to eighth grade (Gau *et al.* 2004). Those children who reported they were "evening people" were more likely to have sleep disturbances, drink coffee and have less parental monitoring. These "evening people" children were also associated with increased moodiness and daytime sleepiness. "Evening persons" were also typically older children who were given more freedom to alter their natural body cycles. It is probably fair to say that once a person's natural body rhythms are disturbed by conscious dietary and lifestyle choices, those interruptions begin to take their toll upon our moods and energy levels.

The 5,000-year-old science of *Ayurveda*—translated as "the science of life"—significantly recognized these daily ultradian rhythms. In *Ayurveda*, the day is broken up into six three-hour ultradian cycles; each governed by one of the three *dosha* behaviors, *kapha, pitta* or *vata.* Each *dosha* relates to a particular type of consciousness, and they blend uniquely in each of us.

The three hours before 11pm, and three hours during mid-morning are each considered dominated by the *kapha* aspect in *Ayurveda.* The mid-day through the afternoon, and the three hours late after about 11 pm through about 2 am are considered governed by the *pitta* aspect. Just before and just after dawn and dusk are considered *vata* periods.

During each of these daily periods, certain activities naturally prevail. Particular foods and liquids are suggested during each period as well. For example, spiced tea, water, and non-mucus-forming foods are said to be good for the morning *kapha* period, while fasting is suggested for the nighttime *kapha* (when we should be sleeping). The heaviest meal of the day is suggested during the *pitta* noon period—when digestive fires are thought to be at their peak. Meanwhile, grain-based meals are suggested for the post-sunset *vata* period and the after-sunrise *vata* period. The pre-sunrise and pre-sunset *vata* periods are also considered significant times for reflection, meditation and prayer in *Ayurveda.* Exercise is recommended by *Ayurveda* during the *pitta* and *kapha* periods of the day, depending upon the type of exercise.

Within these six governing periods, the Ayurvedic science divided the circadian day and night into thirty *ghatikas,* replacing the more arbitrary twelve-hour clock. Each *ghatika* is twenty-four minutes long. In the *ghatika* system, every day and every night consists of six sections of five *ghatikas* each. These appear to uniquely intersect the rhythms of nature's elements and those of the human body. The twenty-four minute rhythm also ties in very well with the estimated forty-five and ninety-minute sleep and REM cycles. Two cycles of 24 minutes equates roughly with the 45-minute and 90-minute sleep cycles, which are rounded to plus-or-minus five to ten minutes.

These are just a few of the many ultradian rhythms and their inter-relationships between nature's rhythms. We find many other cycles documented by this elegant and ancient human science—incidentally also considered one of the safest medical systems in practice today.

Infradian Biocycles

The rhythms of the body that cycle over days, weeks and months have also been the subject of study and controversy for thousands of years. Various Greek, Egyptian, Chinese and Ayurvedic scientists all saw the clockworks of the universe harmonizing with multiple daily and seasonal rhythms of the body. Hippocrates addressed this topic in his teachings, for example, suggesting physicians remain attentive to the good and bad days of their patients.

Western science began to take notice of infradian biowaves when Dr. Hermann Swoboda, a psychologist and professor at the University of Vienna in the early part of the twentieth century—investigated observations of periodic appearances of fevers, swelling, cardiac events, and other illnesses among his patients. Dr. Swoboda's painstaking recordkeeping methodology seemingly uncovered a 23-day physical cycle and a 28-day emotional cycle among his patients. Dr. Swoboda recorded his experiments and results in a number of German books on the subject: *The Periodicity in Man's Life; Studies on the Basis of Psychology; The Critical Days of Man;* and *The Year of Seven,* in which Dr. Swoboda elaborated on the mathematical and clinical foundation of these two cycles.

Dr. Wilhelm Fliess—another late nineteenth and early twentieth century physician most known for his work with Sigmund Freud—was the president of the *Germanie Academy of Sciences* in 1910. Dr. Fliess began to study daily body cycles amongst his patients as well. Through detailed recordings and mathematical record keeping, Dr. Fliess seemingly independently came up with an identical theory: The body cycled through 23-day physical and 28-day emotional cycles. Dr. Fliess was a prolific scientific writer, and recorded his studies in several scientific papers and gave numerous lectures. His books included German titles such as *The Year in the Living, The Theory of Periodicity,* and *The Course of Life.*

The elaborate research of Fliess and Swoboda also brought controversy to the theory of *biorhythms.* Both Fliess and Swoboda unveiled an impressive array of statistics from their studies: Hundreds of family tree histories, numerous case studies; sibling studies; medical treatments; psychological events; traumas; accidents; and historical events were analyzed statistically to establish these two cycles. The theories have been argued against by researchers then and now. Still, many physicians and psychiatrists utilized the two cycles in their daily practice.

In the 1920s, mathematician and engineer Dr. Alfred Teltseher began to observe another pattern among his high school students. Dr. Teltseher launched an extensive analysis of what he called an *intellectual cycle*. His research revealed an apparent 33-day cycle of intellectual performance peaks, valleys, and critical days. Periods where learning is accelerated or delayed, periods of memory recall, and other periodic mental performance were statistically examined by Dr. Teltseher among student performance grading and examinations. His scientific paper on the subject also correlated periodic endocrine secretions with his 33-day intellectual cycle period (West 1999).

A decade later, Dr. Rexford Hersey and Dr. Michael Bennett reported a 35-36 day cycle of intellectual performance by studying railroad workers. The paper was picked up by Colgate University's Donald Laird, who reviewed the research in a paper titled *The Secrets of Our Ups and Downs,* which appeared in a science journal along with *Readers Digest* in August of 1935. Dr. Hersey spent many years thereafter studying this cycle, which apparently included the measuring life statistics of nearly 5,000 men from 1927 to 1954 to provide the data for his 36-day cycle hypothesis (Crawley 1996).

These apparent cycles have been consolidated by a number of writers over the past few decades. Each biocycle is described as a classic sine wave with a beginning point at the zero baseline with a high phase peak one-quarter though the cycle. This follows with a crossing of the zero baseline halfway through the cycle, a negative peak three-quarters through, and ending at zero the starting point ready to repeat the cycle. Interestingly, the focus is not upon the high points and the low points of the cycle. Rather, the focus is upon the transition points when the cycles cross the neutral baseline, going either direction. These transition points are termed *critical days*. The research mentioned above has indicated that these transition days—between the negative and the positive points on the curve—are apparently days when accidents or problems are more likely to occur.

In 1939, Swiss Federal Institute of Technology's Dr. Hans Schwing published a 78-page study of accidents and accidental deaths. This documented a pattern predicted by the three daily biowave cycles. His report consisted of a statistical analysis of 700 accident cases and 300 cases of accidental death. Dr. Schwing covered a 21,252 day period, isolating critical days for the 23-day physical cycle, the 28-day emotional cycle, and the 33-day intellectual cycle. His report concluded that 322 accidents occurred during single critical days (in other words, one of the person's biowave rhythms were crossing the neutral line into positive or negative territory). Seventy-two occurred on double critical days (when two biowave rhythms are crossing the neutral line) and five occurred on triple critical days (when three biowave rhythms are crossing the neutral line). A total of 401 accidents coincided with critical days, or 60% of all accidents. The total number of critical days possible during the 21,252-day period was 4,427 days, or 20% of the 21,252 days. In other words, 60% of accidents occurred on 20% of the days, coinciding with the critical points.

A 1954 report by Rheinhold Bochow of Humboldt University in Berlin studied agricultural machinery accidents together with biowave rhythms. He found that out of 497 accidents, 97.8% of these took place on a critical day of one of the three body rhythms. Interestingly, 26.6% occurred on single critical days, 46.5% occurred on double critical days and 24.7% occurred on triple critical days. This seems to indicate that double critical days—an obviously rarer occasion than a single critical day in any biowave rhythm—appear more dangerous.

The link between these biowave rhythms and accidents has not been without its critics. Winstead *et al.* (1981) reported an analysis of potential biorhythm cycles with dates of psychiatric hospitalization and emergency room visits. They analyzed hospitalization dates for 218 patients and emergency room visits for 386 patients. No apparent correlations existed between these patients' biorhythms and critical biowave rhythm days. The authors of this study concluded the biorhythm theory is *"much too simplistic to account for the complexities of everyday life."*

Nevertheless, there is significant evidence to show human behavior and performance follows rhythmic patterns. According to Peter West (1990), a number of companies in the transportation industry have reduced accident ratios using biowave rhythm critical day analysis in their risk assessments.

The negative phase of all three biorhythms is considered a period of recovery and response rather than a period when lower performance or problems occur. As in all response periods, they also contribute to performance, however differently. For example, the response period for a cycle of breathing occurs when we breathe out. Some might consider this a negative flow when considering the input of oxygen during inspiration. This outflow is a necessary part of the cycle nonetheless—just as necessary as breathing in. Without expiration, carbon dioxide and carbolic acid levels would dangerously build up within the body. Rather, the theory of biowave rhythm performance says that the crossing from the negative or positive part of the cycle to the other—the critical day—is considered more likely for mishap.

Meanwhile, the positive phase of the physical cycle should accompany a heightened sense of coordination and physical performance. This also should be accompanied by faster recovery times and faster healing in the case of injury. This has statistically been confirmed in many case studies of extraordinary performances among athletes. During this phase, the immune system should also be stronger, and thus disease resistance may be greater. Baran and Apostol (2007) studied various physical performance evaluations, revealing biowave rhythm intervals for tests such as neuromuscular efficiency.

The Winstead research investigated psychiatric admissions. Many chronic issues here illustrated distinct periodicity. For example, Leroux and Ducross (2008) reported that chronic cluster headaches have *"circannual and circadian periodicity."* A number of reports have linked various pathologies with different rhythms—many circadian and/or infradian. Respiration and airway resistance in asthma appears to have a rhythmic connection (Stephenson 2007). Incidence of breast cancer seems to be linked with the body's rhythmic behavior (Sahar and Sassone-Corsi 2007). Chronic fatigue syndrome and its associated pain have been linked to biowaves (Perrin 2007). Cardiac arrhythmias, ischemic heart disease and hypertension have all been linked to biowave rhythms (Portaluppi and Hermida 2007). Arthritis has been linked to biowave cycles, particularly with respect to pro-inflammatory cytokines (Cutolo and Straub 2008).

According to the theory, relationships, sensitivity and awareness will be heightened during the positive phase of the emotional cycle. Indeed, mood disorders have been positively linked with the body's rhythms in a number of studies (McClung 2007). Negotiations, exams, meetings, and team efforts would thus bring better results during a positive mental phase. The positive phase of the intellectual cycle would bring stronger decision-making abilities. The ability to learn from difficulties would be thus heightened during this phase. Indeed, studies on memory, executive function and attention capacity have also indicated rhythmic performance (Schmidt *et al.* 2007).

We should add that the rhythmic behaviors found in much of the above research were not necessarily reflecting the specific 23-day, 28-day, and 33-day biowave cycles. This growing database of research illustrates that so many metabolic activities are rhythmic, and these rhythms are all undoubtedly intertwined within the body and with the environmental rhythms surrounding the body. The confluence of these various rhythms obviously combines to create interference patterns and intersecting points of harmonic metabolic activity.

Most researchers agree that the body's systems fluctuate on rhythmic cycles. This fact is difficult to ignore. Pinpointing a strictly common cycle for everyone has proved problematic, however. The assumption that everyone precisely cycles to the same biowave rhythms creates a rather easy calculation process. To calculate ones theoretical cycles to current, we would simply count the number of days since the date of birth, with a day added every leap year. We would then divide the total days of our lives by the number of days of each rhythm. The remainder will be the number of days into the current biowave cycle. Again, this assumes we all cycle to precisely the same rhythmic periods.

It would appear likely that biowave cycles beginning on the day of birth would be subject to variances among the population just as so many other physical cycles are. The potential for cyclic variances seem likely given the proliferation of pre-term births, C-sections, delayed deliveries and other birth anomalies. In addition, we would suggest there is a significant range of events having the ability to influence our cycles. There could be so many possible variables. Logically we could apply one variance due to the location and time of day for our birth—whether this event took place at night under hospital lights, during the day out of doors or perhaps under the duress of an ambulance or even a rough car ride to the hospital. The trauma of a C-section or otherwise pre-term birth would likely apply particular stressors not normally existing in a natural birth as well. Certainly, a pre-term situation would affect the completion of the typical nine-month rhythm occurring for the fetus (incidentally an obvious infradian cycle for both the fetus and the mother). To this we would add the trauma of the birthing event in itself. Might these stressors upon the body affect the initiation or entrainment to a particular rhythm, just as the lack of sleep affects a person's daily entrainment to the sunrise?

It would appear likely the concurrence of various rhythmic occurrences—whether they are stress related, light related, or perhaps related to a particular trauma—should be considered as we analyze the variances among the critical day research. Dr. Schwing's 60% result for accident rates (out of a probability of 20%) may appeal to us scientifically. However, a 40% variance (in other words, why did *all* of the accidents not occur on critical days?) is also quite large when proposing we all cycle to the exact three same infradian rhythms. It appears unlikely all of us each adhere to precisely the same rhythmic cycles, precisely beginning on the same day of our birth. We might add that humans could have cycled in closer proximity in the past than they might today, due to the prominence of natural childbirth and less indoor bright lights, as existed prior to a century ago. We extrapolate this because we know from circadian rhythm analysis that these stressors can significantly alter other rhythms.

Rather, should we correlate this with the many other known rhythmic disorders of the physical body (diabetes, obesity, insomnia, inflammation, and so on); there should be a solid basis for the potential of interference, causing any number of bio-cycles to be distorted. We might consider the heart's rhythms, for example. If a person remains healthy with a good diet and a healthy amount of exercise, the heart rate should remain at a steady resting rate of 60-65 beats per minute during adulthood and possibly until advanced age. It would not be difficult to calculate this to beats-per-day and beats-per-year, establishing a solid pattern of rhythmicity quite similar to the calculation of the biowave rhythms detailed earlier. However, should we consider the rhythmicity of the heart in the case of an unhealthy diet, a chronic lack of exercise or a profuse amount of stress, there is a likelihood the heartbeat rhythm could range from 65 to even 80 resting beats per minute. The stressors applied to the physical body in the latter case changed both the rhythmicity and even the potential duration of the heart's lifetime. Some of this effect may well be outside of our control as well—should we find ourselves in a stressful occupation, for example.

We see similar causal relationships—various traumas or decisions interfering with our natural rhythms—between stressors and so many other types of rhythms, including brainwaves, breathing rate, lifespan, sleep cycles, menstruation, and so on.

There is no reason to believe the theoretical yet plausible 23-day, 28-day and 33-day biowave rhythms are exceptions to these kinds of causal influences. It would appear likely that a number of variables could restart or otherwise alter the rhythm period or cycle of these, just as research has confirmed this among other biological rhythms. Unusual circumstances during our birth (such as a Caesarian section) might affect our start date. A trauma such as a motor vehicle accident or otherwise could cause an abrupt interference that might alter or shift the cycle. In other words, while the research may have illustrated a cycling of rhythms close to these patterns as behavior was examined over large populations; mathematical analysis of each person and each birth date illustrates too much variance to insist we are all have precisely the same cycles.

It is likely that other entrainment influences also create variances. As we discussed, our circadian cycles are significantly entrained each day to the sun's path, which tends to synchronize or tune our circadian cycles. The moon, the stars and the seasonal tilt of the earth all create potential entrainment devices for infradian rhythms. However, the precise mechanisms are larger than our scope of research. In the absence of an entrainment process such as exists with the morning light upon our pineal gland and SCN system, it would seem likely our infradian rhythms would be distorted by unique, personal events.

Simple observation tells us that at least half the population is subject to variable but consistent infradian rhythms. Almost every female body with little variance—excepting cases of significant health disorders—between the ages of about 13 and 50, undergoes a menstrual cycle lasting between 22 and 45 days, with the median being about 28 days. In a study of 130 women at the University Of Pittsburg School Of Medicine (Creinin *et al.* 2004), the average was 29 days, with 46% having a variance of seven days and 20% cycled 14 days or less. While this is a substantial variance, the consistency of cycling among women is quite significant.

This 28- to 29-day rhythm certainly corresponds with the proposed 28-day emotional cycle of Fliess and Swoboda and others. It also appears suspicious that a woman's menstrual cycle is also intimately connected with moods and physical/psychological emotional cycles. Curiously, many modern Fliess and Swoboda biorhythm proponents declare the woman's 28-day menstrual cycle a mere coincidence.

The female cycle begins with the flow of follicle-stimulating hormone (FSH). As named, this hormone stimulates the production of a follicle in the ovary. As the follicle develops and the ovum matures, it produces increased amounts of estrogen. As estrogen's messages are carried to receptors in the uterus, uterine cells begin to prepare the endometrium for the potential of a pregnancy. This means the endometrium begins to thicken and uterine glands elongate.

Estrogen is a complicated messenger—as most hormones are. Within a day or two before ovulation, estrogen will stimulate a spike in luteinizing hormone (LH) which converts a ruptured follicle into the corpus luteum. The corpus luteum in turn produces copious amounts of progesterone, which stimulates incremental growth among the endometrium and supporting tissues. These spikes in estrogen and progesterone also provide an inhibiting feedback response to the pituitary, slowing subsequent LH and FSH release.

Around this time—as if set by an alarm—the ovum slides into the uterus through the oviduct. Here it may or may not encounter a male sperm. If it does, fertilization (also a function of consciousness) may or may not occur. If not, within 2-3 days, the ovum will begin to deteriorate.

The corpus luteum will degenerate, and estrogen and progesterone levels will fall. The endometrium also thins, and small hemorrhages poke through its lining. This causes the bleeding of menstruation. Menstruation will typically last 3-6 days. In Creinin, the average was 5.2 days.

During this time, new cells begin to grow within the endometrial wall. This repairs the hemorrhaged areas. As levels of estrogen and progesterone fall to their negative points on the cycle, FSH is released from the pituitary, feeding back the rhythmic cycle's repetition.

For most healthy women the flow of these hormones; the follicle and ovum growth; movement and eventual breakdown; and the subsequent repair of the system take place every month like clockwork. However, there are significant individual differences. In a study done at Marquette University's College of Nursing (Fehring *et al.* 2006), 141 healthy women underwent testing for cycle consistency. The average of 28.9 days consisted of 95% between 22 and 36 days, while 42% had intracycle variances of more than seven days. For example, while 95% had six fertile days between day four and day 23, only 25% had their fertile days between day ten and day seventeen. The researchers concluded that among other parts of the intracycle, follicular phase seems to be the cause of much of the variation.

There is also significant research indicating groups of women who lived together or spent time in close proximity over a significant period begin to cycle to the same menstrual rhythms. This gradual synchronization of rhythms has been the subject of research between mothers and daughters, roommates and dormitory women. In all three instances, studies have illustrated this rhythmic correlation of physical proximity between women living together (Weller and Weller 1993). In terms of occurrence, Weller *et al.* (1999) discovered among 73 urban households with a relatively high degree of interaction that 51% of menstrual synchrony occurred within families and among sisters, and 30% occurred among friends not living together. This study concluded a correlation between durable intentional proximity and emotional synchrony.

As to the mechanisms of menstruation proximity cycling, there are a number of hypotheses. Some researchers have proposed the existence of an entrainment mechanism through a type of pheromone process. Others have suggested that certain physical and social cues create a synchronized entrainment of rhythms: A sort of subconscious environmental entrainment process. Regardless of the specific mechanism, it appears that emotional consciousness is a function of the entrainment process, and the mechanism appears to be connected to empathic relationships.

We should note there is significant research documenting other interfering influences upon the menstruation rhythms. Multiple studies have confirmed menstrual dysfunction may be significantly affected by light exposure variations (Barron 2007), for example. Disturbance also appears related to melatonin secretion—also related to light exposure. The vulnerability of the cycle to light exposure is exasperated by various psychological and physiological stressors as well. For example, bipolar disorder and polycystic ovary syndrome have influenced a woman's cycle in becoming more sensitive to light exposure. In addition, a woman's menstrual cycle can be affected and altered through poor nutrition or caloric restriction (Elias *et al.* 2007), stress and trauma (Hannoun *et al.* 2007), smoking (Grossman and Nakajima 2006), and surgery (Watrick 2007). In a study of 3941 pre-menopausal women from Iowa and North Carolina (Rowland *et al.* 2002), smoking, depression, increased body mass and other environmental stressors are also strongly associated with irregular menstrual cycles.

These factors, of course, are primarily driven by a combination of conscious choices and environmental conditions. The research significantly indicates that menstruation rhythms act very similar to other rhythms we have discussed. Stress, poor lifestyle choices and toxic environmental conditions can destructively interfere with their cycles—either distorting or depressing them. Meanwhile, nature's environmental rhythms such as the sun appear to constructively interfere with and strengthen menstruation rhythms.

We can summarize our menstrual cycle discussion noting that menstruation cycles are infradian cycles with qualities entrained with the coherence and interference of our environment and our consciousness.

What about the other half of the human population? Is the male body absent of infradian rhythms? In 1990, Chirkova *et al.* reported in the *Laboratornoe delo* that the serum of young healthy men revealed ten different body rhythms of different wavelengths and frequencies. Using amylase testing, several cycles were demonstrated, ranging from eight hours to one month. The authors observed nine different environmental factors that appeared to predicate or influence these cycles. Dr. Peter Celec and associates from Comenius University's Institute of Pathophysiology (2004) concluded that—after using an *analysis of rhythmic variance* test on five healthy males—a strong duodecimal (12-day) rhythm of salivary estradiol levels existed in men.

Dr. Celec and his associates also used this ANORVA system to expose two different cycles of testosterone within the male body in a study published in 2003. Saliva was collected from 31 healthy males between the age of 20 and 22.5 years old for 75 days during the fall of 2000. Using two methods of statistical analysis to remove bias—one a moving average and the other a phase shift variance—the research unveiled both a *ciratrigintan* (monthly) and a *circavigintan* (tri-weekly) rhythm among testosterone production.

Pronina (1992) also found infradian rhythms among testosterone and aldosterone levels. The rhythm frequency for aldosterone was 2.5-5.5 days. Testosterone levels experienced two longer rhythms, one of 5-13.5 days, and another, stronger rhythm with a 21-day period. There was a range between age groups among the amplitudes of secretion levels. The length of the rhythms stayed consistent among different ages, however.

As was noted in the circadian discussion, daily hormone levels are destructively interfered by stress. This correlation is also found among the longer duration of the rhythms, as was discovered in a one-year study of 72 firefighters by Rot *et al.* (2003). Stress cycles were compared with cortisol and testosterone levels within these cycles. It was found during periods of lower stress, cortisol levels increased and testosterone levels decreased. Inversely, during higher stress periods, cortisol levels decreased and testosterone levels increased.

Biophoton emissions appear to cycle in larger infradian rhythms as well. In one of the Cohen and Popp's human trials (1997), a person was measured daily over a period of several months for weak photon emissions. These measurements demonstrated a cycling of biophoton emissions with bi-weekly, monthly and longer cycles of intensity fluctuation. Consistent rhythms of fourteen days, one month, three months and nine months were evidenced by rising and falling photon emission levels. This demonstrated the coherence factor between biophotons and the various messaging pathways conducted via testosterone, estrogen, melatonin, cortisol, LH and all the other biochemical messengers flowing through the body.

Solar Synchrony

Simple observation tells us that seasonal rhythms influence our behavior and the behavior of so many organisms. During the winter, many animals migrate or hibernate. Humans also tend to hibernate indoors, especially in the northern latitudes. This is evidenced by the great incidence of *seasonal affective disorder,* which appears primarily in the winter in higher latitudes. SAD is a sort of depression that typically occurs after a lengthy period spent indoors without natural lighting. Research has shown that SAD is also linked to lower vitamin D production. Vitamin D production is stimulated by the skin's contact with the sun's ultraviolet rays. Seasonal light reduction also results in decreased serotonin levels, as natural light stimulates the production of this mood-regulating hormone. During the winter, our body's messengers also stimulate an urge to eat more. We can also correlate the channeling of messaging pathways that govern the activities of leptin, insulin, ghrelin, amylin, glucocorticoids and resistin; along with all the other energy-related biochemical messengers linked with dysfunctions like SAD and obesity.

As the weather warms during the springtime, our bodies tend to get outside more. We tend to expose more skin to the sun. This time is also associated with romance. The 'spring fling' is experienced primarily by young adults at the peak of their reproductive years. Increased exposure to natural light encourages increased serotonin levels. These messengers participate with vitamin D pathways that render a sense of physical well-being. We can combine these internal biochemical messengers with the exchange of a more subtle messaging system of pheromones. The debate on whether humans exchange pheromones has been settled through research, which included the discovery that androstadienone from human male sweat glands increased female cortisone levels (Wyart, *et al.* 2007).

Spring is also a time of reproduction for many other species. The flowers of many plants produce pollen, which allows the male species to fertilize the female reproductive system through a complex process including the joining of pollen and ovule. This pollination and fertilization process leads to the production of seeds. These seeds blow into the spring and early summer winds to propagate the species. Meanwhile, many animals begin their migration to the more northern or southern latitudes (depending upon their home turf in relation to the equator) for mating in the spring. Hibernating species come out for their first meals in many months during the springtime. These behaviors synchronize with the biochemical messengers prevalent among these organisms.

During the summer, the heat comes on and activity peaks. Most trees come into full leaf, giving shade for other species in need of a respite from the hot sun. The environment tends to become drier during the summer in most northern latitudes. During this period, plant chlorophyll levels peak for maximum photosynthesis. Most animals are in peak activity periods as they hunt, forage and care for their offspring. Humans also tend to increase activity, as we will often vacation during the summer months. We head to the forests, ocean, or lakes for a great escape from our cubicles into the natures our bodies inherently belong. This part of the cycle would then be seen as the tapering off of the positive vector of the seasonal waveform.

During the fall, organisms begin their defensive behavior again. Trees begin to drop their leaves, preparing for another round of rhythmic dormancy. Animals begin their rhythmic migration to warmer climates. School begins, and humans rhythmically return to the partial hibernation of indoor activities. The seasonal waveform crosses the neutral point (the so-called "critical days") during the late fall, into the negative zone of winter lower temperatures, in a full-scale retreat from the elements. This negative cycle peaks as the onslaught of winter collaborates with the sun's solstice.

The seasonal cycles are harmonic with the rhythmicity of nature's conscious organisms. Conscious activity cycles with the off-centered rotation of the earth, which repositions the sun to create the cyclic variation of daylight and solar exposure. Increased daylight accompanies a greater spectrum of radiation: More ultraviolet light, visible light and infrared radiation. With these increased waveforms comes an increase in energy levels. Reproduction is stimulated. Activity is stimulated. During the negative cycle, decreased daylight and lower temperatures stimulates lower energy levels, reproduction and activity. Each cycle creates a balance contributing to the wellness of the organism. Without the combination of the positive and negative portions of each cycle, exhaustion or complete inactivity would result.

The science of *Ayurveda* correlated and classified six seasons of the year with the clockwork rhythms of the body. In the northern latitudes, the late winter season (mid-January to mid-March in the northern latitudes) is known as the *sishira* portion of the year. During this time, there is a predominance of cold and wet weather. The *vasanta* season, lasting from mid-March to mid-May, is the classic spring season. The *grishma* period is the early summer season, until mid-July. The next season is *varsha,* or the rainy season, which in Asia and many tropical areas lasts until mid-September. The *sharat* season is the typical autumn season, lasting until mid-November, and the *hemant* season is the colder early winter season. Each season is connected with predominant lifestyle activities, tastes, types of foods and general lifestyle choices in *Ayurveda.* Each is connected to a combination of the consciousness qualities of *kapha, vata* or *pitta.*

In *Ayurveda,* each season is also accompanied by particular taste associations. The wet winter season is associated with bitter taste, while the spring is associated with astringent taste. The summer is associated with hot taste, the rainy season associated with sour taste, the autumn associated with salty tastes and the winter associated with sweet tastes. Here are some other seasonal tendencies and suggestions detailed in the ancient science of *Ayurveda*:

Wet winter: digestive activity increases and *kapha* is increased. Heavier foods are eaten with more wheat and dairy products. Sweet, sour and fatty foods are also typically increased. Foods and clothing are thicker and warmer. Increased exposure to fire is recommended. Increasing exercise is recommended. Massage is oily.

Spring season: Excess *kapha* is cleansed during the spring but digestion is slowed. Therefore, light and easily digested food is recommended. Yogurts and other fermented foods are recommended. Fruits and vegetables to increase detoxification are suggested. Avoiding sour, sweet and fatty foods is suggested. Massage is dry.

Early summer season: As *kapha* is cleansed, *pitta* begins. Light foods are continued, but sweet and fatty foods can be added. Cold water and fruits are recommended. Cold baths, cool places, light clothing are all suggested. Chandan paste is recommended for body anointing.

Late summer: In rainy areas, digestion is worsened as *kapha* and *pitta* compete in the humidity. In dry regions, *pitta* increases with some *vata* tendencies building late. Cooling foods are recommended, together with cool baths and plenty of swimming. Fruits and light foods are suggested, together with pulses and yogurt drinks.

Autumn/Early winter: The dryness of autumn and the dry cold of early winter aggravate the *vata* element—known for coldness and dryness. Therefore, recommended foods are astringent or sweet. Warm foods are suggested. Grains are good and food should be low in oil. Warm oil massages are increased.

Many of these recommendations—such as light foods in the summer—are natural responses to environmental conditions. Still, many people will not follow these natural behavior rhythms because of stress, training, or intentional decision. The ancient Ayurvedic system is a general guide for appropriate rhythmic behavior, in an attempt to live more harmoniously with our environment. According to *Ayurveda*, atypical habits can interfere with our body's normal cycling through the seasons. The influences of each season also depends upon which characteristics each dominating in each conscious body type. A person with a predominantly *pitta* physical body and consciousness might be aggravated more by the hot weather than a person who is dryer and more *vatic*. The *vatic* person would be more susceptible to variances between the suggested seasonal diets, on the other hand. Meanwhile a *kaphic* person may be comfortable during the winter months as they cozy up to plenty of food and warmth. However, they may also be subject to increased mucus and disease due to an excess of these activities, unless they detoxify properly, according to *Ayurveda*.

Unique seasonal variations are also supported by science. Recent research unveils how seasonal patterns affect birth. In one study of more than 75,000 births in a Pittsburgh hospital between 1995 and 2004, preterm deliveries were 25% less likely for summer and fall conception than for winter conception (Bodnar and Simhan 2007). In an Indiana University School of Medicine (Tweed 2007) study of 1,667,391 Indiana students between third and tenth grade, it was found that students conceived between June and August had the lowest test scores in math and language. A number of theories have been proposed to explain these seasonal differences. Regardless, the link between conscious activity and seasonal behavior is undeniable.

Our bodies also pass through 'seasons' as they age. According to *Ayurveda,* each person's *tridosha* consciousness tends to evolve with each season of the body's lifespan. During childhood, growth and development predominates. As a result, this period is said to be the *kaphic* period, where mucus and anabolism prevails. During young adulthood through adulthood, *pitta* is said to prevail. During this period sexual activity peaks, metabolism peaks, family life prevails and core body temperature heightens. During this period, the person will be less tolerant to hot weather. Then in the body's elderly years, *vata* tendencies become greater. The body becomes dryer, metabolism slows (catabolism), and a period of slow detachment should begin. During this time, the body tends to tolerate heat more—especially dry heat. With each passing *tridosha* time span, certain tastes predominate, changing over time as conscious learning progresses. Children usually avoid spicy or salty foods but crave cold, sweet and sour foods as they seek satisfaction. Adults tend to be attracted to detoxifying spicy, hot, and salty foods as they age and seek purification. The elderly tend to appreciate warm foods with increasingly sweet and bitter tastes as they search inward and backward, seeking wisdom.

The ancient Chinese codification system also connected rhythmic cycles to the passing of years. According to ancient Chinese science, 60-years is a macro cycle consisting of five cycles of twelve years. These cycles are named after animals because each has a distinct predominating quality (for example, the *Year of the Dog*). Each year also has an attribute of either *yin* or *yang* as that cycle is considered to have an emotional effect upon life. Each particular year will be described as either *yin* or *yang*, one of the five elements, and one of the animal-like qualities. The traditional Chinese calendar has a number of other characteristics that are in tune with nature. The months are paced by lunar periods, and the year is calculated using a combination of solar year and lunar year.

Planetary Biomagnetism

A discussion of the nature's rhythms would be truncated without a discussion of the effects of the rhythmically moving planetary bodies. As most of us realize, the heavenly bodies are all rotating within primarily elliptical spiraling galaxies. There are millions of solar systems like ours within each galaxy. There are also millions of galaxies as well. Space is still a mystery to scientists. Our modern telescopes can see a huge array of waveform spectra. Yet still there is still a huge domain of black, unseen space out there. Scientists debate about the composition of this *dark matter,* which appears to make up more than 90% of most galaxies and seemingly is at the center of each galaxy. Some speculate that huge black holes lie at the center of each galaxy, balancing light emission by gradually sucking the galaxy's contents into another plane of existence. Others speculate that these are simply gaseous clouds of chaotic chemicals.

Regardless of these speculations, we know enough to understand that our universe is in full-time rhythmic rotation. All of the planets, solar systems and galaxies are all rotating through distinct yet harmonically congruent rhythms. It is because of this harmonic nature that we can predict the future locations of most of the stars and planets within our visible grasp.

For thousands of years humans have compared behavior with the positioning of these bodies. Almost every ancient culture, including the Indian, Chinese, Egyptian, Greek, Roman, Mayan, Polynesian, Aboriginal and others, has correlated conscious behavior with the positions of the major planets, stars and constellations. Egyptian star charts have been dated at 4200 B.C. Many of the pharaohs apparently utilized the positioning of planetary bodies in decision-making. The Egyptians tracked the sun, Sirius and the planets through the zodiac, as did the Chinese, the Mayans, and the Indus Valley residents. The concept of zodiac houses—the movement of planets through space regions of particular constellations—has been remarkably consistent among various ancient and apparently independent cultures. The understanding and measurement of the positions of particular stars and planets within the houses and their relative positions in the sky were considered important to these societies. Just as our scientists endeavor to understand the effects of particular biochemicals on behavior, these ancient researchers endeavored to understand how our behavior relates to the position of the heavenly bodies. As a result, we find extremely advanced methods of star positioning, and those who understood this science were highly regarded and respected in ancient times. We have thus found curiously sophisticated means of recording the positioning of planets and the moon through the skies among many archeological findings. One of these is the ephemeris. The ephemeris measures and records the relative positions of stars and planets at any particular moment. This advanced tool is thousands of years old and has been used in a number of ancient cultures. It is still in use today.

The ancient *Jyotish Vedanga* of the early Indus Valley culture documents one of the earliest and more advanced forms of mathematical astrology and astronomy. Some date the original written work at 1400 BCE, while other notable Vedic scholars date its origin thousands of years earlier, at 3000-4000 BCE. Regardless, the techniques discussed were in use centuries prior to its recording. The *Jyotisa* formalized a sidereal zodiac, and integrated an ephemeris with the position of the planets and major stars. The ancient *Jyotisa* system calculated the sidereal lunar cycle into a 27-28-day *nakshatra*, with each sidereal day also divided into four quadrants, or *padas*. The total number of *padas* was 108. Each *pada* was connected to the motion and dominance of a principle star. Twelve zodiac houses were defined, and the stars and planets were seen as cycling through these twelve houses. A common use was the ceremonial birthing astrological forecast, which consisted of a *brahmin* astrology expert 'reading' the ephemeris ascendant—the position of the planets and sun relative to each other from the time and place of birth. The ephemeris calculation of the ascendant together with the position of the moon indicated to the astrologer particular personality and activity traits of the baby, for example. Rather than a prediction of the future as most would imagine, this reading would include a discussion of the child's emotional tendencies. This would include the type of work the child was suited for and whether the child was born with leadership or other abilities.

This ancient knowledge that connected ones behavioral tendencies with the position of the celestial bodies was quite advanced. While some have attributed this knowledge to superstition, the approach was actually quite practical and scientific. The celestial positions were considered as a sort of indicator. The *Jyotisa* astrologer had been passed down the knowledge regarding the connection between a specific celestial indicator and a particular characteristic or tendency from previous generations of data collection. These characteristics or tendencies were then connected to the natural order of events that progress or trend towards one result or another. They saw every result as having stages or steps that unfolded along the way, which eventually evolved to the result. The approach was no different from our modern-day weather forecasting tools, which connect visible observations with a long history of result data.

The ancient Chinese culture also used some of the same extensive astrological/astronomical knowledge. Ancient Chinese astrology dates back to at least the Shang dynasty of some 3600 years ago. The Chinese zodiac was also based upon a twelve-year cycle, represented by animals: In order, they consist of the *rat, ox, tiger, rabbit, dragon, snake, horse, ram, monkey, rooster, dog,* and *boar.* As each animal rotated through the cycles of the five elements (earth, water, fire, metal and wood), a sixty-year cycle was created. Twenty-eight constellations were measured and watched as they traveled through the skies. The Chinese were also known to utilize an ephemeris—the interrelationships of angular positions of stars and planets. Planets were also associated with the five elements, and their respective positions were said to influence those elements. According to the Chinese astrological view, each element was also connected to a particular planet. Wood, for example, was connected to the planet Jupiter. Earth was connected to Saturn. Metal was connected to Venus. Fire was connected to Mars. The water element was connected to mercury. These attributes of the five elements to particular planets is also somewhat common among other ancient astronomical models.

Most of the great ancient cultures shared and utilized similar systems. Recordings of star positions have been discovered in hieroglyphs from ancient Babylon dating back to 4200 B.C.E. The Sumerians of 4000 B.C. An indication of the complexity of Greek planetary astrology and astronomy was unveiled recently with the reconstruction of a two-thousand year old Greek astronomical calculator, containing an excess of thirty gears. Called the *Antikythera Calculator,* it was found by divers researching a shipwreck near the island of Antikythera a century ago. The relic has been the subject of curiosity since its discovery, as researchers of various disciplines speculated as to what it was and how it was used. In 2006, researchers from universities in Carkiff, Athens, and Thessalonika used x-ray imaging technology to unravel the relic's purpose. They concluded the mechanism—consisting of upwards of thirty wheels and dials made of bronze—was the world's oldest known computer. A team of researchers from the National Archaeological Museum of Athens was able to reconstruct it. A replica of the relic was developed, which rotated through each planet's position in the sky—accurately predicting the positioning of that heavenly body on a certain day, and its angular relationship to the other planets, the moon and the sun.

The awareness of the effects of the celestial elements on behavior unfolded to ancient peoples over thousands of years, as the data was passed down through lineages of experts. We find evidence that many societies also dispatched seekers to travel and learn the sciences from other cultures. These travelers would return with a wealth of information learned from a far away land. Most indigenous cultures respected and attended to these early scientists. They were considered wise men, and were oftentimes called upon to give guidance to the society's leaders.

This knowledge was advanced with the assumption that the universe was populated with personalities of greater consciousness and increased authority over the environment. Most of the cultures of Mesopotamia attributed many of the heavenly bodies as living personas, just as did the ancient cultures of the Chinese, the Indus Valley inhabitants, the Incans, the Mayans, the Mauri, the Aboriginals, the North American Indians, the Greeks and the Romans. In almost every advanced ancient civilization, we find this model of a conscious universe designed by intention and operated by beings in exalted positions of power, who are in turn governed by an even greater Superior Being.

Greek mythology greatly influenced the current prevailing version of modern western astrology. Archeological findings and the writings of the Greeks have unveiled this connection, which in turn appeared to be gathered from the astrological sciences of the Assyrians, the Egyptians, the Tibetans and the Hindus. The Assyrians of 1300 to 600 B.C.E. developed star maps against the backdrop of eighteen constellations, which were given the names Aries, Taurus, Gemini, and so on. By 600 B.C.E., the Greeks had shrunk the number of constellations down to twelve, consistent with the Chinese and Hindus versions. The movements of the constellations—stars which were associated with each other—were correlated with seasonal changes and the movements of the five central stars through these constellations.

The Greek natural scientist Ptolemy produced one of the most respected scientific treatises on astrology and astronomy. In his groundbreaking work *Mathematike Syntaxis*—also known as *Almagest*—Ptolemy established mathematical relationships between the positioning of the stars and planets, showing how an ephemeris can logically address human behavior. The *Almagest* was composed of two treatises, one called the *Tetrabiblos* and the other called the *Planetary Hypotheses.* The *Tetrabiblos* focused on the astrological elements, and the *Planetary Hypotheses* focused on a cosmological positioning of the universe. His proposal consisted of a nesting of spherical shells in which the planets moved. The works of another early Greek astrologer, Hipparchus, were used extensively in Ptolemy's works. Hipparchus was known as a great mathematician, often given credit for the founding of trigonometry. The *Almagest*—like the other works of Ptolemy—was embraced by Arabic, Roman and European natural scientists until the sixteenth century. His calculations used angular measurements extensively, correlating the angles between heavenly bodies with natural occurrences. It was during this era when Ptolemy's *geocentric* view (the earth being the center) of the universe was gradually replaced with the *heliocentric* model proposed by Copernicus, Kepler and Galileo—of the earth encircling the sun. Though Ptolemy's model was stricken, most of the relationships he described are still recognized as accurate.

The Arabic astrologer-astronomers of the medieval era combined the various systems into twelve houses, with angular measurements of each of the major stars and planets positioned within these houses measured in relation to each other. This modified version of the skies was extensively taught at the major universities throughout the Middle East and Europe during the middle ages. Eventually it was embraced by the scientists of the Renaissance period, where it commingled with the works of Regiomontanus—or Johannes Muller von Konigsberg—of the fifteenth century. Regiomantanus' was held in high regard as an astronomer-astrologer all over Europe during that era. It was his ephemeris that was used by Christopher Columbus. The new Babylonians, the Greeks, and the medieval Europeans gradually redirected this wealth of astrological understandings towards personal forecasting—frowned upon by religious conservatives. Even renaissance astronomers such as Kepler resorted, albeit hesitantly, to giving astrological horoscopes occasionally. He produced natal charts for various nobles. He performed personal astrological services for Pope Paul II, Matthias Corvinus, King of Hungary and many others. His prolific writings also influenced many of Nicolaus Copernicus' views. Frenchman Nostradamus was also a highly regarded astrologer-scientist of the Renaissance era. Nostradamus uncannily forecasted daily and annual futures of various nobles and dignitaries around Europe. This forecasting focused towards personal prediction astrology during the Middle Ages was frowned upon by the Church during this era. Soon thereafter, the Church condemned astrology in its entirety.

The Church of England and the Vatican both launched efforts at different times to dissuade the populace from a fixation upon events of the future. The legitimacy of astronomy was nonetheless by that time infused into many areas of medical science. The ancient sciences of *Ayurveda* and Chinese medicine were heavy with astrological influences. Astrology also influenced the many advances of Arabian medical sciences—known as one of the world's more advanced systems for thousands of years. This also influenced the Greek and Roman medical sciences, and carried into the medical disciplines of the Middle Ages and the Renaissance era.

These early medical sciences utilized the angles and locations of the planets and stars in their discussions of both disease and anatomy. Parts of the body and their infirmities were associated with different houses, and said to be governed by particular planets. Various medical manuscripts in use during these centuries included anatomical drawings of the body associated with the zodiac. Phases of the moon and the convergence of planetary paths were associated with various medical procedures. Many physicians of that era were also respected astrologers-astronomers.

Modern medicine scoffs at such a relationship between health and the motions of the universe. Yet we might pause before we dismiss thousands of years of behavioral observation and health science so easily. As evident from some of the research laid out here, modern science is only just beginning to realize the interplay between the rhythms of the sun and moon and the various biochemical messengers like melatonin, cortisol, dopamine, serotonin, estrogen and others as we have discussed. As these messengers are linked to behavior and pathology, there is little stretch to apply the movements of at least our major heavenly bodies to the topics of anatomy and pathology.

The various physiological influences of the sun are well established. In addition to the sun's pervasive radiative influence over our metabolism through the direct ultraviolet and visible light spectrum, we find evidence for significant effects from the solar sunspot cycles. The scientific endeavor into solar cycles is due largely to the research of Russian scientist Alexander Chizhevsky, also known for his groundbreaking research on ionized air during the earlier part of the twentieth century.

In the early 1920s, Chizhevsky analyzed the timing of wars, battles, riots, and revolutions among the histories of 72 countries from 500 BCE to 1922. He discovered that 80% of these critical events took place close to a sunspot activity peak. In an attempt to explain the data, Chizhevsky proposed that strong magnetic fields might be emanating from these intense solar storms. He suggested that magnetic influences from solar storms could trigger mass behavior changes among large populations simultaneously. These magnetic stimulatory effects, he thought, could affect mental propensities, predisposing aggressive or violent behavior. Considered a novel and controversial concept at the time, recent science has confirmed many of important effects of *geomagnetism* upon behavior and disease.

Chizhevsky's studies demonstrated similar patterns between solar sunspot cycles and mortality rates caused by epidemic and spikes in births. The relevance and conclusions from his research have recently received confirmation in research by Musaev *et al.* (2007), which studied demographic data together with infectious disease mortality between 1930 and 2000. Disease and mortality statistics related to cardiovascular, psycho- neurological, oncological, bronchopulmonary, and various infectious epidemics were included. The data indicated a clear relationship between these pathology statistics and solar storm activity cycles.

Recent research has also focused upon the pathological effects resulting from the influence of auroras, sunspots and solar storms. The Cardiology department of Israel's Rabin Medical Center (Stoupel *et al.* 2007) studied the occurrence of acute myocardial infarction together with the timing and measurement of solar activity. They differentiated the effects of higher cosmic ray activity from periods of higher geomagnetic activity (magnetism resulting from sunspot activity). This study found myocardial infarction rates inversely correlating with monthly solar activity, and positively correlating with increased cosmic ray activity. Low geomagnetic activity days and higher cosmic ray days were both separately linked with significantly greater rates of fatalities due to myocardial infarction.

Marasanov and Matveev also reported in 2007 that among lung cancer patients having surgery, complications occurred more significantly during geomagnetic solar storm periods than during geomagnetic "quiet" days.

Stoupel *et al.* (2006) also compared levels of immune system strength by measuring IgG, IgM, IgA, lupus anti-coagulant, clotting time and auto-antibody blood levels of subjects. These levels were correlated with periods and strengths of solar activity as measured by the U.S. National Geophysical Data Center. This research found that immune system biomarker levels significantly decrease with solar geomagnetic activity.

This research confirmed studies done at Canada's Laurentian University (Kinoshameg and Persinger 2004) which concluded that rats exposed to induced geomagnetic activity had immunosuppression, resulting in higher rates of infection.

Vaquero and Gallego (2007) confirmed the connection between immunosuppression, outbreaks, and sunspot cycles in research studying pandemic influenza A outbreaks. In 2006, Yeung analyzed pandemic influenza outbreaks from 1700 A.D. to 2000 A.D. Significant correlations were found between outbreak periods and sunspot cycles.

A 2006 study from researchers from Kyoto University in Japan (Otsu *et al.*) reported that correlations between sunspot activity, unemployment rates and suicides existed between 1971 and 2001. Both unemployment and suicides were inversely proportional to sunspot rhythmic periods.

Another study from 2006 (Davis and Lowell) using the birth dates of 237,000 humans found a positive correlation between the births of genetic mental diseases like schizophrenia and bipolar disorder with solar activity. They also found similar correlations between solar activity cycles and diseases like multiple sclerosis and rheumatoid arthritis. These diseases were also closely correlated with being born in a particular season.

In another study done in Israel (Stoupel *et al.* 2006), 339,252 newborn births over a period of seven years were compared to monthly cosmic ray and solar activity. Significantly more babies were born of both genders during higher cosmic ray periods. Significantly fewer newborns were born during solar activity periods as compared with non-solar activity periods.

The Rabin Medical Center (Stoupel *et al.* 2005) also studied Down syndrome cases among 1,108,449 births together with solar activity. With 1,310 total cases of Down syndrome in the data, a significant inverse relationship between solar activity occurred (r=-0.78). In other words, Down syndrome—long considered a genetic defect—occurs more often during the periods between solar activity, and less often during periods of solar activity.

Researchers at the Universidad de Chile's Clinica Psiquiatrica Universitaria (Ivanovic-Zuvic *et al.*) presented a study in 2005 of increased hospitalizations of depressive patients and manic patients conjunctive with solar activity periods. In this study, depressive hospitalizations correlated with periods of lower solar activity, while manic hospitalizations positively correlated with higher solar activity periods.

A study at the Augusta Mental Health Institute in Maine (Davis and Lowell 2004) established that excessive ultraviolet radiation from the sun combined with solar flare cycles correlated positively with mental illnesses resulting from DNA damage.

It also appears from research as reported by Davis and Lowell (2004) that human lifespan correlates with solar activity. From this research, chaotic solar cycles (as opposed to typical cycles) coincide with increases in mutagenic DNA effects. Further exploration into lifespan and birthdates around solar cycles found disrupted solar cycles correlating positively with shorter lifespan.

In an Australian study (Berk *et al.* 2006) of suicides between 1968 and 2002, both seasonal and geomagnetic solar storm activity were investigated using 51,845 male and 16,327 female suicides. Suicides among females significantly increased in the autumn, concurrent with increased geomagnetic storm activity. Suicides were lowest during autumn for males and lowest during the summer for females. The average number of suicides for both males and females were the greatest during the spring.

This seasonal and geomagnetic activity rhythm connection with suicide was also confirmed in research on 27,469 Finnish suicide cases between 1979 and 1999 by Partonen *et al.* (2004).

As Kamide (2005) commented in his paper in *Biomedical Pharmacotherapy*, *"the earth is located within the solar atmosphere."*

The moon waxes and wanes with a tilted elliptical orbit around the earth, reflecting sunlight with different trajectories. Though controversial, a respectable body of research correlates behavior and biological metabolism with the position of the moon. Thakur and Sharma reported in the British Medical Journal (1984) on the incidence of crimes reported by police stations in three different Indian towns from 1978 to 1982. One town was rural, one town was urban and the other was an industrial town. Crime rates were higher on full moon days in all locales. Crimes were also slightly higher on new moon days. In 1978, the *Journal of Clinical Psychiatry* (Leiber) reported a computer analysis on human aggression, homicides, suicides, traffic fatalities, and psychiatric emergency room visits in Dade County Florida. There was a significant clustering of these events around the lunar synodic cycle. In 2000, the *British Medical Journal* published a study by Bhattacharjee *et al.* showing that of 1621 cases of animal bites to humans, incidence rose significantly during full moons.

On the other side of this coin, there have also been a number of studies published confirming no correlation between extraordinary events and the full moon. One study also published in *BMJ* reported no correlation between dog bites and the full moon in 1671 cases in Australia (Chapman and Morrell 2000). A study of traffic accidents over nine years showed no correlation between the moon's cycles and traffic accidents (Laverty and Kelly 1998). Owen *et al.* (1998) showed a lack of correlation between the lunar cycle and violence in two studies. A Canary Island emergency room was studied by Nunez *et al.* in 2002, which showed a lack of correlation between emergency room entrance and the moon's cycles. Psychiatric admissions of 8,473 patients between 1993 and 2001 for a Navy Medical Center in San Diego also showed no correlation between the moon's synodic phases and psychiatric admissions (McLay *et al.* 2006).

As to the discrepancy between these results, we can only offer the possibility of a differentiation between the methods of lunar calculation. The differences between the sidereal lunar cycle and the synodic cycles are significant. While the sidereal month measures the path of the moon relative to the stars and constellations behind it to form a cycle of 27.21 days, the synodic path is measured relative to the sun's path. Because the earth is in rotation, it takes the moon about 29.5 days to cycle back to the same position when referencing the position of the sun.

Gender may also be a variant that might explain the contradictory results. In a study (Buckley *et al.*) published in a 1993 edition of the *Medical Journal of Australia,* self-poisoning of 2215 patients between 1987 and 1993 were studied. Self-poisoning among women was greatest during the new moon, at 60%. However, the result was significantly lower for men. In addition, while the mean illumination of the moon was 50.63% at the time of overdose for women on average, for men it was 47.45%.

In a study by Kollerstrom and Steffert (2003) from England, four years of telephone call frequency data was compiled from a crisis call center. The new moon brought a significant increase in women callers, with a swing of 9%, and a decrease in callers by men during the new moon. This makes sense, noting the timing of the female menstrual cycle.

Anthropological studies have indicated a link between the new moon and menstruation among the female population (Bell and Defouw 1964). In this study, the authors also discuss the discrepancy between the various lunar cycle calculations, noting that while some have used a 30-day monthly cycle in their calculations, others have used a 28-day lunar cycle, and still others have calculated using the 29.5 synodic cycle.

Research on animals also demonstrated physiological patterns seemingly related to the moon's cycles. For example, Zimecki (2006) confirmed that lunar cycles correlate with cycles for circulating corticosterones, melatonin levels, taste perception, sleep quality, as well as pineal and hypothalamus gland activity in animal research.

No one versed in botany can deny the moon's effects upon plant growth. Farmers generally plant with phases of the moon, timed also with seasons, temperatures and moisture. These rhythmic effects of the moon on plant growth have become obvious over thousands of years of trial and error. Observation has led us to understand that the waxing moon typically stimulates plant growth as compared with a waning moon. Hence, farmers are likely to plant crops that bear aboveground fruits during the waxing moon and root crops during the waning moon. Most trees, even fruit trees—are considered root-oriented so tend to be more vigorous when planted on the waning moon. For example, grass tends to grow faster when planted during the new moon.

Studies in 1939 by Kolisko on wheat found that seeds sprouted better if they were sown during the full moon. Poor sprouting resulted from new moon plantings. Other studies have followed confirming these findings. Northwestern Professor F. Brown found that with equal temperatures, sprouting seedlings absorb greater water at full moon. This seems to indicate that plants hold more water during the full moon as well, and consequently have less during the new moon. Even when Brown shielded the plants from the light of the moon, they still responded to moon phase (Brown and Chow 1973).

From 1952 to 1862, biodynamic grower Maria Thun performed research on moon phases on her farm in Darmstadt, Germany. She sowed row crops systematically over sidereal-measured moon positions. She weighed crop yields using this system after each harvest. Thun found that potatoes planted when the moon was in Taurus, Capricorn and Virgo had better yields than when the moon was in the other constellations. Conversely, root crops did not produce well if they were planted when the moon was in the houses of Cancer, Scorpio and Pisces. Though controversial, these results were replicated by later researchers (Kollerstrom and Staudenmaier 2001).

It appears evident that modern science has yet to fully grasp the orientation and extent of influence on behavior and biology by the various rhythms of the universe around us. Thakur and Sharma mention in their analysis that the body contains at least 50-60% water; and the tidal gravitational pull upon water by the moon is evidenced by the ocean's tidal rhythms. Various environmental measurements have indicated that the moon's gravitational pull is about 23% less than its pull on full moon days.

Certainly, science's overwhelming interest to understand the potential influence heavenly bodies have upon our bodies has been cause enough for the volume of research sampled here. Many of the ancient astronomers were also leading researchers, respected mathematicians and physicians. Still, modern medicine opted to throw out this body of observational research and start from scratch. Gradually, we are accumulating the evidence that illustrates these ancient physicians might not have been the crackpots we assumed they were. We are also hopefully learning that double-blind controlled research is not the only path towards knowledge.

Modern science currently questions how planetary bodies millions of light years away from earth could affect human activity. If we consider that simply the ability to see these stars requires the reception of the electromagnetic radiation emitted from every star, it seems at least remotely viable that the radiation of these stars may also have some sort of subtle influence. We might suppose this influence is geomagnetic, electromagnetic, or gravitational—or perhaps a combination thereof.

When we look at the billions of stars on a clear night, we are often overwhelmed by the majesty and the largeness of it all. As we look with amazement at a swirling universe billions of light years away, and ponder black holes that appear to contradict the rules of matter, we have good reason to pause and wonder. The effects these bodies have upon consciousness may be subtle. Perhaps the combined effects of the sun, moon and planets together with the various thermal, atmospheric, genetic and clockwork biochemistry within the body create a confluence of biological influence. The central question is whether these influences disregard or dismiss our ability to make conscious choices. Certainly not. We can see simply by observation of human behavior that people influenced one way or another still have the ability to make conscious decisions to move in a manner contradictory to those influences.

Epigenetic Intention

In 1869, the Swiss Dr. Friedrich Miescher isolated an interesting conglomeration of molecules extracted from discarded surgical bandages. Believing this substance was derived from the nuclei of human cells, he called this substance *nuclein.* Two decades earlier the Swiss botanist Karl von Nageli observed this same material dividing in plant cells. They were named *chromosomes* because they so conveniently received identifying colored dyes, making them very visible (chromo) when peering through a microscope. In a series of discoveries from 1905 to 1929, Dr. Phoebus Levene demonstrated the existence of ribose and deoxyribose linked together in phosphate-sugar base units. Dr. Levene was convinced, however, that these units were isolated and did not contain any kind of coding information.

In 1944, physicist Erwin Schrödinger proposed in a book called *What is Life?* that the cell contained an information element within the chromosomes, which he surmised, scripted the activities of the cell and life in general. This consideration lay dormant until in 1948, using x-ray diffraction imaging, Dr. Linus Pauling pointed out that most proteins inside the cell were made not only of complex 20-amino acid combinations, but were often curiously helical in shape. These observations led to a deepening curiosity regarding the nucleus' protein content, and a suspicion they provided the instructional foundation for cellular growth and metabolism. Between 1950 and 1953, again utilizing x-ray diffraction, Dr. Rosalind Franklin and Dr. Maurice Wilkins independently developed scans of base pairings that demonstrated the possibility of a much larger helical molecule with numerous base pairings. Working from these unpublished results, Dr. Francis Crick and Dr. James Watson were the first to publish a presentation of a double-helixed deoxyribonucleic acid, or DNA, in a series of articles for *Nature* magazine.

Proteins are the primary biochemical structures involved in the execution of nearly every cellular process throughout biological life. Proteins are the body's soldiers: Some proteins act as enzymes and catalysts to assist in metabolic reactions. Some proteins are hormones. They stimulate cells and various organs to perform certain activities. Other proteins will assist in cell growth, energy production, or immune systems. Most other proteins are made up of a distinctive arrangement of up to twenty different amino acids. A typical protein molecule will contain hundreds of different combinations of these twenty amino acids. Many protein molecules are twisted, helical or semi-helical molecules. An example of this is the interleukin-6 molecule, a complex immune protein produced by the body's T-cells.

DNA is actually a very large protein. DNA might be aptly considered a protein library, as its sequencing and transcription with RNA predicates the formation of specific proteins. DNA is a very complex molecule. It is elegantly designed, made up of long sugar-phosphate chains linked to combinations of four possible purine or pyrimidine nucleotide pairs. The DNA molecule has two complementary strands bound between the pairs, which form its double-helix structure. The two strands are not precisely identical. They are described as complementary because they have a slightly different polarity. This polarity bends DNA into its beautiful spiral structure.

The order of nucleotides on the DNA chain and the particular amino acid each nucleotide associates with creates distinctive sequencing combinations. These are typically called the *genetic code,* or the *hapmap.* Portions of a hapmap or sequenced combinations are referred to as *alleles.* It has been estimated that one human DNA molecule can have over 3 billion base (purine or pyrimidine) pair and amino acid combinations. Together, the combination of sequences is called a *genome.*

The DNA pairs making up the sequencing are connected by weak electromagnetic hydrogen bonds. These electromagnetic bonds allow the DNA molecule to quite easily separate its framework under stress, depending upon the length of the strand. Shorter DNA strands will fall apart more easily in a heated solution or from radiation for this reason. These weak bonds are easily breakable, but their sequencing combinations provide a framework for a translation mechanism for information. Several decades of progressive genetic research has confirmed that DNA sequences match up with unique characteristics and functions within individual cells and organisms.

The reason for DNA's mysterious complexity is not its double helix shape or its intricate coding system: Its coding system is actually rather simple. The incredible complex nature of DNA lies primarily with ribonucleic acid or RNA. RNA molecules are very similar to DNA molecules, except most are single-stranded. Most RNA are still helical, however. RNA also have slightly different chemical base systems, but their sequencing is programmed via the copying—or *transcription*—of sections of the DNA's hapmap.

RNA transcription allows DNA to be replicated—or copied to make a new DNA molecule with the same coding sequences. To accomplish this, special DNA enzymes such as DNA polymerase will split apart a DNA strand. RNA strands are then somehow stimulated to wrap up against the DNA strand to extract and record the code. Once it records the coding, RNA uses this to help make another DNA set by transferring the coding on to structures that assemble proteins.

RNA is the molecule implicitly required not only for the survival of DNA, but also for the production of the millions of proteins, which in turn perform most of the body's metabolic processes. The various types of RNA will translate selected sections of the DNA's sequencing information for different purposes: Transfer RNA (tRNA) transfer amino acids to protein sequences to assemble active proteins. Messenger RNA (mRNA) are considered metabolic information carriers: They communicate specific action plans from DNA sequencing to specialized ribosomes—where many proteins are assembled. This process of making proteins in the ribosomes is also assisted by another RNA type, the ribosomal RNA (rRNA). Catalytic RNA or ribosymes are catalysts for specialized biochemical reactions. Double-stranded RNA (dsRNA) appear to be intermediaries for another active double-stranded RNA called small interfering RNA (siRNA) which apparently interfere with the expression of certain DNA sequences. This seems to create a protective function in circumstances where invasion or mutation is possible.

A number of other RNA types have been classified as non-coding RNA (ncRNA). These include micro RNA (miRNA) and germline RNA. These were proposed by Rassoulzadegan (2006) as being heritable—or able to be passed through to new generations. Non-coding forms of RNA provide the new frontier in understanding RNA function.

In essence, RNA appear to provide the mechanisms to copy and transmit the informational coding contained in the DNA. After copying the DNA master hapmaps, RNA seem to effectively pass on that information into executive form by enabling protein mechanisms to perform their particular activities. RNA enable the process of manufacturing specialized protein molecules, and even contribute particular amino acids themselves. RNA's activities also provide a storage and retrieval function for DNA's coded sequencing, thereby guaranteeing the DNA's survival as cells divide and become replaced.

Noting that RNA provide a form of information biocommunication, most researchers have assumed that all of this information is chemically transmitted through the transcription process. Recent research from Stanford Medical Center's John Rin and Dr. Howard Chang (2007) has confirmed that RNA can also communicate their instructional messages remotely. RNA can remotely silence individual genes by interfering in their expression, for example. ncRNA were observed regulating and suppressing genes on remote chromosomes at remote distances within the cell.

Over the last two decades, geneticists have focused on assembling the combined gene combinations that together would make up the genome of particular organisms. The human genome research combined with an institution-wide focus on establishing the genome of other species. The assumption in the beginning of this research project—which involved hundreds of scientists from different specialties over two decades—was that we would find within the genome the answers to all the mysteries of the body, disease, evolution, and our ultimate identity. Surprisingly, none of this was found. The evolutionary assumption, for example, was that they would find an increasingly complex assembly of genes up the evolutionary 'hierarchy' of species. This fell on its ear as the research revealed that humans only have about 25,000 gene combinations—about the same amount that a small fish or a mouse has. Plants contain more genes than humans. In other words, gene combinations were no more complex in humans than they were in many other creatures.

Furthermore, the initial assumption was that the combination of genes in humans would unfold and unlock the key to all disease pathologies. Preliminary research connected certain gene combinations or gene expressions to particular diseases. It was assumed that every disease had a particular genetic trait to match. This worked out pretty well until researchers began discovering that sometimes two or three diseases were connected to the same genetic trait or expression. For example, Angelman Syndrome and Prader-willy Syndrome both relate to the same chromosome 15 deletion. This revealed some further factor involved.

The other mystery for geneticists, which we will discuss later in more detail, was that identical twins—which have the same DNA at some point, seemingly at conception—do not develop the same diseases. Identical twins, in fact, often have very different physiological outcomes. This was apparently related to whether the genes were switched on.

This has forced a calibration of the genetic theory with the concept of *epigenetics.* In general, epigenetics is the acceptance of additional factors that affect the switching of gene expression and non-expression. It was hypothesized—and confirmed by the research—that ones DNA was not as important as how gene expressions—or *phenotypes*—were turned on or off. If the genes were expressed, particular metabolism consequences resulted. If they were not expressed, there would be other consequences.

The original concept of epigenetics was penned by geneticist Conrad Waddington in the early 1940s to explain in general how environmental circumstances could effect ones genetic instructions. The concept, however, was given increasing focus in the 1990s and early 2000s as geneticists discovered the various many holes genome assumptions contained.

The biochemical relationships between gene expressions have focused upon the action of DNA methylation or histone regulation. These biochemical messengers were observed switching alleles on or off. Experiments on mice at McGill University's Douglas Hospital Research Center (Szyf *et al.* 2008) found that phenotype switching could be turned on and off with the exchange of increased nurturing from the mother. Those baby mice receiving the nurturing from mama would switch on genes differently than those mice that received less nurturing from mama.

Biochemical mechanisms like phosphorylation, sumoylation, acetylation, methylation, and ubiquitylation appear to be mechanically responsible for phenotype expression—which connects them to the availability of nutrients like vitamin B and Co-Q-10. Even so, a critical element of the *epigenome* bridges these messaging systems with consciousness.

Non-environmental epigenetics provides the missing bridge between the conscious operator and the body. Like the rest of the various messaging systems of the body, genetic expression is a coded assembly allowing an informational transmission system between the functions of the body and the conscious intentional operator of the body—the self within.

Chapter Two

The Real You

Before we can fully understand the intentional and conscious nature of the body and its anatomy, we must understand its driving force. What is the source of the energy and life of the body? Where is the generator? Who or what is running the body? This also relates to the concept of identity: Is each of us simply a temporary physical body? Are we simply cellular machines that decompose after a few decades?

If we ask someone their identity, they will most likely describe their body's physical features. Or perhaps their body's country of origin. They might say "I am American" or "I am black" or "I am five feet tall, weigh 125 lbs, and female with brown eyes." The logical question here is: Am I this physical body? If so, what happens if the body gains 100 lbs of weight or becomes disfigured? Does my identity change?

Most of us believe our identity runs deeper than our physical body. A person with a black body wants equality with a person with a white body because that person considers that beneath the skin, we all have equality. Similarly, an obese person wants to be treated equally with someone of a more slender stature. Why would we request equality unless we are assuming we have deeper identities?

As science has debated this topic, there have been two general views (Popper and Eccles 1983): The first assumes a machine-like information-processing generating system with various modules of activity, all competing for control. This "chaos-machine" theoretically builds upon a system of learning and evolution without any central person or actor.

The other, more prevalent view historically, portrays the body as driven by an inner self or life force, central and governing to the body's existence. Among proponents of this inner self model, there is also some debate regarding the characteristics of the inner self. Some suggest it is a small part of the living organism. They refer to the "soul" as a type of "moral organ." Others refer to the soul as part of some kind of trinity: *"body, mind and spirit."* Still others consider the inner self as the central component of life. Debate on this topic continues, but empirical information and clear research data clarifies the conclusion.

The Lifeless Body

By any physical observation made in the death of any living being, life leaves the body during death. When we see a living body full of life, movement, energy, personality, and purpose, we understand these symptoms of life are residing within the body. When death arrives, suddenly those symptoms of life leave: There is no movement, no energy, and no personality remaining within the dead body. The body becomes lifeless. There is no growth, no will, no personality and no purposeful activity.

For thousands of years, doctors and scientists have autopsied, dissected and otherwise examined millions of dead bodies. No one—not even modern researchers with technical medical instruments—has been able to find any chemical or physical element missing from the dead body that was present when the body was alive. The dead body has every physical and material component the living body had. All of the cells are still there. The entire DNA is still there. All of the nerves, the organs, the brain and central nervous system—every physical element—is still resident in the cadaver.

The claim of a 21-gram weight difference at death was weak at best and never corroborated. In 1907, Massachusetts physician Dr. Duncan MacDougal attempted an experiment where six patients were monitored as they died upon a table rigged with a scale. MacDougal's experiment consisted of monitoring six patients as they died upon a table rigged with a beam scale. Of the six, two were eliminated because of technical issues. Three subjects died of tuberculosis. Two of these were losing weight before and after death by "evaporation and respiratory moisture." One subject died from "consumption" and seemingly lost ¾ of an ounce in weight as he was dying—later converted to 21.3 grams. Dr. Mac-Dougall admitted that it was difficult in some cases to know at what point the patient had died (MacDougall 1907).

A fellow doctor in Massachusetts, Dr. A. Clarke, immediately debated this single finding, arguing the typical sudden rise in body temperature before and subsequent cooling without circulation upon death could account for slight weight changes due to evaporation. Especially noting the patient had lethal tuberculosis. One of the other problems with the research was that the moment of death was difficult to ascertain. Dr. MacDougall assumed it was when breathing stopped. While clinical death has confounded the issue, currently, death is considered to take place when brainwaves cease.

Until his own death in 1920, Dr. MacDougall tried to repeat the results and could not repeat his finding. In one test, he killed fifteen dogs while weighing them and found no weight loss. No other study has substantiated such a theory of weight loss upon death. The 21-gram concept should be officially remanded to the urban legend category for once and for all.

With the exception of these weak findings, many centuries of cadaver research and autopsies have carefully examined organs, bones, nerves, brain, blood, neurochemistry and other vital body parts. None has substantiated any structural or biochemical difference between a live and dead body. The dead body is simply missing an immeasurable element of life that once animated the body: An invisible force that gives the body personality, energy, motivation, and the will to survive.

The life force of the body has never been seen under a microscope or by any other physical piece of equipment. Furthermore, since this living force separates from the body at death, leaving an intact physical body with no life, it is obvious that this life force is not part of the body. Since the personality is also gone when this life is gone from the body, it would also be logical that our personality is part of this life force, and not part of the physical body—again since the physical body including all the DNA and neurons remains. Just as the driver is not the car, he or she may be driving. The driver can step out of the car at any time. Therefore, the driver logically has a separate identity from the car.

This concept pervaded during the time of the Greek philosophers. Plato, Aristotle, Ptolemy, Socrates, Hippocrates, Pythagoras and others all ascribed to this notion. Hippocrates professed that the life within the body was due to a "vital spirit" within, which acted through four different humors, for example. When one of Socrates' students asked him how he wanted to be buried, Socrates gave them a clear reply: They could do whatever they wanted with the body, because he would be long gone by then.

What Body Part are You?

Following an arm amputation due to an infection or other injury, no one would claim the amputee is any less of a person. This is because the same personality is there despite the massive structural change in body. This logic can be extended to even severe cases such as the loss of both arms and legs or other major parts of the anatomy. An explosion or other traumatic accident might leave ones torso intact while amputating both the body's arms and legs. Regardless of losing these appendages, the person is still perceived as a whole person—the same person as before—even though their body cannot function the way it did before. The person who operates the body still contains the same conscious being with the same personality. This is why paraplegic and quadriplegic rights are protected by law, and why quadriplegic Stephen Hawking was considered a great theoretical physicist despite physical handicaps. Physically disabled people are given equal rights because society considers these persons equal in all respects, despite any deficiencies in their physical bodies.

The physical organs can illustrate the same logic. It is now commonplace in medicine to surgically remove and replace organs such as kidneys, livers, hearts, hips and other parts in order to preserve the healthy functioning of the body. Some parts—like hearts and hip sockets—are now replaced with artificial versions. Modern medicine has illustrated through many years of organ transplants that a person's identity does not travel with the organ. Otherwise, we might have—as a few comedic theatrical performances have suggested—people whose personalities reflect their organ donors. Imagine someone receiving a heart transplant and assuming part of the personality of the dead donor.

We might compare this to an auto accident: Let's say a car is brought into a repair shop after a collision: The shop determines the car needs the tires changed, the engine rebuilt and various other parts of the car replaced before the car can be put back on the road. These changes and new car parts do not affect the driver of the car. The driver will still be the same person no matter how many new parts are put on the car. After the engine is rebuilt, the new tires installed and the other parts replaced, the unchanged driver gets back into the car and drives it away.

Living versus Nonliving

The difference between the physical body and the living personality requires a clear differentiation between matter and life. This investigation has been captured by science under the term *autopoiesis*. Autopoiesis is the study of the characterization of a complete living system as it compares to either a part of another living system or non-living matter.

To investigate this we could first analyze the difference between a living organism and a piece of matter without the component of life. An easy comparison would be between single-celled bacteria and a dead cell separated from a living body. A single-cell bacterium is a complete living organism. Studies have shown bacteria indeed respond to stimuli, avoid death, and avert pain. As we know from medicine, bacteria will intelligently mutate and adapt to antibiotics. New antibiotic-resistant *superbugs* are examples of bacteria who have intelligently evaded death. Living bacteria also conduct all of the activities required for independent survival: eating, digesting, reproduction, movement, response to stimuli, sense perception, the intention to survive, and self-organization. In Dr. Backster's work and others, bacteria were observed sensing the endangerment of other bacteria through a subtle means of communication.

Non-living objects display none of these characteristics independently. While a machine may digest and respond to stimuli, it will not have sense perception and emotional response. A machine relies upon a living person to program its tasking and response. Once a cell has been disconnected from a living organism like a human body, the cell ceases independent function. A single cell can be put into an incubating Petri dish and kept alive, however. This *in vitro* survival makes the cell now dependent upon the environment of the lab equipment, driven by living lab operators. The cell has thus become a surrogate of the lab, just as it was formerly a surrogate of the living body. It displays no independent sense perception, the desire to survive or independent emotional response. While the cell is part of the living body it maintains the body's *self-concept.* Once detached, it displays metabolic continuation, but no separate self-existence. Dr. Backster's research illustrated this as well.

Over many years of animal research, test results have demonstrated that like humans, animals also have this self-concept awareness, which prevails through their responses to various environmental challenges. The functions of their mechanical physiology has also confirmed that this self-concept pervades through all living tissues, reflected by the display of episodic memory—remembering specifics about past events and past sensations. For this reason, we see animals learning quickly which activities result in pain and which activities result in pleasure. They immediately respond simply because every living being seeks pleasure (Dere *et al.* 2006).

Bitbol and Luisi (2004) sum up the distinction between living organisms and non-living matter to be grounded within the principle of *cognition.* A definition of cognition as proposed by Bourqine and Stewart (2004) is, *"A system is cognitive if and only if sensory inputs serve to trigger actions in a specific way, so as to satisfy a viability constraint."* Bourqine and Stewart also contend *"A system that is both autopoietic and cognitive is a living system."* Bitbol and Luisi clarify that *"the very lowest level of cognition is the condition for life,"* and *"the lowest level of cognition does not reduce to the lowest level of autopoiesis."*

When we consider the element of cognition, we bring into focus the nature of awareness. Cognition is the awareness of *self* and *non-self.* The awareness of self and non-self are required for a living organism to consider survival important. Without an awareness of self and non-self, there is no intention for fulfillment. Without intention and the awareness of self, there is no consciousness. Without consciousness, there is no life.

Are You the Cells?

Throughout its physical lifetime, our body is continually changing, yet we continue to maintain our core identity and consciousness. Research has shown all living cells in the body have a finite lifespan, ranging from minutes to days to years.

It is thought a few cells of the body—such as certain bone marrow stem cells and brain cells—may exist through the duration of the body. Still there are only a handful of these cells compared to the estimated 200 trillion cells making up the body. By far the vast majority of cells in the body will participate in cell division. Following division, older cells time out and are broken down by the immune system and discarded, leaving the newly divided cells in their place. Using this process the body constantly sloughs off older cells from the body, replacing them with new ones. Different cells in different parts of the body have different death clocks. For example:

- Intestinal cells are replaced between two and five days
- Stomach lining cells are replaced between two and ten days
- Neutrophil and eosinophil blood cells are replaced within five days
- Lung alveoli cells are replaced within eight days
- Blood platelets are replaced within 10 days
- Epidermis skin cells are replaced within a month
- Osteoplast bone cells are replaced within 90 days
- All liver cells are replaced within 18 months
- Most stem cells are replaced within 3-5 years
- All fat cells are replaced within 8 years
- All bone cells are replaced within 10 years
- All heart cells are replaced within 10 years
- All bone cells are replaced within 10 years

Nerve cells and retinal cells can live for decades, and some over the lifetime of the body. In 2005, research from the Lawrence Livermore National Laboratory and Sweden's Karolinska Institute utilized carbon-14 analyses to examine cell lifetime in the brain.

They discovered that many of the brain's cells are generated when the body is young, and many brain and nervous system cells will be replaced over the body's lifetime.

They found that these longest-living cells will still recycle much of their atomic composition: The exception is some of the nucleotides within the brain cells' genetic matter, which turnover more slowly.

However, the composition of all cells will turn over. Every cell is made up of ionic and molecular combinations. The atoms that make up these molecular combinations are constantly being replaced. Our cells' cytoplasm, organelles and membrane will thus be composed up of recycled atoms.

This is all supported by the science. Research in the 1950s led by Dr. Paul Aebersold at the Oak Ridge Atomic Research Center concluded that approximately 98 percent of the atoms composing the body are replaced every year.

Furthermore, as we'll discuss later in the book, our body contains more bacteria than cells. Microbiologists have estimated that the typical human organism contains ten times more bacteria than cells. The typical body may contain about 200 trillion cells. But our body will also contain about 2,000 trillion bacteria units, of hundreds of different species.

Each of these bacteria are single-celled living creatures. Yes, like our cells, bacteria have cell walls and cytoplasm and organelles. They also typically have a short lifespan. Our body's bacteria will reproduce by division anywhere from a few minutes to a few hours. So like most of our cells, the precise makeup of our bacteria is also constantly undergoing change as well.

However, unlike our cells, bacteria are also living organisms in themselves.

As we'll discuss later, bacteria have consciousness. They will communicate with each other using quorum sensing along with biochemical secretion. Indeed, bacteria also communicate with their host (our bodies) utilizing cytokines and other biochemicals. In this way, they can stimulate the body's immune system and also help regulate the body's moods and biorhythms.

Our body cannot survive without these bacteria. They are critical to the body's health. But these bacteria are not us. They are independent living entities.

Understanding our bacteria are separate from us; our physical bodies change nearly every cell within days, weeks or years; and every atom and molecule is replaced from the food we eat, the water we drink and the air we breathe; *the body we were wearing five years ago is not the same body we are wearing today.* We are wearing a completely recycled body. In effect, we have each *changed bodies.* Every rhythmic element of matter—every vibrating atom—has changed.

This might well be compared to a waterfall. The water within a waterfall is always changing. From moment to moment, the waterfall will be made up of different water. Therefore, the waterfall we see today is not the same waterfall we saw yesterday.

Since each of us is the same person from moment to moment and year to year within an ever-changing body, logically we each have an identity separate from this temporary vehicle. We cannot be the body, since the body has been replaced while we are still here. Should we look at our photograph taken five years ago, we will be looking at *a completely different body* from the one we are wearing today. The eyes looking at the eyes in the picture will be different eyes.

Our body is a fluid structure. It is a complex recycling mechanism that supports life. Not only does it support trillions of microorganisms. This mechanism supports a living entity within - a living being separate from the body's ever-changing cells, molecules, atoms and bacteria.

Are You the Brain?

One might propose that since we have yet to transplant someone's brain maybe we are the brain. Most of us have heard of the famous neurosurgical experiments first documented by Dr. Wilder Penfield, where he stimulated the temporal cortex and stimulated particular memories in subject during brain surgery. These results and their confirmations left scientists with an impression that life must reside in the brain since emotional memories were stimulated with the electrode testing.

This assumption is disputed by other brain research over the past fifty years on both humans and animals, however. The assumption that the emotional self is contained in the brain has been conflicted by the many cases of intake emotions and memory following the removal of brain parts and even a majority of the brain. Mishkin (1978) documented that the removal of either the amygdala or the hippocampus did not severely impair memory. Mumby *et al.* (1992) determined that memory was only mildly affected in rats with hippocampus and amygdala lesions. According to a substantial review done by Vargha-Khadem and Polkey (1992), numerous hemidecortication surgeries—the removal of half the brain—had been conducted for a number of disorders. In a majority of these cases, cognition and brain function continued uninterrupted. A few cases even documented an improvement in cognition. Additionally, in numerous cases of intractable seizures, where substantial parts of brain have been damaged, substantial cognitive recovery resulted in 80 to 90% of the cases.

These and numerous other studies illustrate this effect—called *neuroplasticity*. In other words, the inner self is not reduced by brain damage or removal. The same person remains after brain parts are removed. The same personality remains. Many retain all their memories. The majority of stroke patients go about living normal lives afterward as well. Even in cases where memory, cognitive and/or motor skills are affected by cerebrovascular stroke, the person within is still present, and though handicapped, remains unaffected by the physical changes in the brain.

Memory, sensory perception and the emotional self-concept are not brain-dependent. Many organisms have memory and sensory perception without having a brain. Bacteria, for example, do not have brains, yet they can memorize a wide variety of skills and events, including what damaged or helped them in the past. Other organisms such as plants, nematodes and other organisms are living replete with memory and recall without having brains.

MRI and CT brain scans on patients with various brain injuries or stroke have shown that particular functions will often move from one part of the brain to another after the original area was damaged. We must therefore ask: Who or what is it that moves these physical functions from one part of the brain to another? Is the damaged brain area making this decision? That would not make sense. Some other guiding function must be orchestrating this move of the function. Who or what is guiding this process?

The retention of memory, emotion, and the moving of brain function from one part of the brain to another is more evidence of a deeper mechanism; an *operator* or *driver* within the body who is *utilizing* the brain—rather than *being* the brain. The driver is the continuing element. Physical structures continually undergo change, while the driver remains, adapting to those changes.

The Contradiction of Aging

Consider how most of us perceive the aging of our body with respect to our identity. Most of us try to deny the age of our body in one respect or another. Teenagers want to be older and more mature, while older adults want to be younger and more youthful. Most adults refuse to accept getting old. As any birthday party will illustrate, adults are surprised at the body's age as it gets older. We try to disconnect ourselves from the physical age of our body somehow. This denial is often joked about, but to most of us—as we are faced with an ever-wrinkling body—it is no laughing matter. We are often embarrassed by our body's age as we get older. For this reason, many older adults do not want to state their age. They are embarrassed by it. They want to distance themselves from it. Furthermore, many of us dress the body with make-up, hair dyes and/or trendy clothes in an attempt to hide the body's age.

For this same reason, many in our society undergo forms of surgery in order to achieve a younger looking body. Plastic surgery, hair-removal, hair transplantation, breast enhancement, and various other medical interventions are examples of attempts to reconcile our identity with the aging nature of our temporary physical body.

In recent years, maintaining the youthfulness of our physical body's appearance has taken a variety of less extreme forms. These include processes for removing wrinkles, special creams and lotions to preserve a youthful complexion, facilities to remove bags from the eyes, injecting Botox (OnabotulinumtoxinA, from the botulism organism) and other facilities to keep the body's skin looking plump and youthful.

Many also use other, more common facilities to change the appearance of our bodies. Many use, for example, hair coloring agents to remove gray hair or to simply take on another hair color to appeal better to others. Some of these hair coloring agents expose us to caustic chemicals. (It should be noted that natural hair coloring agents do exist—some that have been safely used for centuries such as henna.)

This does not mean that all attempts to change ones appearance are necessarily issues of self-identification. Many women, for example, will wear makeup, make hair color changes or otherwise make changes for the purpose of maintaining an appearance acceptable to others in today's competitive business atmosphere. Both men and women will gear their clothing, hair styles and hygiene for acceptance in a business atmosphere in order to maintain their positions of employment. This is a matter of survival rather than an issue of self misidentification.

Still, it is quite easy to confuse the line between maintaining a suitable appearance, and the conflict between our body's age versus our identity.

After a certain age, very few in modern society try to look older. Most of us want to look younger. This is because we innately do not feel that we are aging. Our body may be becoming older, but we do not relate with that age. We do not feel that we are old, despite our body's age.

This simply indicates a deeper identity. It indicates that we are not these rapidly aging bodies.

Biochemical Identification

Over recent years, various researchers have proposed from one basis or another that our identities are chemical. They have proposed that emotions and personality are seated within the chemicals (such as hormones and neurotransmitters) that flow through the bloodstream, basal cell network and the synapses of our nervous systems. Could our identities simply be a mixture of complex chemicals? A logical review of the scientific evidence would indicate otherwise.

Emotional responses to environmental stimuli will initiate any number of biochemical cascade pathways to occur within the body as we have discussed. We have pointed out that a cascade occurs when one chemical release stimulates the release of another biochemical, and that biochemical in turn stimulates the release of another. The biochemicals in the cascade might stimulate a particular cell, tissue or organ response. With each cascade, there is a particular initiating stimulus and particular end responses from various tissues and nerves.

Because neurologists and other researchers have seen these biochemicals involved with emotional response, some have proposed that these biochemicals contain the emotion. They propose that chemicals such as endorphins, dopamine, serotonin, epinephrine, or acetylcholine each contain the particular emotions they reflect, and are thus the sources of the emotion. They propose that these signaling biochemicals connect with receptors positioned at the surface of the cell; the response by the cell is the emotion being released from the chemical. An example some have used is the famed *opiate receptor,* linked with the cell's reception of morphine or endorphins, and subsequent feelings of euphoria. The idea is that the feeling of euphoria is produced when the ligands like endorphin connect with the receptor.

One problem with this speculation is that no two organisms respond identically to the same chemical. With opiates for example, some may hallucinate while others may only respond casually. On the other hand, some may have nightmarish experiences. If these structurally identical neuro-chemicals *contained* the emotion, why would each person respond differently to the same chemical and dose?

Another major problem with this thesis is the experiencer: *Who* is observing that the body feels euphoric feelings? *Who* observes the hallucinations from certain chemicals? *Who* observes the positive or negative sensations of the body? The fact is, without an observer, there is no way to have an objective view of the event. A physical body that is experiencing a physical emotional response with no observer could not objectively observe the experience. Therefore, there could be no discretion regarding the event. There could be no judgment available as to whether the experience was positive or negative. There could be no available decision on whether the experience should be continued or curtailed. These elements require an objective observer of the experience.

The perception of pain may offer some clarity. In 2005 Dr. Ronald Melzack, co-author of the now-standard 1965 *gate control theory* of pain transmission, updated his theory of pain from a simple gateway effect to one of a multidimensional experience of *neurosignatures.* His new theory—which he calls the *"body-self neuromatrix"*—explains that the consensus of clinical research over thon acute pain, behavior and chronic pain indicates an independent perceptual state of self; observing and exchanging feedback and response with the locations of injury. This *neuromatrix* indicates that pain requires an interaction between the nervous system and what Melzack calls the *"self."*

Elaborating, pain requires two components: 1) The sensory transmission of pain and 2) the observer or experiencer of that pain. Once that pain is experienced, there may also be a feedback response from the experiencer. This feedback may either be: 1) take action to remove the cause of the pain; or 2) if there is no apparent cause then become extra-sensitive to the pain until the cause is determined (Baranauskas and Nistri 1998). This increased sensory elevation may lead to what is called *nociceptic pain*—pain not appearing to have a direct physical cause. Some might also refer to this type of pain as being *psychosomatic,* although psychosomatic pain is often considered not real. Noiceptic pain is considered real, but its cause is not obviously physically apparent.

Regardless of the name, this type of pain is very difficult to understand and manage, especially for doctors and patients dealing with chronic pain appearing unrelated to trauma or inflammation. Because the self naturally seeks pleasure, we would propose the current cause of that pain is always real, from either a gross physical level or a more subtle level. Regardless of the level, the self experiencing the pain would certainly be considered separate from the pain, along with any biochemical messengers assisting in its biocommunication. After all, how could the self escape something that it was a part of? For this reason, medications that interrupt the messaging system for pain transmission are a multi-billion dollar business.

Since these biochemical messengers like *substance P* among neurons are present during pain responses, it is logical that these chemicals have a *role* in the physical responses to emotions or memories. However, the proposal that memory and emotions exist *within* the chemicals is not supported by logic or observation. If the chemicals contained memory or emotion, these characteristics should exist in the chemicals both inside and outside of the living mechanics of the body.

Illustrating this, scientists and doctors regularly remove the biochemicals in body fluids from one subject and transfer them (or their components) to other subjects. The biochemical-self theory is tested thousands of times a day by hospitals who transfuse blood from one subject to another. In none of these cases are emotions or feelings transferred from one person to another.

Researchers have observed an increase in biochemicals like dopamine, serotonin, and various endorphins in the bloodstream during feelings of love or compassion. The question being raised is whether the emotions stimulated the biochemicals or the biochemicals stimulated the emotions.

The implications of proposing the limited view that the emotion was created by the biochemicals are many. This would be equivalent to saying love comes from biochemicals. It would open the door to a murder suspect pleading that his body's chemical balance was responsible for his committing the fatal crime.

We must severely question the logic of this proposal altogether. Dopamine, serotonin and endorphins are circulating at heightened levels following activities such as laughing eating, sex and post-traumatic stress. These biochemicals are also circulating at other times, albeit at different levels. If they were creating the emotion, they would be present only in and prior to specific emotions. Instead, they are present during a variety of emotions. We also sometimes see emotions related to specific neurotransmitters in people who are low in those particular neurotransmitters.

In other words, these biochemicals carry the emotional self's response. This is the same logic of current traveling through an electric wire. There is a generating source of the current.

Like current in an electrical wire, neurotransmitters carry sensory feedback messages to the self as well as carry emotional responses from the self. The self is the observer of the input messages, and stimulates feedback responses utilizing the same biochemical pathways.

We must therefore conclude that there is someone inside who is either—directly or indirectly—stimulating and responding to the body's neurochemical messengers. In all cases, in order to stimulate any emotional response, there must be a conscious stimulant. Fuel may ignite a spark in the cylinder of an automobile engine causing combustion, which will push the rods into motion, exerting force on the axel cranks. Fuel is not the original stimulant, however. Nor does fuel contain directions or guidance to achieve an intended destination. Rather, it is the driver of the car who consciously turns the key and drives the car using the steering wheel, accelerator, and brakes. The driver stimulates the flow of fuel through the injection system.

We can test this at the time of death. After the moment of death there are no emotions exhibited in the dead body. Yet all the hormones, neurotransmitters, genes and cells—all the ligands and receptors—are still contained within a newly dead body. Still, the body supports no memory or emotional response because there is no longer a conscious driver present. The conscious driver who drove the feedback and response neurochemistry has left.

Emotions elicited from a response to an observation or other sensual stimuli would logically come from someone who separate from those stimuli. Because emotion is integral with interpreting stimuli, an observer would be necessary for that interpretation. Without an observer, there could be no decision-making: There would be no optional behavior. We would essentially all be robots.

This does not mean that all physiological responses require conscious interpretation and decision from the self. For example, should we touch the burner of a stove there is programming in place within the neural network to instantly react by pulling the hand away. This will often happen before the self has a chance to make a decision. However, this programming does not mean the self cannot engage in the decision to resist that reaction of pulling away. A firewalker may intentionally walk on the coals despite his sympathetic system's programmed response to jump away onto the cool sand. These observations lead us to understand that the self can be involved in almost any sensory reception should there be determination and intention.

Other stimuli might require the emotional self to respond on the other hand. Otherwise, no action would occur. This is where intention comes in. Upon hearing the alarm in the morning, the self could choose to do nothing—lying in bed for the rest of the day. The self could also intend to accomplish something that day, and rise to begin the day's activities. The self creates the intention and impetus for action.

Once sensual stimuli are pulsed to the neural network after being received by one or many of the biochemical receptors, the body forms specific information waves. We have discussed these waves. At any particular point in time, there are billions of brainwaves of various specific frequencies moving around the brain. As the different waves collide—or interfere—they create different types of interference patterns. The neurological research headed up by Dr. Robert Knight at the University of California at Berkeley and UC at San Francisco illustrated that the interaction of these interference patterns together formulate a type of informational mapping system.

This mapping system forms a type of observational screen from which the self can view incoming waveform information. Using this mapping system, the self can view the sensory information coming in from sense organs, and combine these with the feedback from the body, creating a total perception of ones environment and situation.

As the self views these waveform image patterns, we can respond with intention. Intention from the self is typically translated through the prefrontal cortex and medial cortex to create response brainwave patterns, although other cortices are also often involved. These response brainwave patterns are translated through the hypothalamus and pituitary gland to produce master hormones such as growth hormone, adrenocorticotropic hormone, follicle-stimulating hormone, oxytocin, luteinizing hormone, and others, stimulating the cascade of biophysical response. For example, waves in the delta frequency range have been observed stimulating the production of growth hormone.

To suggest that any one of these biochemicals is responsible for a particular emotion would be to ignore its physiological relationship with the rest of the body's biochemistry. Almost every biochemical process in the body is cyclic, with various operational conclusions. The notion of 'biochemical emotion' ignores the optional selection of choices by an intentional "decider." In other words, if we were simply biochemicals, we would all respond without exception to the same inputs. Any variations would be predictable. Personality would be impossible. We would be chemical machines.

The Biofeedback Observer

Consider biofeedback. As was discussed earlier, sensors are attached to various parts of the body to monitor physical responses like heart rate, breathing, brainwaves, skin response, muscle activity, and so on. These sensors are connected to a computer, which displays the various response levels onto a monitor for the subject to see. The heart rate amplitude and frequency readings will be displayed on the monitor in waves, bars, and/or numbers.

With a little practice, most people—once they see their heart rate with graphics clearly on the monitor—can consciously lower their heart rate with intention. Biofeedback has thus been used successfully to teach people to alter physical functions such as muscle tension, hunger, physical stress, and other autonomic functions. Biofeedback training gives the subject the ability to directly control a variety of physical responses including stomach cramps, muscle spasms, headaches, and other occurrences—many known to be part of a biochemical cascade.

The reason why the biofeedback subject can learn to control certain biochemical messenger driven autonomic functions is that the self ultimately exists outside the biochemistry of the body. The self is the key participant who influences physical functions. Once the person intends to make a change, the mind will facilitate the stimulation of the biochemicals by the appropriate glands to produce a physiological response.

Sometimes this can take time, discipline or practice. Even without biofeedback, a person can initiate various autonomic responses. Most of us have experienced how a physiological fear response may be initiated by simply imagining a dangerous event or situation. This happens every day in the professional world, where executives stress over events that have not happened nor may never happen. This stress increases the heart rate and stimulates stress-biochemical release. Most of us have experienced being worried about an event that may never happen. The resulting increase in our heart rate indicates our body's autonomic response to an over-anxious self.

If the self can affect the body's biochemistry with anxiousness, the self is separate from the biochemistry. Furthermore, if the self can affect the body's biochemistry intentionally, there is no question of the self's ability to direct the body through intention. The range of control the self has over the body is limited by design. Still, there is no doubt that intention initiates the sequencing of instructional messaging through the body.

This neurochemical process would be analogous to a computer operator operating a computer. A computer will tabulate, calculate, and memorize data. It will display various graphics and perform various functions, based upon the input or direction of the operator. The software and hardware are designed in such a way to coordinate computer functions very quickly and automatically within particular limitations. Regardless of the programming, the operator is required. The computer operator must decide to turn on the computer and must decide to input into the machine certain intentional commands to initiate the computer's programming functions. In the same way, the physical body, with all of its functional chemistry and various physical responses, is ultimately being steered by the personality within: this is the self, the living being—the operator of the body.

It is difficult sometimes to separate the self inside the body from the various physical and biochemical operations of the body. This is because the feedback-response system bridges the self with the physical body. For example, breast-feeding is now being rediscovered. Researchers have discovered breast-feeding not only gives the child better nourishment and a stronger immune system, but also renders a better temperament and brain development due to some of the biochemistry of breast milk. This notion is consistent with the observation of various nutrients or drugs altering moods and behavior.

Chemicals influence behavior because they not only stimulate physical tissue response, but they also give feedback to the self about what is going on in the body. For example, the feeling of thirst is a neuro-chemical signal to the self that the body needs water. The combination of hormonal, osmotic, ionic and nerve signaling all integrate to stimulate *osmoreceptors* located among brain tissue (such as the anteroventral third ventricle wall). Once stimulated, these receptors initiate waveform signaling through the hypothalamus, which converts into the more subtle waveforms of the mind. Through the reciprocation of the mind, the self observes this feedback, and responds by initiating action to find some water.

A computer will also feed back to its operator in the same way. The computer is not only designed to perform operations based upon the input of the operator, but also its programming is designed to feed back to the operator the results of those operations, signaling a need for new responses from the operator.

This process is called a feedback loop. The body's feedback system is designed to respond to environmental and physical changes around the anatomy. The system is designed to signal to the self on how the body is functioning. This is one of the purposes for serotonin release in the body: To feed back the presence of balance within particular organs and tissue systems. A diet balanced in proteins, carbohydrates, and fats, along with physiological activities stimulate the conversation of tryptophan to serotonin. This conversion is also stimulated by such activities as relaxation, laughter, and exercise. These are all positive activities for the body's metabolism. This combined state of balance and activity results in a normal flow of serotonin, which feeds back through the brain's translation systems to the self the presence of physiological balance among certain parts of the body.

Pain, on the other hand, indicates quite the opposite: Some imbalance exists somewhere. Pain feeds back to the operator the need for an adjustment among certain functions or activities. This necessary adjustment could be to the diet, fluid intake, sitting posture, lack of exercise, or perhaps an infection of some sort. Chronic pain indicates an unresolved lack of balance in the body, requiring an appropriate response to fix the issue.

Just as an instrument panel on an automobile informs the driver of the running condition of car, we can monitor the condition of our body through these and other neurochemical feedback mechanisms. Just as the car driver slows down when the speedometer shows the car is over the speed limit, the self—directly through conscious control or indirectly through the autonomic system—can make the needed adjustment when the body's feedback systems indicates a problem.

Clinical Death Research

Evidence concluding our identity as separate from the body has been presented by a number of respected medical researchers over the past four decades. With the advent of resuscitation and medical life-support technologies has come a proliferation of patients whose bodies have clinically died prior to resuscitation. Author and researcher Dr. Raymond Moody pioneered this research in the 1960s, and introduced us to the *Near Death Experience* (or NDE). Dr. Moody presented hundreds of cases documenting common experiences among patients declared clinically dead in a clinical setting. Dr. Moody's research reviewed a cross-section of thousands of cases of patients with a variety of religious and socio-economic backgrounds. Dr. Moody discovered a common experience: After separating from the body, the self often floats above it, viewing the various resuscitation efforts taking place on the body. This is often followed by the self remotely traveling to and viewing loved ones. Often traveling at the speed of thought to their homes or locations, the self often tries in vain to communicate with their loved one.

Afterward, many subjects detailed being drawn into a darkened tunnel with a bright light at the end. At the end of the tunnel, many encountered a dazzling light and/or person. Many reviewed their lives in an instant. Some spoke with this personality. In some cases the personality indicated it was "not their time yet." Following this, they instantly returned to their body. This usually coincided with the revival of the body, often while being resuscitated. While specific details of the experiences were different, nearly all NDE subjects experienced the separation from their physical body and felt at least peaceful (Moody 1975).

Naturally, this research had its skeptics. A few questioned Dr. Moody's protocols such as patient selection and interview techniques. This gap was quickly filled by Kenneth Ring, Ph.D. In a well-received peer-reviewed study published in 1985, Dr. Ring randomly selected 101 patients who had experienced an NDE. Dr. Moody's patients were collected as their cases were presented to him. This offered some but not complete randomness. By contrast, the 101 patients studied by Dr. Ring were chosen randomly to eliminate any bias, imagination, hallucination, inconsistency, and other elements possibly affecting the objectivity of their after-death experiences. Of the 101 subjects, a third reported out-of-body experiences, and a quarter reported entering the darkness or tunnel with the light at the end. About 60% reported at least a positive, peaceful experience. Those NDE subjects whose death was the result of a suicide attempt experienced no tunnel or light. The suicide NDEs in this study experienced a "murky darkness" after feeling separated from their body, but did not proceed any further. The rest had little or no recollection of the experience (Ring 1985).

Ring's findings—though not in the exact same percentages—were substantiated by professor of medicine and cardiologist Michael Sabom,

M.D. in a 1982 work called *Recollections of Death: A Medical Investigation.* There have been several other studies confirming NDE experiences as well (Blackmore 1996). Dr. Elisabeth Kubler-Ross documents researching some twenty thousand cases of near-death in her 1991 book *On Life After Death*, confirming the same primary conclusions of the research done by Sabom, Moody and Ring.

Upon review of the other various explanations, it appears unlikely any of the possible physical causes could suitably explain NDE. The only reasonable explanation is that the self is not the body. The sheer cross-section of people with this same experience provides too much variance to provide any other rational explanation. The common NDE experiences regardless of the level of religious reverence, expectation levels, drug-administration, knowledge of NDE and brain or biochemical stimulation provides few alternatives.

Additionally, when both Moody and Sabom tested the observations of NDE out-of-body observations with hospital staff, they almost without exception confirmed the observations the NDE subjects made from outside of a body clinically unconscious. While unconscious and with eyes closed, the patient could hardly be expected to observe those events—even if by subconscious hearing. This is evident from the detail of the NDE subject descriptions. Nonetheless, a few skeptical researchers have suggested some sort of paranormal experience involved in NDE experiences. However, we must ask these skeptics: How rational it is to accept the radical notion of a paranormal experience yet not accept an out-of-body observation? Either scenario requires an independent observer.

Again by far the most logical and scientific conclusion to the evidence presented is that the self is truly a separate entity, and once the body dies, the self departs—a conclusion also shared by many of the researchers.

Remote Viewing

For twenty-three years, the Stanford University Research Institute studied *parapsychological phenomena* (also termed PSI—after the Greek letter *psi,* or *psyche*) such as *remote viewing* with a grant from the United States government. Two physicists named Dr. Russell Targ and Dr. Harold Puthoff teamed up for much of this research, and they conducted controlled experiments under the watchful eye of the CIA. Much of this top-secret research was not released to the scientific community due to its sensitivity to international security. Part of the research consisted of sealing talented subjects into guarded rooms with observers. From the sealed rooms, the subjects remotely viewed and described in detail events and locations thousands of miles away. Their viewing documented minute details of the locations, down to the current weather conditions. They described specific geographical facilities, the locations of specific buildings, and activities taking place—years before internet use was common. The locations and specifics of these observations were controlled and confirmed as being otherwise unavailable to the viewer. Two particular viewers, Pat Price and Ingo Swann, were able to identify military installations around the world, including then-secret Soviet bases on the other side of the planet, including accurate weather conditions at the time of viewing. Other experiments included placing objects on a table in a remote room. From a sealed room located thousands of miles away, the remove viewers were able to describe the objects in detail, including their positioning and orientation (Puthoff and Targ 1981; Puthoff *et al.* 1981).

Other remote viewing experiments over the years have since confirmed that many of us have this ability to "see" things not within our physical sensory range. Moreover, it seems this skill can be developed. Targ and Katra (1999) describe being able to develop that skill by attempting to "separate out the psychic signal from the mental noise of memory, analysis and imagination."

These controlled studies illustrate the existence of a seer existing outside of the realm of the physical senses and neurons of the brain. If seeing was merely a biochemical and physiological experience driven by a mixture of molecules and cells, then who is it that is able to see things beyond the physical range of the eyeballs? Who is it that can visualize and describe material objects half way around the world?

The limitations of our physical senses have been well established by science. As humankind has progressed technologically, we continue to gain new information about things we previously did not perceive through our gross sense organs. This growing technical facility increasingly makes it clear that our physical senses only perceive a small portion of the vast spectra of waveforms around us. Outside of the physical spectrum lies the *conscious spectrum*. Our physical eyes and physical instruments simply are not equipped to see into this spectrum. The spectrum of the living dimension must then be transcendental to physical sense perception.

Mind versus Self

There has been a great movement over the last century proposing the mind is the all-powerful entity, and thoughts have the capacity to manipulate the physical world. This was proposed a century ago by William Walker Atkinson in the book *Thought Vibration or the Law of Attraction in the Thought World* (1906). The proposals put forth by Atkinson in this and almost one hundred other books—some under a variety of pseudonyms—are similar. Atkinson's theory has formed the framework for a multitude of self-help books in the decades following and to the present day. Atkinson's theory attracted a number of followers, including influential writers such as Mary Baker Eddy of *Christian Science* fame and Wallace Wattles, author of *The Science of Getting Rich* (1910). The *governing mind* philosophy of the late Mr. Atkinson and Mr. Wattles has also influenced various other works, such as *Think and Grow Rich* (1937) by Napoleon Hill, *The Greatest Salesman in the World* (1968) by Og Mandino, and the wildly popular book and movie *The Secret* (2006), by Rhonda Byrne.

These works have attracted the masses because of their promise of material successes such as wealth and admiration. These appeals to our more narcissistic natures appear to be grounded in the idea seemingly first proposed by Atkinson: The self is the mind, and the mind ultimately drives and controls the physical world. This has led to the unfortunate proposition that nothing real exists but the mind, and the mind is the creator of the universe.

The interesting part of this very seductive proposal is that while the mind is proposed to be the all-pervading controller of existence, the intent of these numerous self-help writings is to theoretically help people by *changing their minds.* The techniques proposed may vary slightly, but the intent is generally to help the reader gain greater wealth, fame, success, attention and influence by *changing* their thinking.

The problem with this proposal is that if the person is the mind, then *who* is it that decides to *change the mind?* In order to change the mind there must be a driver and observer who can intend and initiate that change. Furthermore, as noted in these works, the process required in order to change the mind is quite difficult. *Who* is the constant force making the determination to change the mind; despite all of its former thinking habits? Lastly, *who* remains to reap the rewards once the mind has been changed? If the self is the mind, and the mind has changed, that former self is gone once the mind changes. Therefore, no one remains to realize any reward, since the last mind—the one who initially read the book—is gone, replaced by the changed mind.

The notion of the power of thoughts has prevailed among ancient philosophies for thousands of years. In this respect, thoughts and the mind have been seen as vehicles of a living self or soul. Like the body, the mind is an instrument of an intentional self. The mind is a subtle sorting, translating and recording device. The intentional self is the driver of the mind. The mind reflects and categorizes incoming waveforms onto its mapping system, while the self is the viewer of these images. Using these images, the self can concoct particular desires and intentions for the mind to execute through the neural network.

We can observe how the mind records this information when a vision or piece of music can be recalled minutes, days and even years after first being seen or heard. We can see it immediately by looking at an image, closing our eyes immediately afterward, and seeing that image imprinted onto our mind. Our mind can also associate and compare stored waveform data with incoming sensory images of tastes, sounds, tactile sensations and other images our senses collect over the years. As the mind imprints these images, the self subtly directs the mind through intelligence to record these images, cataloging them according to priority. The mind is thus like a software program, designed to utilize the biochemical bonds within the neurons to resonate waveforms for storage and playback. This system might be compared to the recording capability of magnetic recording tape or diskettes, which store music, images, and data through magnetic arrangement.

The mind's operations transcend the body just as the operating system software of the computer transcends the actual hard disk or other hardware of the computer. Just as the operating system software provides an interfacing language between the various hardware devices of the computer, the mind interacts closely with the limbic system and neural networks of the body to execute commands, and feedback regarding the condition of the body.

The mind is a changeable, subtle mechanism, yet is distinct from the self. The separate existence of the mind can be easily shown in practical behavior: We can each observe the workings of our mind. We can watch images on the mind and see how sensory inputs become recorded and recalled. After watching a movie with special effects, we can close our eyes and watch a scene's mental imprint on the mind. We can also replay music recorded by the mind. We may hum or sing the words of a song we heard previously, with the tune replaying in our mind long after the song was heard. Like a television or a radio, we can also turn and change the mind's images. We can decide to change our focus from one image to another. In other words, we can each *change our mind.*

Reflective Genes

A newer version of the biochemical identity put forth by modern scientists over the last few decades is the notion that the self is the genetic information, or DNA of the body. Admittedly, the total mapping of the genome and further mapping of the individual allele locations within codons—their haplotypes and collectively, their hapmaps—reveals a complexity of design beyond our current understanding. Over the past three decades, tremendous research efforts have gone into creating statistical models to match the physical traits of humans and other organisms with particular gene sequences. As a result, thousands of species genomes have been tabulated and connected with physical characteristics. In addition, different diseases have been connected to certain sequences. Although these efforts are laudable, science has unfortunately succumbed to a blurring of the relationship between these genetic traits and life itself. The erroneous assumption is that specific gene sequences—the particular arrangement of alleles or nucleotides at different positions of the DNA molecule—are the *cause* of those physical or behavioral traits. That somehow, those sequences together make up the identity of the individual.

While some might call this a chicken-and-egg problem, the solution is certainly clearer than this. This assumption that the self is the genetic hapmap would be equivalent to saying a telephone is the source of the voice we hear through its speaker. It is elementary: The voice on the line is coming from a remotely located person. We may not be able to see the person while we are speaking with them, but we know a person is out there because we exchange personal communication and perform a type of voiceprint analysis as we hear their voice. In addition, the voice on the other side responds to our statements with a clarity that can only come from a conscious speaker. Even computerized voice greetings are clearer if they are recorded by real people.

The sequencing of genetic haplotypes indicates its complex structure. This complex coding indicates programmed design. As with any programming, there must be an underlying motive for the program. It is not logical to assume that a complex, well-designed code with specific rules comes from a chaotic and accidental design process. Just as we can connect the lucid voice on the phone to a personal consciousness, we can tie the sequencing of genes to a living, intentional component, ultimately driving its design with intention.

If we were to extract a DNA molecule from our skin or body fluids, and place it onto the table or even in a test tube, we will find there is no display of life. Just as the body after death is lifeless, DNA or RNA molecules extracted from a living body become lifeless. We should also clarify that RNA transcription and genetic mutation is impossible without a living being driving the process. We can certainly force a mutation upon an organism or its seed through the vehicle of a virus. Yet the mutation will only become duplicated through an organism if there is a living force present in that organism. In other words, we cannot insert a mutated gene into a dead body and see that mutation replicated through the dead body.

The proposal that personality is determined by genetic code is refuted by children who have inherited genes from parents. Children are each born with distinct personalities, talents and character traits not necessarily portrayed in their parents or grandparents. While we are quick to notice similar physical traits among our children, each has their own character and personality. We can easily observe children behaving significantly different from their parents in similar situations. We can also witness the many conflicts that arise between children and parents. We have also observed that the extraordinary talents of child music geniuses or savants are not passed down genetically. In most musical savant cases, the parents have relatively little or no musical gift whatsoever.

If personality and behavior were genetically driven then genetically identical twins would live parallel lives and have identical personalities. They would make the same decisions, leading to identical histories.

This is not supported by the research. Twins live dramatically unique and individual lives from each other. Depending upon how much time they spend together, they will make distinctly different choices in life as well. In general, they display significantly unique and often diverse behavior. Hur and Rushton (2007) studied 514 pairs of two to nine year old South Korean monozygotic and dizygotic twins. Their results indicated that 55% of the children's pro-social behavior related to genetic factors and 45% was attributed to non-shared environmental behavior. It should also be noted that shared environmental factors could not be eliminated from the 55%, so this number could well be higher if shared environments were removed. In another recent study from Quebec, Canada (Forget-Dubois *et al.* 2007), an analysis of 292 mothers demonstrated that maternal behavior only accounted for a 29% genetic influence at 18 months and 25% at 30 months. In a study of 200 African-American twins, including 97 identical pairs, genetics accounted for about 60% of the variance in smoking (Whitfield *et al.* 2007). In a study done at the Virginia Commonwealth University's Institute for Psychiatric and Behavioral Genetics (Maes *et al.* 2007), a large sampling revealed that individual behavior was only about 38-40% attributable to genetics, while shared environment was 18-23% attributable and unshared environmental influences were attributable in 39-42%. These studies are also confirmed by others, illustrating a large enough variance from 100% to indicate the presence of an individual nature within each twin.

Distinct identity despite genetic sameness is further evidenced by the fact that identical twins will have distinctly different fingerprints, irises and other physical traits, despite their identical genetics. Many twins also differ in handedness and specific talents. Researchers have found that twins will make significantly different lifestyle choices later in life such as sexual preference, drug abuse, and alcoholism.

Say two people purchase the exact same make, model and year automobile at the same time. Comparing the two cars in the future will reveal the cars had vastly different engine lives and mileages. They each had different types of breakdowns, and different problems. This is because each car was driven differently. One was likely driven harder than the other was. One was likely better taken care of than the other was. They may have been the same make and model, but each had different owners with different driving habits.

Because twins have the same genetics—just as the cars shared the same make and model—the unique factors related to the eventual circumstances of their lives stem from the fact that each body contains a distinct driver. This distinct driver is the realm that scientists are now grasping at with epigenetics research. Discovering that even the same genes or the same genetic abnormalities will not render the same pathologies, epigenome researchers want to peg the environment and biochemistry as the sole instigators of differentiated gene expression. This too falls short, as even twins who shared the same diet and environment will still have vastly different disease pathologies. This means there is a missing element the researchers are not considering: A distinct inner self.

Evolution of the Living

The evolutionary theory has dominated biological sciences for over one hundred years. This theory has also been the subject of intense debate over that period, primarily because of its conflicts with certain religious teachings. The original evolutionary theory of Darwin has been revised to accommodate recent research on genetics, and combined with a chemical basis for life—which some refer to as the *primordial soup theory*.

We do not debate the concept of evolution. Still, we must clarify this theory assumes the human organism is likened to a machine undergoing extrinsic accommodation based solely upon environmental factors and an inherent quest for survival. The underlying premise remains an assumption upon an accidental existence and an incidental environmental accommodation. According to the basic theory, every creature supposedly evolved from the accidental and spontaneous birth of a single living unicellular organism. This original organism theoretically became more complex incidentally through the processes of *genetic mutation, survival of the fittest* and *natural selection*.

Though widely accepted, many still debate the theory. Fossil evidence and diversity among species certainly present a compelling case for the progressive improvement of certain species. Breeding observations also show that mutations develop through generations. Still there are some weaknesses in the theory. There is little evidence of any genetic connection between humans and dinosaurs, for example. Yet the assumptions of the theory would necessitate that these life forms were either ancestors of humans, or at the very least, cousins. The other critical problem seems to be the sheer improbability of all the mutations necessary for the evolution from a single cell to a human within a few hundred million years occurring *accidentally*.

The basic dilemma of the theory, however, is that there is no consideration of the unique consciousness residing within each body. Where did this consciousness come from? Evolution is based upon an erroneous assumption that there is no distinct living driver within each physical body. This is inconsistent with the evidence. Even the smallest of organisms such as single celled paramecia have illustrated conscious behavior, with problem-solving abilities and an individual desire to survive.

In order to appropriately understand our past and the past of other living organisms, we must be able to view it within the context of the living portion of the organism. If we accept that each living organism contains a unique spark of consciousness, the discussion of evolution without a consideration of this individual consciousness would be akin to proposing that the earth is populated by walking chemical robots.

We could also study the development and evolution of racing cars over the last 100 years. We could describe how they mechanically evolved from slower cars into faster cars. However, without a consideration of the car drivers who raced them, the builders who designed and built them and the executives who financed and promoted the industry, we would be ignoring the functional elements within the racing industry. The evolution of the shape and performance of the cars would simply be the byproduct of these developments. After all, the cars did not build themselves.

Because each living organism contains a unique personality, complete with independent feelings, emotions, desires and the need to love and be loved; it is essential this living element not be ignored. Similarly, as we review human history we typically attempt to understand the emotional elements involved. We want to know the emotional reasons behind the decision of a particular king to go to war. We want to know what personal issues were behind a rivalry between an Egyptian monarch and another ruler. Perhaps an offense of to his wife was behind this event, for example. Historians understand how the personal and emotional elements of humanity direct history. Should historians follow the incidental evolutionist model, they might resign these historical events as being solely 'survival of the fittest' events and ignore the personal histories.

The accidental evolution theory has been grounded within the *primordial soup* theory. As most of us know, this theory states that following a theoretical big bang, life spontaneously arose from a random pool of chemicals. This theory requires a process called *spontaneous generation.* Unlikely as it seems, the spontaneous generation of life theory was debated by scientists for hundreds of years, as they observed molds and bacteria seemingly growing from barren flasks. Finally, Dr. Louis Pasteur refuted spontaneous generation by illustrating that growth within an isolated liquid chamber was due to the presence of tiny bacteria in the original chamber environment. For many years following, other researchers attempted to create life from 'primordial' chemicals without success.

A truly fantastic assumption about the evolution theory relates to this spontaneous creation of life and intention. It is assumed that chemicals combined and somehow developed the *desire* to survive. These chemical combinations somehow developed the intention to improve their chances of survival. Have we ever observed chemicals desiring survival? Chemicals simply do not display this characteristic. No scientist has ever found the intent to survive outside of a living organism. No chemical desires survival unless part of a living organism—hence the name *biochemicals.* Chemicals may react and form various substances, and certainly will change structure when heated or cooled. Having a desire to survive is another matter altogether.

The desire to survive is connected to the desire to improve survival factors and eliminate threats to survival. The need to improve survival requires that *someone* values survival. This would require chemicals valuing their existence somehow, which in turn requires the chemicals to somehow recognize a difference between living chemicals and dead chemicals. This in turn requires that chemicals have awareness, because the desire to survive requires an awareness of self-existence. It also requires a fear of death—an illogical consciousness for a chemical.

In other words, in order to desire to survive, a living organism must be aware, consciously or subconsciously, that it is alive. A living organism must be able to differentiate itself from others and other chemicals. If there is no distinction between life and lifeless chemicals, why avoid death? Why desire life without a distinction between living and nonliving chemicals? Certainly it would be easier for a batch of chemicals to remain dead chemicals than to struggle for survival in the midst of all the environmental challenges to remain living.

A small unicellular organism could be killed by so many environmental challenges: Freezing, direct sun exposure and any number of natural enemies. If there were no distinction between living or dead chemicals, then the path of least resistance would be to remain dead chemicals. If there were no awareness and desire for survival in the face of all this resistance, no living creature would bother to avoid death. This in turn would mean no incentive for survival—the opposite premise for evolution.

Put more simply, if a living entity could not distinguish itself from a nonliving entity there would be no urge to survive. Without the urge to survive, there would be no motivating factor to encourage adaptation or mutation. There would be no impetus to evolve because survival is not valuable without an awareness of life.

In his 1977 book *The Selfish Gene,* Dr. Richard Dawkins proposed that genes themselves somehow became not only selfish in their orientation, but also somehow acted upon their selfishness. Certainly, we can all agree that in order to become "selfish," there must be a "self." Without a self, how could something be selfish? How could there be an orientation towards oneself (i.e., self*ish)* without there being a self?

We must also ask, logically, just *who* would be available to recognize life in a chemically based existence? We are being asked to assume a batch of chemicals developed a state of consciousness, yet there is no individual present to be conscious of being alive.

The accidental and incidental evolution theory as it stands today simply has no logical basis. An organism cannot desire survival, mutate, or make changes without a conscious self present within the organism. This living being must be aware that it is alive, and must therefore value survival. Once the self values survival, it has a logical basis for making genetic and physiological adjustments to better adapt and survive. Because the self is fundamentally alive, when it is inserted into a temporary physical body, it naturally strives to survive within that organism.

Note we are not contending with the proposal that living organisms have not undergone a historical evolutionary process. The basic premise the original and modern-day evolutionary theory rests upon is the similarities between species. We suggest this process is driven by the development of a transmigrating self rather than a random process of incidental evolution.

To analyze the likelihood of even one typical protein molecule to have been randomly developed, we can reference Dr. Francis Crick's statements in his 1981 book *Life Itself: Its Origin and Nature.* Here Dr. Crick calculates that the chance of even one conservative protein molecule of two hundred amino acids coming into existence is one chance in 10^{260}—the number one with two hundred and sixty zeros behind it. He furthermore states that this would be analogous to a billion monkeys typing onto a billion typewriters and somehow typing one sonnet of Shakespeare.

The chance of a 1,000-nucleotide chain DNA molecule forming accidentally is more remote. Both Dr. Dawson and Dr. Crick agree with this. Lester Smith (1975) calculated the probability as about one in 10^{600}.

The probability of genetic mutations accidentally leading to a new species is even more remote. Dr. Lee Spetner (1998) calculates that a new species (one positive mutation step) would have a negative probability of 2.7×10^{-2739}, using Stebbins' (1966) estimation that five hundred intermediate mutations would be required to establish one positive mutation step.

In the 1950s, a fox breeding experiment directed by Dr. Dmitry Belyaev of the then-Soviet Union's Institute of Cytology and Genetics in Novosibirsk studied mutation in breeding. The intent of this forty-year long study was to determine the genetic role humans played in the domestication of animals, particularly dogs, which theoretically evolved from foxes and wolves over the improbable period of ten thousand years. Most importantly, Dr. Belyaev wanted to study how contact with humans might bring about new behavior and changes in body features and physiology. The prime subjects of the study were silver foxes, who were caged while they and their offspring were put through various degrees of contact with humans.

The results were revealing. After over thirty generations of foxes were handled and petted by humans, profound changes became apparent when compared to undomesticated controls. One of the most apparent physical changes was the development of droopy ears among the domesticated foxes. Rather than the perky upright ears seen among wild wolves and foxes, these domesticated foxes developed floppy ears. One cannot help but be reminded of the sight of domesticated killer whales, who also mysteriously tend to develop floppy dorsal fins during their capture and domestication in public aquariums.

Other observed effects of domestication include the fact that domestic foxes developed rolled up tails rather than tails pointing straight up. This appears analogous to the floppy ear characteristic. Dr. Belyaev speculated that the pointed ears and tails were possibly used by the foxes both as defense (to stand tall against challengers) and to sense the external environment more acutely. During captivity within protective dens provided by humans, these facilities were no longer necessary for survival.

Other significant differences were seen among neurotransmitter and hormone biochemistry. The domesticated foxes had significantly higher levels of serotonin in the bloodstream, and their corticosteroids would cycle differently than their wild relatives.

Behavioral changes were also consistently observed as the foxes became domesticated. Over generations, they became increasingly relaxed and comfortable around humans, responding positively to petting and other touching. Their ability to respond and communicate with humans also increased over the generations.

When we consider the central difference between the domesticated environment and the undomesticated environment of Dr. Belyaev's fox studies, the central difference outside the possibility of attack was being in the company of an organism (humans) of higher consciousness. If we consider that at least part of the physical and behavior alterations were specifically related with the rate of being in the proximity and care (and protection) of humans, then we must logically connect their genetic and behavioral changes also with their proximity to organisms of a higher consciousness. Rather than being left to their own devices to defend themselves in the wild, the foxes were protected and fed daily. This encouraged the foxes to see the humans as advocates. As the foxes gradually got closer to humans, and began relating with their human handlers through touch and behavior, they began to trust the humans. As a result, their behavior and physical features changed because they learned to rely upon the humans. This was accompanied by biochemical changes and genetic changes. This is also consistent with an animal of one species being raised by another species. There are behavioral and physical changes resulting from a relationship between conscious individuals.

Consider for a moment how our bodies can also change and adapt with our changing desires, activities, and relationships. A long-distance runner who trains and races for several years will most likely become slender with well-built calves and thighs. These developments, along with better-conditioned lungs, give the runner an edge over the untrained runner. These changes will be accompanied by subtle genetic changes that govern metabolic responsiveness. On the other hand, a person who tends to overeat will probably develop a larger stomach, enabling more eating. Assuming a lack of exercise, this will probably accompany the creation of more fat cells and corresponding genetic changes, possibly including surtuin-related sequence alteration.

The physical body changes are a result of our intentions, decisions and activities. The shape of the body will reflect our choices in life: This is a net change due to consciousness. Should we decide to become a boxer, after partaking in that activity for a while we will probably end up with a broken or twisted nose and a puffy, scarred facial countenance. Likewise, a hardened violent criminal will probably have a number of scars and injuries because of his or her choices in life. His body may also end up dead because of his consciousness. On the other hand, an accountant will probably have more delicate physical features, and probably smaller, weaker muscles as a result of his intentional choices and subsequent activities. Though we can easily connect stronger muscles with more exercising, the determination to exercise arose from an intentional self.

We can easily see how our physical features reflect our consciousness in so many different ways. Considering our consciousness to be a combination of our current desires and past behavior, we can see how our accumulated situation reflects either decisions we may have made in this lifetime or a past lifetime. As our consciousness changes, so does our body. We can scientifically and logically conclude that our various bodies (and species) reflect our evolution of consciousness.

Hypnotherapy research over the past twenty years has accumulated a large amount of data indicating that most of us have occupied previous physical bodies. The procedure, called *past-life regression*, was in part developed by Dr. Ian Stevenson, a medical doctor and professor of research at the University of Virginia, Department of Psychiatric Medicine. Over several decades of research, Dr. Stevenson and his associates clinically put subjects under hypnosis, easily drawing them into a recall of a previous lifetime. This research was soon corroborated by the results of many other researchers. Actually, this result was only accidentally discovered. Being a conservative psychiatrist and professor, Dr. Stevenson had no prior belief in the transmigration of the self.

The research documented hundreds of subjects who detailed previous lifetimes as historical persons, describing events with a clarity and experience only possible from having lived personally in that situation. The research did not stop there. The scientists then researched the historical accuracy of the statements heard during hypnosis, to confirm whether (1) the subject could have known these facts otherwise, and (2) whether the facts can be confirmed as being historically accurate. In both instances, the evidence clearly supported transmigration.

Though undoubtedly controversial, the research has been thoroughly peer-reviewed and clinically supported. Some thirty scientific books and hundreds of scientific papers have been written to document studies by hypnotherapists, many of whom are M.D.s and/or licensed psychiatrists. Dr. Stevenson's research itself spanned over thirty-seven years, and documented hundreds of cases of previous life recognition by children who remembered their past lives. His corroborated research indicated that past life recollection fades by about age seven. Before that age, children will often speak spontaneously about their previous lives as historical individuals, recalling historical details decades old and otherwise unknowable. Dr. Stevenson and his various associates meticulously documented these recollections along with the research confirmed their historical accuracy. Dr. Stevenson himself has written several books on the subject, presenting the evidence in a clinically rigorous and scientific manner (Tucker 2005; Stevenson 1997). As mentioned, a number of other scientists have documented regressing patients into verifiable past lives, including Dr. Helen Wambach (1978), Dr. Morris Netheron (1978), Dr. Edit Fiore (1978), Dr. Bruce Goldberg (1982), Dr. Joel Whitton (1986), Dr. Brian Weiss (1988), Dr. Christopher Bache, Dr. Winafred Lucas (1993), Dr. Marge Rieder (1995; 1999) and a number of others.

Some of the studies targeted particular periods or events among subjects. Dr. Rieder, for example, documented regression sessions with certain patients that revealed historical information regarding Millboro, VA—a pivotal village during the Civil War. Dr. Rieder's patients accurately described many detailed elements of the war and the town, including the uncovering of previously unknown hideaways and tunnels used during the war in Millboro.

To this, we can add the research of Dr. Michael Newton, a psychologist and master hypnotist who regressed patients into the period between their last body and the current body. Dr. Newton's patients consistently tell of inter-life judgment scenarios, karma and other topics in his 1994 *Journey of Souls: Studies of Life between Lives,* and his 2000 work, *Destiny of Souls: New Case Studies of Life between Lives.* Dr. Newton was a clinical specialist in pain management who stumbled into the reality of past-lives while treating patients. His texts document some fifteen years of clinical research.

The Real Self

Empirical evidence reveals the existence of a transcendental inner self operating the body. This is the true "I" of our existence. The self is the source of personality and life, which the body expresses through physical activity over its lifetime. Since there is energy, personality and movement in a living body prior to death, followed by a lack of movement, personality and energy afterward, the source of the energy and personality must leave the body at death. Contrary to the proposals of many, since each personality is unique and different from all other personalities, each self must be an independent, individual being.

Many philosophers have proposed that after death, the living being either fades into "nothingness," or expands into "everything." This philosophy proposes that the living being does not have an individual identity after death: Instead, the now individual self simply vanishes and evaporates into space. This is often described as merging into "nothingness"—also called the void—or merging into "everything"—sometimes referred to as the white light. Still others contend that after death we merge into a vast ocean of consciousness. These two assumptions are the same proposition, because in either case the individual self loses individuality.

Rather, each individual self is a unique and distinct personality. This individuality is expressed by the special talents unique to each of us. These special talents also point to an individual existence prior to birth, as confirmed also by Dr. Stevenson's and others' work. If the self existed as an individual prior to birth and throughout a lifetime of an ever changing body, is it logical that the self would lose that individuality after death?

The inner self is the underlying source of our personality; our feelings, emotions, desires, the ability to love, and the desire to be loved. This personality is distinct from the mental programming taking place through the brainwaves and neural network of the physical body. Beyond the physical programming, each of us retains an independent, active inner self with a central objective of happiness, and receiving and giving love. Does it appear logical that this active being—continually seeking happiness and loving relationships—would suddenly abandon these propensities and permanently merge into a state of nothingness or mass consciousness?

What should the purpose of a temporary separate existence be then? Could a collective vague consciousness or nothingness separate into a multitude of individual purpose and will? Furthermore, the living self has maintained a consistent existence throughout many decades of a changing physical body. This equates to surviving a body that is continually dying. Does it seem logical that the fatal death of the same body would then remove our inherent will to survive and prosper? Should the death of this temporary body abruptly end our desire to love and exchange love?

Purpose and activity are the key distinctions between living and dead matter. Both of these elements (purpose and activity) indicate the existence of individuality. The very definition of *consciousness* requires individuality. Consciousness requires *awareness.* Awareness of something or someone requires an individual consciousness separate from that object or person being *aware* of. Thus, an 'ocean of consciousness' would logically be an oxymoron.

Consistent with the ancient teachings of all major religions, the ancient philosophers and the vast majority of western scientists prior to the emergence of the concept of an incidental accidental evolution of species, we propose the existence of a unique individual being transcendental to the gross physical plane who evolves through lifetimes of learning experiences in different physical bodies. As the inner self evolves, each progressive physical body reflects that current evolution.

Plato, Socrates and most of the ancient Greek philosophers referred to this inner self as the *soul.* The translation is thought to originate with Aristotle, who described the self with the Latin *telos.* Rather than a vague spirit-like organ, *telos* most accurately translates to a personality with purpose, will, and character. In this context, we would emphasize that each of us does not possess a soul: each of us *is* a soul, accessing the physical plane through a temporary physical body.

Chapter Three

Conscious Pathways

Five thousand years ago, the oldest healing science was recorded. Archeologists confirm this with findings from the ancient Indus Valley of India—many dating well over 5,000 years ago. Its texts documented a science that had been previously been handed down from master to student for thousands of years prior. Today we know this knowledge as the science of Ayurvedic medicine. Its language was Sanskrit—understood to be the world's oldest complete written and spoken language.

The Ayurvedic healthcare system has been clinically applied throughout these five thousand years among billions of people throughout the world. The primary writings regarding the practice of *Ayurveda* were presented within the texts of the *RgVeda* and the *AthrvaVeda.* Additional texts followed over the centuries, authored by various Ayurvedic physicians, focusing on various specialties within *Ayurveda.* Among other topics, these various texts explored the human and universal anatomy together, providing a process for achieving harmonic balance between the two.

Ancient texts from other cultures indicate the Ayurvedic science attracted early physicians and philosophers from ancient Egypt, Arabia, Greece and Rome. As these other medical sciences evolved, we find many *Ayurveda* principles ingrained in their treatments and knowledge.

Today *Ayurveda* is the world's oldest existing clinical medical science. Thousands of years before the Europeans began leeching, bloodletting and other grotesque surgical techniques in the Dark ages, Ayurvedic doctors of the Indus Valley civilization performed diseased organ removal and even brain surgery as early as 2500 B.C.E. Long before the European pharmacopeias came into being, Ayurvedic medicine had already developed centuries of clinical herbal and biochemical experience. Early *materia medica* of herbal extract treatments and various techniques such as *pancha karma* and *tridosha therapies* set early standards for health care and detoxification.

Ayurveda may well outlive the current western medical "pharma-sorcery" as well. Ayurvedic medicine has proved, through empirical and raw population evidence, that its application has little if any negative side effects. *Ayurveda* is not only practiced by billions of Indians, Indonesians and Asians today. It is also practiced by millions of Europeans, Americans, Australians, New Zealanders, South Americans and Africans. The reason *Ayurveda* has outlived most other medicines of the world is its foundation upon the bigger picture of our universe combined with a rational grounding in human physiology. This is compounded by

Ayurvedic medicine's utter respect for the power of nature, leading to an understanding of her curative powers. Today Ayurvedic healing methods and botanical treatments have been the subject of controlled research on several fronts—with overwhelmingly positive results. While often not delivering the treatment speed expected from pharmaceuticals, *Ayurveda*—if practiced appropriately—has a history of gently delivering therapeutic results without dangerous side effects.

Closely related to and following the Vedic medical system arose another great medical science from Asia: *Traditional Chinese medicine* (TCM). Silk scrolls dating from the fifth century B.C. document the application of TCM herbal medicines and the manipulation of various energy channels through which currents called *Qi* moved. Early texts included the Emperor Huang's internal medicine classic *Huang Di Nei Jing* and *Yin Yang Shi Yi Mai Jiu Jing* from over 2100 years ago. Two earlier texts excavated in 1973 focused on stimulation with hot herbal swaths, or moxibustion: *Moxibustion Classic with Eleven Food-Hand Channels* and *Moxibustion Classic with Eleven Yin-Yang Channels.* These early texts described the location, use and treatment of various disorders and diseases by manipulation of particular energy channels, now referred to as *meridians.* The treatment of numerous diseases through the stimulation of these channels has been extensively recorded over the centuries. Today TCM has become widely used throughout the world in numerous clinical settings, including many hospitals and emergency rooms. Traditional Chinese medicine and acupuncture has a long history of effectiveness and safety. TCM has been the subject of many controlled clinical studies. TCM also has been used as a treatment for billions of people with a myriad of disorders. Little or no side effects have been the norm for traditional TCM medical treatments.

The wisdom of these traditional medicines played an important role in the Greek, Roman and Egyptian views of the body and health. Hippocrates' concept of disease closely mirrored the Ayurvedic and TCM views. Hippocrates believed that health required a balance of "humors," of which he professed there being four. When these humors were out of balance, he thought, disease resulted. As Hippocrates' influence on medicine is well known, this concept pervaded much of the perspective of health and medicine for centuries in the region. Though the humor count might have been slightly different, the concept of disease resulting from an imbalance between the humors of the body had been promulgated over thousands of years in *Ayurveda* and TCM.

It is with this strong foundation of science and tradition between these ancient medical systems that we present a unified basis for describing the flow of conscious information throughout the human anatomy. We describe this waveform information channeling system as laid out in both the ancient Ayurvedic and TCM versions using a practical application within the realm of western anatomy and biology. Because much of the conscious anatomy is beyond the reach of the physical eyes or instruments of the eyes, we will attempt to bridge with some of the science presented in the first chapter.

Information Channels

From the *RgVeda* texts, we find elaborate descriptions of a system of waveform conducting nodes and channels, referred to as *chakras* and *nadis.* From the TCM texts, we find elaborate descriptions of what appears to be a sub-section of the *nadi* system flowing through the organs and nerve plexus—commonly termed the *meridian* system. *Meridians* and *nadis* may also be technically referred to as pathways, channels or conduits, and *chakras* as conversion centers—to better elucidate their operational functions.

The existence of *chakras, nadis* and *meridians* has been disputed by modern allopathic medicine. This is because this network of conduits and conversion centers cannot be observed through anatomical dissection. For this reason, a certain level of disbelief of this technology exists within modern western medicine circles. In defense of this western view, the presentation of these channels and centers has yet to satisfy peer-review. We find several post-era texts written on these subjects, many of which appear too deeply entrenched in the ancient descriptions to deliver the information into the context of modern science. We hope to offer some new perspectives to this debate.

As we discussed in detail in the first chapter, researchers have discovered a variety of pathways through which the body relays information waveforms between cells, tissue systems, the outside world, and the inner self. Western science has documented and confirmed the existence of these informational pathways through highly technical *in-vitro* research, *in-vivo* research and clinical human research. Ion channels, brain waves, peristalsis, sensory nerve conductance, microtubules, hormones, neuro-transmitters and DNA-RNA are a few of the physiological technologies the body uses, as unveiled by scientists over the past few decades. All of these fall within the spectrum of informational conductance and messaging as also perceived by the ancient physicians. Just as modern researchers utilize language such as *cascades* and *pathways,* the ancient physicians utilized a language of *meridians, nadis* and *chakras.* The basic difference between the two descriptions of the anatomy is that modern research has uncovered the biochemical and electromagnetic detail regarding these channels, while the ancient physicians utilized an intuitive approach to reveal a broader scope of the network: what types of consciousness are being transmitted within each channeling system, and the general location of the conduits. However, the lens and magnification of modern research is sharper and more myopic. Therefore, the ability of modern science to step back and see the bigger picture from each of these discoveries is hampered. The ancient sciences already had this wider lens open—allowing a bigger picture that, if understood correctly, may provide a useful tool for understanding the larger purpose and potential application of some of the research findings over the past few decades.

Controlled and double blind research using acupuncture and various electrotherapy techniques have confirmed the efficacy of stimulating key points along a network of *meridian* channels. Over the past three decades, acupuncture has been successfully applied in clinical environments throughout western medicine. Thousands of randomized, double-blind studies have illustrated acupuncture's ability to reduce pain, increase healing times, and provide acute therapy for many disorders. These studies have been performed around the world, successfully proving predictable and repeatable responses in patients being treated with channel therapy. Controlled research showing acupuncture's effectiveness typically entails forming two groups of subjects with the same condition. One group is treated with acupuncture while the other is treated with needle insertion at non-channel points (called *sham treatment*) or simply not treated. The comparison of the groups, considering the placebo effect, requires a large threshold of success. Using these strict controls, acupuncture research from around the world has confirmed TCM's legitimacy as a healing medical science.

In addition, there has been a growing body of positive research results and clinical use with electronic trigger impulse therapy. Electrostimulation technologies such as the *transcutaneous electrical nerve stimulator* (or TENS) units have shown positive results in patients with various nervous system and/or muscular disorders. *Spinal cord stimulators* (or STIM units) have also shown effectiveness for damaged spinal columns and nerve systems in many studies and clinical applications. A STIM is implanted into body with wires inserted into the epidural spaces of the spinal column. Some STIM units are coupled with radiofrequency receivers. Use of the *cranial-electro stimulator* (also called cranial electrotherapy stimulation or CES) is also increasing. Among other effects, CES has been shown to stimulate the flow of serotonin. All of these therapies stimulate the body's conduits existing within nerves and tissues, modulating key messaging pathways within the body. Each of these methods infuses particular waveforms into specific locations of the anatomy—locations found to have the most effective response. Interestingly, most of these positions are also points described in both Ayurvedic and TCM texts. Many acupuncturists today utilize electrostimulators in their work to stimulate or reduce waveform flow through the *meridian* channels. When the correct waveform is utilized, the channel circuits are properly stimulated. This in turn provokes a healing response, and in many cases the modulation of pain gateways.

For example, microwave (30-300 gigahertz) stimulation therapy was applied along acupuncture *meridians* at 1500 treatment centers in Russia and the Ukraine in the 1980s. More than 500,000 patients with over 60 pathologies participated in the study. The results were overwhelmingly positive (Jovanovic-Ignajatic *et al.* 1999).

Research by Kandel *et al.* (1991) showed an increased electrical conductivity at the skin along *meridian* and *nadi* points when compared with surrounding tissue. This skin conductivity confirms an increased waveform potential within *meridian* and *nadi* pathways. Increased ion resorption along these points has also been observed. In addition, newer research into the nerve intercellular channels called *gap junctions* has illustrated significant ion concentration levels inside acupuncture points and *meridians*. The research shows these gap junctions are each made up of two cylinders, called *connexons*. These connexons meet in the gap junctions between pre-synaptic and post-synaptic nerve cells.

Connexons conduct waveforms in volts through the modulation of pH and calcium ions. These connexons seem to provide a gateway shuttering system as well, allowing electromagnetic waveforms to pass or be blocked. This waveform channel gateway has a range of 3.5 to 20 nanometers of separation. Within this gated channel system flow ions, hormones and metabolites between cells. The connexons act as communication pathways between nerves. Testing with electrostimulation equipment has confirmed these particular gated channels resonate with both 50-80 gigahertz and 2-4 hertz ranges. This means these channels conduct at frequencies in the ultra-low (seismic) range along with the significantly higher microwave range (Jovanovic-Ignjatic 1999). This was confirmed by Schlebusch *et al.* (2005) as well: After light stimulation of the body in the 3-5 micron range, *"light channels"* appeared on the body precisely in the locations of the *meridians*.

Further research by Yang *et al.* (2007) found among thirty healthy volunteers clear evidence of *meridian* channels consistent with TCM *meridian* charts, using infrared thermal imaging. Previously Hu *et al.* (1993) conducted forty-nine passes over another thirty healthy volunteers, revealing 594 channels of *"radiant track"* using infrared beams. Thirty percent of these tracks were consistent with the fourteen traditional *meridians* of TCM, confirming not only the existence of the TCM *meridians* but of others. The others, we would conclude, would be part of the larger network of *nadis*.

Biochemical messengers like hormones and neurotransmitters are intimately connected to the flow of instructional waveforms through these subtle channels. Electrostimulation of acupuncture points with two-hertz electrodes was found to stimulate endorphin release, while serotonin and norepinephrine release were stimulated at 100 hertz (Ulett, 1998). Others have stimulated endorphins at four hertz, and serotonin and norepinephrine at 200 hertz.

Further research providing the scientific basis for the existence of these *meridian* channels was led by Dr. Hiroshi Motoyama—author of over fifty books and numerous scientific papers. In the 1970s, Dr. Motoyama began experimenting with electrocardiograms to detect the electrical potential and/or energetic change along *meridian* channels. In order to gain enough sensitivity, (the EEG was not sensitive enough for this type of energy exchange) Dr. Motoyama invented a machine called the *AMI machine*—or *Apparatus for measuring the functioning of the Meridians and the corresponding Internal organs.*

Dr. Motoyama applied his machine on thousands of subjects. In a study published in *Science and Medicine* (1999), Motoyama applied a painless rectangular waveform pulse to the skin of subjects. Following the pulse, sympathetic nerve responses rendered a significant change in potential within milliseconds at the traditional *meridian* points. There was no potential change at the non-meridian locations. Furthermore, he found that while *yang meridians* recorded positive potential changes, *yin meridians* recorded negative potential changes to the waveform pulse from the AMI.

A few years later, Dr. Motoyama designed a second machine, which he named the *chakra machine.* This more sensitive machine took readings of the changes in static field potentials between the environment and the skin. The level of the energy disturbances rendered an "energy shadow" over the *chakra* region. Dr. Motoyama's research included both control subjects and subjects advanced in controlling physiological states. The higher electromagnetic disruptions occurred around the *chakra* regions in all cases, but varied in intensity from person to person. The results also indicated a greater energy displacement at the *chakra* centers among subjects who were proficient in *kundalini* (the ability to raise the life air through the *chakras*) (Jackson, 2007).

University of California at Los Angeles researcher Dr. Varie Hunt evaluated the existence of *chakra* regions with *electromyography* (or EMG) electrodes in 1978. Her research found sinusoidal waveforms extending from the *chakra* regions ranging from 100 to 1600 cycles per second (Hunt 2000).

Schwann cells and other *glial* nerve cell systems have been shown to conduct electrical impulses through current potential shifting. Through a variance of voltage, waveform information is conducted through exchanges between ions within and around the neurotransmitter fluid. As nerve impulses move through these nerve cell connection systems, the characteristic waveforms of each voltage shift forms a unique waveform pulse of information. When these voltage-shifted waveforms are received through receptors, their circuit is completed through a biocommunication synchronizing mechanism. This biocommunication system serves to connect the conscious source of the instruction (the self) with the physical activity intended.

Physical movement is seismic in nature with cycles of 1-4 per second. Brainwaves range from 10 to 100 cycles per second, with a predominance of 30-hertz speeds. Muscular activity stimulation from the central nervous system will range up to 225 cycles per second. Here we see a boosting of frequency as information moves from brainwave to nervous system conductance. Following this boost, the muscles translate and reduce the waveform frequencies to the seismic level. This can be compared to a computer system. Information is translated from keyboard input to machine language through a software conversion. Once in machine language, the computer can execute the hardware operations, screen imaging and execution.

We might remember from our discussion on waveform mechanics that frequency or cycles per second is not the only characteristic of a waveform. Other characteristics include amplitude, wavelength, and multi-dimensional waveform aspects including as wave shape, slope, angular momentum, and spin. As we break down the electromagnetic spectrum as it translates through the medium of the conscious anatomy, some waveforms may be better described as spirals or helices. This is reflected in many biomolecular structures. As we investigate the anatomical holography of the physical body, we can also correlate different types of organ activity with these distinctive waveforms. Each primary *chakra* region resonates with a particular waveform, and thus each resonates with particular organs and thus specific physiological functions. The primary *chakra* regions are also each positioned anatomically close to particular organ systems. For example, we find *chakra* regions located near the gonads/ovaries, the adrenals, the spleen, the digestive system, the liver, the heart, the thyroid and larynx, the pineal gland/hypothalamus and the limbic system, respectively. Because each of these organs has characteristic physiological functions, we can undoubtedly make the case—regardless of whether the notion of these primary *chakra* regions is accepted—that each organ system functions within a distinct range of functional connectivity with the rest of the body.

Biophysical Layers

According to the ancient texts of *Ayurveda*, both the universe and the body are comprised of eight basic layers. The origins of these layers come from three basic consciousnesses: goodness, passion and ignorance. From these spring the three basic physical elements or *doshas: vata* (goodness), *pitta* (passion) *and kapha* (ignorance). From these basic elements arise the five physical waveform layers or planes: Solids, liquids, gases, thermals, and the plasma-electromagnetic plane. These five relate to each other in the *tridosha* system: *Vata* combines solids and liquids. *Pitta* combines liquids and thermals. *Vata* combines gases and aether-electromagnetics.

Just as the earth is layered with chemical elements stratified by density and waveform function, our physical body is also layered by these elements that conduct waveforms of particular frequencies and amplitudes. The gross physical world is made up of five states, which include the solid elemental state, the liquid elemental state, the gas elemental state, the thermal elemental state, and the plasma-aether-electromagnetic elemental state. Each elemental state contains a medium of different density, and as the density decreases, the types of waveforms radiating within that elemental state change.

Solids, liquids and gases are the standard elemental states taught in any college chemistry course. Yet physicists told us decades ago that molecules are electromagnetic in essence, and consequently, "solids" per se are actually non-existent. While quantum physics has been accepted by science as defining the substance of matter, most agree that atomic matter is composed of "stuff" with waveform dynamics and characteristics.

Indeed, most physicists agree that electromagnetic waves govern the orbitals between electrons and their nuclei, and atoms and their molecular structures. The *strong forces* and the *weak forces* combine to maintain bonding and repulsion structures according to modern physics theory. These are all forces with electromagnetic waveform characteristics. The particle portion of the *particle-wave model* is still considered "inconceivable."

Quantum physics is thus completely compatible with the waveform-density nature of the five-element concept.

The elemental state with waveforms with frequencies that induce heat is categorized as the thermal elemental state. This element is often referred to as *fire* in the ancient texts, and that waveform density-state of matter housing the electromagnetic spectrum is often translated as *space,* or *aether.* A more technical term for the later from a scientific viewpoint, would be the *plasma-electromagnetic* state.

These five basic elemental states are each mediums that maintain a particular structural density and range of waveforms. Solids provide the medium for the seismic waves. Liquids provide the medium for water wave frequencies. Gases provide the medium for air pressure waves. Thermals provide a medium for the radiation of temperature change, which can also be byproducts of infrared, microwave and other electromagnetic waves—although thermal conduction moves within molecular matter outside the range of the classic electromagnetic spectrum. The plasma-aether medium provides basis for the higher frequency electromagnetic waves, which include microwaves, radiowaves, x-rays, cosmic rays, gamma waves and others—some of which are likely not yet measured by our equipment. To this, most scientists agree that we have only found but a small percentage of the total electromagnetic spectrum.

According to the ancient science of *Ayurveda,* beyond these five physical waveform layers lie three subtle facility layers: The mind, the misidentification of the self as matter, and intelligence—the bridge between the mind and the self. The mind is considered the subtle programming center of the physical body and its elemental layers. The mind translates intention into emotional waveforms, which stimulates the signaling mechanisms of the limbic system, nerves and biochemicals. These intentional mechanisms should also be considered the sources of remote viewing and any psychokinetic ability. This waveform realm is also the medium within which the self transmits intentions through dreaming.

The misidentification feature (translated from *Ayurveda* texts as *false ego*) is a design feature that instigates a veil or governor feature between the self and the mind. The false ego is the interfering element that shields the mind from a real perception of the self. We might compare this to turning down the lights in a movie theater so we can focus on the movie.

This misidentification feature effectively allows the inner self to falsely perceive our identity as physical. Sigmund Freud hinted to this as he described the *id* as the identity component driving people towards particular behaviors. In the same way, the Ayurvedic concept of misidentification drives us to behave (or pretend) as if we are the changing physical body. When our body is young, we believe that we are young and strong. When our body is old, we believe that we are old and weak. We are the same personality in either body. We may have learned and evolved from experience, but our core being has not changed. We are still the same personality. This is why we become surprised as our body ages. The body is aging, but we do not feel any older.

We could compare this false state of identity to a person sitting in a dark cinema theater for two hours watching a movie. The largeness of the screen combined with being isolated in a dark theatre causes the moviegoer to begin to identify with the virtual characters of the movie. For those two hours, the moviegoer temporarily forgets his or her "real" identity and "real life" outside the cinema building.

Intelligence and false ego are considered counter-balancing. Intelligence counters the assumption of physical fulfillment with issues relating to logic, morality, forgiveness and understanding. This is because these are fundamental characteristics of the self.

Each of the eight Ayurvedic elements is considered a layer or medium because each also corresponds to a particular waveform density—ranging from the extremely dense to the extremely subtle. The solid element is denser than the liquid element, as it contains more molecular matter per area than gas does, for example. With each successive layer or medium, we find a decrease in density. At the same time, we find an increase in energy potential and information potential with each layer. This makes sense because higher frequency waveforms are capable of transmitting more information in the same amount of time. To illustrate this, a knock on the door (a seismic waveform) can communicate information, but the amount of information is limited. Morse code, for example, can transmit thoughts and feelings, but very crudely and time-consuming. On the other hand, a radiowave (an electromagnetic wave) can communicate voices and images—a greater amount of information—almost instantly, as we see in case of television and radio transmissions.

Our bodies utilize all these waveform mediums. Each is designed to support transmission of particular types of information. Together these elemental waveform states provide a type of layering system, covering the inner self with layers of interacting waveforms. This hierarchical layering of waveforms essentially provides both a vehicle and a barrier between the external physical world and the self within. Just as a building or automobile is built with a layering of different elements to give its structure strength to protect the driver from the outside world, the human body is also built with a mix of layers. In our crude analogy of the moviegoer, we might compare the paint on the cinema wall to one layer, and the drywall, building framing, electrical wiring and insulation to other layers—all effectively separating the moviegoer from the 'real' world outside the cinema. We might take this analogy further to say that the movie screen could be compared to the mind, the blackness of the room might be compared to the *id* or false ego, and the seats—which ground the moviegoer to the reality of not being inside the movie itself—to intelligence.

The layering of densities and waveform mediums equates to an elemental structuring of the physical body according to *Ayurveda*:

- The bones nails, and supporting tissues (solids)
- The blood, bone marrow, lymph and cellular fluids (liquids)
- The lungs, oxygen transport and flatulence (gases)
- The digestive, lower endocrine and liver organ systems (thermals)
- The senses, nerves, neurotransmitters and hormones (electromagnetics)
- The brain cortices, pineal, pituitary, thalamus, and hypothalamus (mind)
- The immune system and genetic system (intelligence)
- The reproductive system and epigenetic system (*id* or false ego)

Though each layer may have its solid physical organs and attributes among the other elements (liquid, gas and so on), the predominating element is driven through that particular facility. Each elemental state interacts with the various structures, architecture and specific waveforms moving within those parts of the body. These are best described with the understanding of the body's biomolecular structures as waveform converters and messengers. Each of the body's different anatomical systems transmits and conducts waveform information. This conduction is verified simply because we can make a decision to move in a particular direction, and our body follows immediately by moving. The motion we see indicates that all of those ions, cells, nerves, hormones and neurotransmitters involved were part of the messaging and execution system that translated our intent to move into action.

This might be compared to discerning the wire cable itself from the electricity network and energy generator. Without the wire cable that connects the utility company to the houses, electricity would not have anything through which to transmit. Therefore, the wire cable is included when we describe an electrical system, although we understand that the current itself is not the physical wire. We can simply unplug the wire to understand this. Within our body, the various biochemical molecular components are also part of the conducting system for the body's energy systems. They exist to provide useful pathways and transformers for the 'current' of waveforms originating from conscious intent.

Just as the solid layer corresponds with the earthly elements of rock, mountains and soils, the solid layer relates to the bony structures of the body. The solid layer also connects the molecular elements within the muscles, ligaments, organ systems and outer skin tissues. These parts of the body are primarily mineral and carbon-based, and provide the harder 'shell' architecture of the body. They also allow the body a grounding vehicle for the magnetic fields of the earth. Without this grounding, the body could not plant its feet solidly onto the ground. Nor could it lie down restfully and sleep. The earth's seismic waveforms thus harmonically 'flow' through the bone and tissue cells of our body. Because the solid layer vibrates at lower frequencies, its movement is slower and more perceptible. Our solid body layers resonate with these seismic frequencies.

The solid layering of our molecular biochemistry is in motion at all times, however. Our bones may not look like they are circulating, but they are. They are absorbing and resorbing elements like calcium, silica and boron while excreting these in a constant flow of molecular recycling. This circulation of the bones compares favorably to the circulation of soil or elements of rock through oceans, lakes and streams. Soils and rocks circulate their contents slowly through adjoining waters, which form channels of rivers and streams through them. Soil and rock runoff in turn helps nourish aquatic organisms. Bones circulate nutrients and water through small channels that flow between osteocytes, ridding toxins to the lymph and blood stream. We might question the ability of solids to transmit information. A simple knock on the door or tap on the floor will answer that question. Rhythmic waveforms transmitted through the solid elemental state can be quite clearly informational.

At the macroscopic level, the liquid element relates to the movements of the various fluids around the planet. This includes the rivers, streams, oceans, lakes and aquifers of various substances, including water, lava, oil, and other natural fluids of the planet. The liquid layer of the body also deals with the rivers and streams of the blood and lymphatic systems, as well as the fluid-filled cavities located within cells, organs and basal cell membranes. Fluids also provide a means for transferring various messaging biochemicals such as hormones around the body via blood circulation. The blood also provides structure via dissolved ions as they circulate amongst cells and organs. The physical body's fluid nature also provides the body with its ability to detoxify and nourish. Fluids give the body the ability to respond with flexibility. This means that water is a means for the body to adapt and alter course. Solidity tends to be stable and stubborn, while liquidity tends to be adaptive and compromising.

Emotions are often expressed with liquid movement. The formation of tears expresses certain emotions. A person might spit to express another emotion. Some people react with shock when seeing their own blood, as we identify emotionally with this fluid. The fluid layer also provides a turnover of nutrients and toxins, which drive metabolism and detoxification. Proper liquid movement through the body is critical for the body's balance.

The gaseous layer moving through the living organism is less dense and even more motion-oriented than the liquid layer. On the macro basis, this element covers our planet and provides several layers of protection—including blocking some of the dangerous radiation like cosmic rays pulsing into our atmosphere. The gases inside the atmosphere also provide the elements of oxygen and nitrogen for mammals, and carbon dioxide for plants and algae. Our ability to see into this medium as we do with the solid and liquid elements is hampered by the density of the medium. Our eyes cannot perceive spectra from other mediums outside the primary sensory receptor abilities of the rods and cones. At the same time, the gas state provides a good medium for the transmission of sound.

The gaseous elemental state exists throughout the body. Gases travel through the bloodstream in the form of oxygen, nitrogen, carbon dioxide (in the form of carbolic acid) and others. Gas states of various molecular structures are present throughout every tissue system, cell, organ and of course the lungs and digestive tract. While cadaver dissection does not reveal much in the way of the gas element, we can see the gas state interacting through respiration and digestion. A simple belch or 'passing of gas' will quickly illustrate the role gases play within the digestive system. Gases circulate within our body through channel systems just as the other elements do. The gas elemental state also provides balancing mechanisms within the body just as do the other states. The gas state also forms a means for expression. Breathing patterns and digestive efficiency reflect emotions quite well. Heavy breathing tends to reflect anxious moments, and we tend to belch when we feeling comfortable after a fine meal.

Thermal currents conduct through our environment within the water, the atmosphere and even through the earth. Weather systems provide an expression of the movement of thermals through the atmosphere—reflected by pressure and temperature change. The thermal element within our body is easily identified with thermal-sensing equipment. This can be done by the casual observer with a thermometer or more precisely with thermal sensing units available to medical facilities. These units allow us to see that the body is not necessarily the temperature of the environment, and not one temperature throughout. Rather, temperature gradients tend to flow through the body just as water or gas circulates. The body thus will have different temperatures in different locations, and these gradients will interact with a variety of metabolic and physiologic functions.

Certain instruments can "see" these thermal waveforms. Heat detectors such as thermographic cameras image temperature radiating from a hot surface in distinct gradients. Occasionally we will also see thermal waves rising up from a heated asphalt road. Infrared and microwaves might present some confusion because these are electromagnetic waves, yet they also appear to transmit thermal waveforms. Actually, these electromagnetic waveforms do not conduct or transmit thermal waveforms. Rather, their interaction with a particular substance creates the thermal waveforms. A number of electromagnetic waves can excite the quantum elements of a substance to a point where the substance radiates heat, often along with other electromagnetic radiation and possibly even an altered molecular structure.

Research has indicated that thermals are one of the primary waveforms moving through many of the *meridians*. Thermal waveforms will transmit through the nervous system and the bloodstream as well. Thermal waveforms also circulate through the spaces around the cells—the intercellular spaces or basal membrane. Thermal waveforms transmit information that influences a suitable environment for muscle exertion, organ activity, and cellular response. In addition to this channeling of information, heat-producing molecules like glucose, cortical and thyroid neurochemicals transmit thermal potentials, as they produce reactions that convert intention to kinetic energy. The citric acid ATP-transfer (or Krebs) cycle is an example of a thermal waveform-producing energy reaction working within a catalytic (conversion) environment.

Together these pathways provide heat conduction within our bodies, which in turn drive the various enzymatic and metabolic activities. We also identify greatly with the thermal element, as we connect with our body's energy levels. Most of us will comment that a person has "good energy" or perhaps "low energy." We may also call someone "dynamic" or "hot," indirectly reflecting on his or her thermal waveform expression. This is because thermal waveforms directly influence metabolism. Faster metabolism typically produces a more attractive and shapely body figure and radiation due to the increase in energy utilization and activity. When we describe someone as a dynamic person, we are usually referring to someone who is active and radiates with responsive radiance. These characteristics relate to their thermal conductivity, because the thermal waveforms also transmit passionate feelings and emotions, and the intentional self's drive for achievement.

Incidentally, many incorrectly relate the layer of thermal energy directly to the self. It is true that without the host of the inner self within the body, no heat can be generated. Therefore, many interpret the result of thermal contact with photographic paper—rendering the famous *Kirlian corona*—as a vision of the soul or self. Again, while we can easily connect the inner self with the body's ability to transmit thermal waveforms, the visual observation of Kirlian photography would not be any more "spiritual" than seeing the color of ones skin or hearing a person's voice. Rather, this image simply reflects photographic thermal waveforms generated from the spread of intentional consciousness through the thermal elemental state.

The use of these elemental layers is illustrated as we investigate their relative frequency levels. Pure electromagnetic transmission provides a higher frequency informational waveform. As such, conscious information requiring immediate and precise instructions tend to travel through the body's electromagnetic pathways. The nerves provide the primary pathway for electromagnetic waveform biocommunication. We might call the nerves the electromagnetic racetrack. This is not to say that electromagnetic waveform transmission only travels through the nerves, however. Electromagnetic information is also transferred between cells, tissues, organs, blood, lymph, ion channels, hormones and others. The biocommunication of information through the ligands and receptors is electromagnetic. Even if the transmission requires the chemical binding between the ligand and receptor, the actual biocommunication is electromagnetic.

Some solids may delay, distort or muffle various electromagnetic waveforms. Others, such as crystals, may convert and disburse them. These alterations will also result in particular information being transmitted. The interaction between pure electromagnetic waveforms and the covalent bonds between the atoms and molecules of a substance creates a new waveform interference pattern—another platform for communication. Liquids tend to refract electromagnetic radiation, altering their waveform transmission. Gases tend to diffuse electromagnetic radiation, but this also depends upon the content of the gas. Electromagnetic radiation may refract through gas as well. Both are seen among the sun's different electromagnetic rays as they enter our atmosphere. The thermal energy state will often magnify or intensify particular electromagnetic radiation. Electromagnetic waves can also produce thermal waveforms, as seen in microwaves and infrared waveforms.

Using the facility of the mind, the intentional self utilizes these various interactions between the waveforms conducted through the body to form interference patterns of information. This might be compared to a person utilizing a flashlight and hand to create a particular hand puppet on the wall. The light would have no meaning without the intentional interaction by the person manipulating his hand in front of the light. Without the interaction between the two, there would be no image.

This manipulation of waveforms is precisely what the inner self learns to do using the facility of the mind. The various waveforms transmitted within our body relate to information. The transfer of information from our physiology and sensory system to the brain cortex region and into a format that can be utilized by the self requires a sorting and conversion process. This is what the mind does. The mind assembles the various waveforms from the five elements into interference patterns that most closely match the goals and intentions of the self. These interference patterns are then imaged by the self, whereupon the self responds by driving intention back through the mind. The mind then converts these intentions back into physical instructions via waveform conversion.

When we speak, for example, we are broadcasting something that was translated by the mind. We might ask how did the thoughts and intention find their way to the voice box? We know there is an electromagnetic conduction between the brain and the voice box. Intention and thoughts are translated to vocal cord activity. The translation device is the mind.

The reception and translation of logic, hope, intuition and morality come through another medium, however. People often refer to our sense of morality or intuition as coming from a deeper place than the mechanical (translational) nature of the mind. This is true. Intelligence is channeled through the mind from a deeper source. Once viewed by the self, it can either be ignored or focused upon. This is the choice of the intentional self, who views the input from the body and senses and either sorts them using intelligence or the filtering device of the false ego.

Intelligence also provides the foundation for the storage of our environment, decisions and intensions into our genes. Intelligent information is stored within the DNA and RNA though their sequenced electromagnetic bonding patterns. These form a basis for coding, just as a byte of a machine code contains an assembly of bits (1s or 0s): The combination of bits making up a byte conveys a distinct piece of information. DNA and RNA retain and convey our history of decisions and consciousness within their sequenced molecular combinations. Through the facility of RNA, the information is translated to processes that govern cellular behavior. In this way, the combination of our past decisions and our consciousness combines to form and translate our karmic balance within our DNA and RNA.

The *id* or false ego is described as a subtle filtering layer in *Ayurveda.* While we cannot see it, we can see its effects. Even though we should logically realize that we are not the changing body, we continue to do so. One look at a childhood picture should indicate our not being the body (i.e., that body is now gone). This would be analogous to a person continuing to drive his neighbor's car to work even after he was told the car was not his. Why would he keep driving it around thinking he owns it? It does not make sense. Logically, something must be influencing our continued erroneous assumption that each of us is a changing body.

The five elements of solids, liquids, gases, thermals and electromagnetics are easy to understand and relate to. The more subtle layers of the mind, intelligence and false ego require another perspective of reality. These subtle facilities exist on a platform that lies beyond the senses. We know the mind exists because of its sorting, translation and conversion effects. We know intelligence exists because we have all drawn upon a deeper sense of morality or logic, often beyond what the senses present. As for false ego, it presents as somewhat of a counter-intelligence. While we might know that something is morally right, we are teased by the possibility that we might become happy if we just did it. This comes from a mis-identification of the nonphysical self with physical matter.

The layered waveform elements of the physical body are classified appropriately within the unique *Ayurveda tridosha* system. The grosser elements of solids, liquids and gasses reflect a more grounded consciousness, called *kapha.* This is more closely identified with the characteristic of consistency and predictability. *Ayurveda* generally classifies thermal activities as characteristic of *pitta* consciousness. *Pitta* reflects the characteristics of activity, passion, anger, and responsiveness. On the other hand, the higher frequency electromagnetic waveforms pulsing through the body and the mind are considered primarily *vata,* reflecting a consciousness of sensitivity, intensity and anxiety.

Broadcasting Life

We could compare the informational biocommunications of the body to the operating of an automobile. A modern car is made using a variety of materials including steel, plastic, rubber and even fabric. Each of these functional layers of different materials compares to the elemental layers existing within the physical body. Each layer has a different density and function. Using this analogy, we can touch on how the body interacts with the environment and the self within.

The car driver instructs and gains feedback from the car using specific levers and instruments. Turning the key is necessary to start the engine. The gearshift engages the engine in one direction or another. The gas pedal accelerates the car. The instrument panel enables feedback from the car's operations. A radio and maybe a CB radio broadcast receive communications from the outside world. Both have a power button and tuning dial to locate the correct frequency. A GPS system gives the driver location and direction information. The climate is controlled by still other buttons, enabling the driver to turn on the air conditioning or heater. Or perhaps these are preset with a thermostat. In any case, the driver will then direct the car using still another lever system—the steering wheel.

The self operates the physical body using a similar system. Rather than turning knobs and levers with fingers and hands as the car driver might, the self operates the 'knobs and levers' of the physical body through the waveform expressions of the mind. The mind sends waveform instructions through several key translation centers (the 'knobs and levers') within the brain and central nervous system—such as the prefrontal cortex, hypothalamus, amygdale, and pituitary. These translation centers convert the intentions of the inner self into physical activities within each of the body's elemental levels. The specific 'knobs and levers' might include particular brain loci. However, the physical waveform translation points of the physical body (comparable to the car's gearing systems) are located within the neural network. The central pathway of the neural network is located along the spinal column and cerebral region. These centers or regions also correspond with the points of sympathetic nerve response along the spine. These also coincide with the *chakras.*

There are seven primary *chakra* centers located vertically within the neural network according to *Ayurveda.* Each of these translates intention a little differently and through a slightly different elemental medium, just as each knob and lever in a car translates the driver's purpose differently. As such, each of these *chakra* centers also stimulates particular organs and tissue systems within the body.

The original meaning of the Sanskrit work for *chakra* means *wheel.* This literal translation relates to the *chakra*'s ability to radiate its translation of intention through a particular pathway or network of the body. Another translation of the word *chakra* is *vortex.* This word relates to the multi-dimensional aspect of *chakras*, and their ability to convert intention from another plane of existence into physical expression.

In the western world, *chakras* are often discussed as though they are some type of strange organ system within the body. Some have offered sayings such as *"balancing the chakras"* or *"subduing"* or *"correcting"* a *chakra* in order to bring about a better physical result or emotional outlook. These descriptions may have validity on a certain analogous level. Still, they misconstrue the *chakras* true structure and function. Such concepts might be equivalent to the car driver blaming the car's speed and direction on the gas pedal and steering wheel. *"That damn pedal needs to be fixed,"* the driver might complain upon receiving a speeding ticket. He actually just made some bad decisions regarding his speed. Or perhaps he simply did not watch the speedometer.

Of the seven major *chakra* regions within the human body, the lower four are aligned vertically within the spinal region, and the upper three align with key loci in the brainstem and cortex systems. There are five general body regions overlaying these *chakra* regions. They are in the pelvic region at the base of the spine, the navel region, the solar plexus region, the throat and cervical region, and the brain region. Each of these centers provides a control or lever of influence into a particular elemental state, a particular organ system, and particular sense organs. The brain region contains three different *chakra* regions, however. The last two rise above the plasma-aether of the electromagnetic, into the waveforms of the mind, intelligence and subtle false identity field.

Here we clarify that these *chakra* centers are made up principally of neurons, ganglia and their supporting cell networks. These together form a region that provides a conversion or translation mechanism for waveforms. Collectively, these effectively which translate the intentional purpose and consciousness of the inner self into biophysical instructions and activities. Each of the centers is designed to convert particular types of conscious intentions into particular waveforms. These translation centers simply provide a bridge between consciousness and the physical body.

We might wonder how this process works on a practical level. The body performs millions of processes automatically. The inner self is not consciously aware of most of these (autonomic and sympathetic) operations. They are automatic processes that have been programmed into the system, yet they still trace back to the objectives and inclinations of the inner self. This becomes obvious in biofeedback. In biofeedback, the inner self can somehow direct many of the body's autonomic processes through direct intention, taking conscious control over the physical function. In sympathetic functions, the self utilizes the programming capacity of the mind and *chakra* system to accomplish what we would call pre-programmed functions. This might be compared to a computer operator setting up programs that automatically do certain *if-then* operations.

To illustrate this further, let us say a person is afraid of the body's death—as most of us are. As the inner self runs the mind through (or is taught) the various scenarios of how the body might die (usually at a very young age of the body—the initial programming stage), programming is initiated. The mind is programmed by the self's intentions, which in turn emits subtle waveforms through to the *chakra* linkage down the spine. This *codes* or programs the *chakra* system to respond to particular dangers. Let us say the eyes see a tiger. The programming will determine particular responses. One automatic response might be to begin running as fast as possible. Another might be to begin yelling for help. Another might be looking back and checking for the distance between our body and the tiger's. These requirements then set up subsidiary response programs within each *chakra*, according to its link to particular organ systems and particular biomolecular elemental states. Ultimately, the inner self is driving the body with a fear of death, and the mind initiates the *if-then* programming of the lower physical *chakras* through the release of special electromagnetic pulses stimulated through particular brain cortices. These create unique interference patterns, which are held within the ionic and molecular arrangements within the nerves' gateways. In other words, specific waveforms are generated from the mind's stimulation of particular brain centers, which in turn send subtle messenger waveforms through the neural network and down the spine. These waves are bound within—or better, crystallized within—regional neurons, setting up the necessary internal programming.

These *chakra*-held programs are assembled via the particular waveform interference patterns crystallized within neuron biochemical structures and DNA sequencing. The network of nerve cells that innerve particular organs and tissues in that region of the body thus resonate with particular waveform frequencies. Programming instructions from the mind set up informational interference patterns with certain waveforms, which are collectively held or crystallized by these arrayed neurons. These crystallized (standing) interference patterns form gateway states that together create response patterns to incoming waveforms (from sensory inputs) with particular characteristics. A series of these gateway states would be analogous to the on-off (1-0) states of computer machine language bits coming to form *if-then* statements in bytes. These gateway-triggered responses include stimulating particular endocrine glands to release neurotransmitters and hormones, or initiating immediate motor responses in key muscle fibers in certain conditions, for example.

In this way, the neural network cells and supporting tissue cells within and surrounding that *chakra* region are all programmed to respond in particular ways to sensory perception. Seeing the tiger would initiate a response within key *chakra* programming for the various endocrine glands to produce adrenaline, vasopressin, cortisol, insulin and a number of other messengers to initiate and support immediate motor response, along with immediate skeletal muscle responses like running. This would be analogous to the car's air bags automatically releasing upon a collision—as long as the car was properly equipped and programmed, and the driver had the airbag switch turned on.

Further to the car analogy, just as the driver of a car simply sits and turns the wheel to steer the car within a pre-programmed range of directions through its gearing and steering mechanisms, the self sits aloof of the body, steering physical activity using a pre-programmed range of choices while steering the wheels of the *chakras*. To make the car analogy better, we would imagine that the car and its particular features was selected by the driver, and some of its more detailed functions (like the airbag for example) were programmed in by the driver.

Remember that the mind also utilizes a *chakra* network to translate its waveforms. These "master" waveforms then program and stimulate the lower physical *chakras* along the spine.

It is for this reason that some people respond differently to others during a stressful or life-threatening situation. Research shows that while some people will spring into action in a life-threatening situation, others will freeze, scream, or otherwise make illogical decisions. What determines this difference in response? It is the self within utilizing the mind, which programs the body's response centers in preparation for emergencies.

Research has illustrated that in order to be properly prepared, we need to run the mind through the scenarios necessary for survival in the event of the emergency *prior to the emergency*. If we are on an airplane, for example, we might consider what will happen if the plane goes down. We might find the exit door, and see how it might open. In this way, we run our mind through how we might deal with the emergency. This 'running through the scenarios' ultimately creates the programming necessary for the body to react. Again, this takes place through the facility of the mind. The mind subtly programs the *chakra* centers for their necessary responses. The research has illustrated that it is those who prepare themselves and run through the disaster scenarios who appropriately spring into action. They are the ones who help others during a disaster. Those who did not perform any preparedness find their body and mind unable to respond appropriately to the disaster. The mechanism for training the body takes place through a mental programming of the *chakras*.

The seven *chakras* also align with the self's consciousness to form a ladder of evolution and growth. Here is an explanation of each *chakra* region and its specific characteristics according to ancient Vedic texts:

The Foundation

This is considered the first and *root* energy *chakra*. It is also referred to as *muladhara,* which means *foundation.* Within the body, it is located in the region at the base of the spine near the pelvis, in a lateral position between the anus and the genitals. This center resonates with the waveforms of the solid element and the *kapha* consciousness. It is thus considered connected to the earth, and survival.

This *chakra* region is often referred to as the *seat of the vital energy,* because it is the most grounded region of the body. This region controls the activation of survival instincts, and this is translated through the activities of the lower adrenal system or the adrenal medulla gland, which releases adrenal hormones like epinephrine and cortisol. These hormones stimulate physical activation of the survival and fear responses.

This *chakra* region also activates the muscles that control ejaculation and orgasm, and thus form the basis for our attraction to the physical forms of the opposite sex. This *chakra* region is often referred to as the *coil* for procreation and physical perpetuity.

The foundation *chakra* region resonates with the olfactory senses. This also relates to survival, as the body becomes a tool for seeking out adequate food and refuge. The primary work organ this *chakra* region is tuned into is the anus. This of course is located between our sit bones, so it is also appropriately positioned for grounding when we sit. The bony skeletal system is the primary rhythmic tie to this *chakra* region, and the condition of our bones is often a reflection of our issues as they relate to the family and the survival of the physical body.

The net of these physiological functions indicates this *chakra* region stimulates concerns of survival: Maintaining adequate food and shelter. This of course ties into other concerns relating to survival: money, jobs, and family, for example. Whatever environmental component may be connected with the body's physical survival will resonate with the foundation *chakra* region.

The flow of waveform energy through this *chakra* region is primarily linear and one-pointed. Some might say narrow, but when someone is focused upon survival due to some threat, this can be an overwhelming scenario requiring clear focus. This tendency forms the foundation for much of the stress that we bring upon ourselves, should we have an innate fear and attachment for the physical survival of the body. When we see how too much stress relates to adrenal exhaustion, we are able to connect the relationship between fear and this particular region.

This *chakra* region is also the prevalent translator of intention for the self between the body's first and seventh years. Children display tendencies that are related to one-pointed survival and insecurities. These insecurities result in the outcries of children that we often hear. Many of these cries are too quickly mended with food or drink, which can send the wrong message to the inner self during these formative years. Instead of learning to deal with and understand our needs and fears, we are led to believe that material things will satisfy us. This creates a cycle that is hard to break later.

We often find that those who become overly concerned with survival have a tendency to over-eat: An attempt to save up for a day when less food might be around, or simply an attempt to fill our emptiness. This survival instinct translates from an over-concern regarding the body's future survival. This concern will eventually translate to various metabolic disorders, along with muscular and spinal issues related to obesity.

Fear is often an emotion that the inner self channels through this *chakra* region. This is because insecurity is reflected by fear, and insecurity is bred from fear because protection is sought after. Fear can also breed violence if survival is seemingly threatened. When someone becomes fearful for the survival of their physical body, they may—in an attempt to protect the body's survival—become violent towards someone else. We might refer this to an animalistic mentality.

The root *chakra* region is also an important aspect of the inner self's evolution. Being "grounded" is a necessary platform from which to expand. However, should a person become overly focused upon the survival aspects of the physical world, our personal evolution will be stunted. Realizing for example that the Almighty has provided the necessary components for physical survival for even the less developed creatures will allow us to expand our scope beyond the animalistic survival mentality. Raising our consciousness beyond these concerns can begin a path towards self-awareness.

One of the central hormones the adrenal system produces is cortisol and related glucocorticoids. These neurochemicals mobilize physical response during stressful times by stimulating an increase in blood glucose and fatty acid levels. This mechanism increases the potential for metabolic response. These neurochemicals also balance the immune response after an injury by inhibiting the immune system's histamine, lymphocytes, and macrophages. Without these balancing hormones, our immune response could launch an all-out attack against our entire physical body with little control (autoimmunity). The adrenal cortex also releases mineralocorticoids like aldosterone and androgen steroids. These neurochemicals increase muscle size, stamina and power, especially during critical times when extra response potency is required. We have all heard of these steroids increasing power and stamina among athletes. Androgen production is stimulated through a renin-angiotensin cycle, which is related to blood vessel constriction and expansion during times of stress.

In addition, the adrenal medulla produces epinephrine and norepinephrine. These two important neurochemicals stimulate blood flow into skeletal muscle regions of the body. This in turn helps stimulate greater heart rates in a fight-or-flight response. If we were to face a tiger in the wilderness for example, our pre-programmed *chakra* response based upon the fear for the body's survival is translated into these neurochemical messengers.

The Dwelling Place

The second *chakra* region in the human body is called *svadhisthana,* meaning the *dwelling place,* because many of us focus our intentions upon our physical passions and physical family. The location of this *chakra* region is at the sacral region of the spine, in the region of the groin. Intentions related to passion translate their energy into the activities of the testes and the ovaries. This energy translation thus resonates with inner self's desires for fulfillment, translated by the mind into sexuality, procreation, fantasy, family, intimacy and emotional physical relationships. The primary shape of this center is said to be circular, symbolizing the evolving and circular relationship between lust and love.

The elemental aspect of this *chakra* region is liquid. The radiation from this center resonates through the liquid elements within the body, allowing intention to stimulate the ebb and flow of the bloodstream, tissue fluids, bone marrow, lymph, cell membrane fluid, and intracellular fluids. The waveform effect of the fluid layer is expressive, which is why emotions are often expressed through tears, stomach acids, sweating and spitting. Because neurochemicals often circulate through the body's fluids, this *chakra* region echoes emotional responses through the endocrine system into the bloodstream—circulating responsively throughout the body.

The human organism resonates more predominantly through the second *chakra* region between years eight and fourteen. New emotional drivers bring varying states of awareness during this period. During this period, the inner self also begins to translate friendships into sexual relationships, which also stimulates hormones and brings initial instability and mood swings.

The second *chakra* region resonates with the sense of taste, so it is tied to the activities of the tongue along with genital function. The tongue and the genitals are considered the two loci where the inner self connects most with passion in the physical plane. Thus, most of us consider the taste of food and the activity of sex to be critical to our enjoyment of the physical body. For this reason also, we often see passionate couples combining sex with food. We can also see this reality as we look around us at the various advertisements competing for our attention. We find at least one of these two elements in practically every advertisement. Many ads will contain both enticements.

This *chakra* region is said to reflect light blue. As the liquid layer is connected to moods, we find that the moon's lunar cycles influences emotional ups and downs, just as the moon affects the ebb and flow of the tides. The woman's menstruation is therefore also connected to the moon's cycles and this *chakra* region. For this reason, we often see a woman's emotional cycles moving pacing with menstruation and the moon's cycles as well. Many medical researchers have connected these mood swings to estrogen/progesterone imbalances. In reality, these hormones are simply messengers whose release was stimulated through the *if-then* programming set-up between the inner self, the mind, and this *chakra* region. Imbalances in these hormones thus stem from conflicts between the inner self, the mind and the body's aging and procreation mechanisms.

The City

The third *chakra* region is called *manipura,* meaning *the city of gems.* This term is used because this center is connected with ten key nerve endings that distribute the waveforms translated and/or programmed in this *chakra* region. The location of *manipura* is at the spinal region between the solar plexus and navel region. It resonates with the frequencies related to thermal waveforms, and thus is coherent with the radiating heat energy of the sun and the thermal nature of the digestive process.

This *chakra* region directly stimulates the adrenal cortex and the liver. This cortex portion of the adrenal system is strongly related to the ongoing processes of the digestive system, and many other metabolic processes of the body involved in thermoregulation and activity. These work hand in hand with the liver's multifarious tasking, as will be discussed in more detail later. Various glucosteroids work in tandem with pancreatic hormones such as insulin, which monitor and guide energy conversion and glucose utilization within cells.

The sense organ connected to this *chakra* region is the eyes, and thus its sensory conversion is sight. The air of this *chakra* region is the upper abdominal air. The rhythmic shape of this *chakra* region is said to be triangular, reflecting reddish frequencies.

Simply put, the self accesses the thermal state of the body through this *chakra* region. The thermal state reflects the pace of energy conversion and metabolism, which is expressed with emotions of pride, fashion, control, anger, and manipulation. When a person dominates through this *chakra* region, they may exhibit a fiery or hostile personality—one imbued with arrogance and haste. Balanced relationships of this *chakra* region trend towards constructive activity. Exercise, bursts of physical energy, determination to accomplish a particularly difficult task, and a tendency to rush things are notable aspects of one who expresses through this *chakra* region in a more balanced manner.

One of the most profound aspects of the third *chakra* region is its connection to will power. The intention of sticking to something, or finishing what we start, is defined by the self's purposeness, discipline and stability. Continuing through hardship with determination, even though the odds are against us in order to accomplish a particular goal is considered an act of will, and a display of will power. This *chakra* region tends to resonate with these intentions, translating them to physical activity.

The third *chakra* region also tends to focus one's prideful energies into activity. Those absorbed in how others perceive us will translate that intention into actions meant to impress others. When we are focused though this *chakra* we might be constantly concerned about what others think of us. We are concerned about our appearance. We are concerned about how we come off. We are concerned about how well we fit in. When we think we are not getting what we deserve, we may feel angry, feeling life is unfair to us. This anger, rooted in our frustrated desires, is often referred to as being 'hot-headed,' and a person known to explode with anger easily will often be referred to as a 'hot-head.' It is more than coincidental that heat is related to anger, and redness is related to heat. The channel to these activities is through the third *chakra* region.

Years fourteen through twenty-one tend to be expressed more heavily through the third *chakra* region. This is one reason why we see more competitive and volatile behavior during these years. The inner self is developing the ability to become stable amongst an array of choices, and some of these choices are expressed with passion and more easily result in frustration.

The Balancer

The fourth *chakra* region is located along the spine in the region of the cardiac plexus, known within the medical community as the heart. This *chakra* region is referred to as *anahata,* which translates to *"unstricken."* This center connects the inner self to aspects reaching beyond the mundane, into areas related to relationships of caring and compassion with those around us.

This fourth *chakra* region connects to the organs of the heart and lungs. It is therefore circulatory in nature, and the waveforms it resonates with lie primarily within the gaseous elemental state. As air is taken into the lungs, oxygen is bound to hemoglobin within the boundaries of the alveoli—small sacs that line the lungs. The alveoli draw the hemoglobin from the bloodstream. Oxygen's attachment to hemoglobin is stimulated with pressure—a waveform. The binding between oxygen and hemoglobin increases as the pressure approaches the most efficient 104mm Hg level. Meanwhile, the normal atmospheric pressure of oxygen is 159mm Hg.

As the oxygen-attached hemoglobin is drawn back into the blood, oxygen is transmitted through the body's cell network through thousands of blood vessels and capillaries. This process of pressurized attachment of oxygen is reversed as oxygen is released from hemoglobin into cells around the body. Cellular tissues maintain pressures typically around 40mm Hg—far less than atmospheric pressure. At this lower pressure, oxygen disassociates from hemoglobin bonds, releasing the oxygen into the cell. Here oxygen is used in the oxidative phosphorylation portion of the ATP-electron transport chain, which is the key to the cell's production of energy. This phosphorylation process upgrades adenosine-di-phosphate (ADP) to adenosine-tri-phosphate (ATP), releasing kinetic energy and heat. This energy is translated into muscle contraction and other cellular functions.

Here we can see how the gas layer imposes its rhythmic effects upon movement. As the oxygen gas is used for energy production, carbon dioxide is released as a byproduct. Carbon dioxide is carried to the lungs via water molecules in the bloodstream, forming H_2CO_3. These molecules are brought to the lungs, whereupon the carbon dioxide is released into the lungs, again through the alveoli. This also illustrates how the standing gaseous waveforms resonate through the liquid layers as they move to their operational directive of exhalation. Incidentally, through the process of respiration, toxins are sloughed off, which helps purify the body.

This fourth *chakra* region also translates immune response programming from the mind's waveform range to stimulate a variety of messengers that spread the body's immune cells throughout the body. The thymus gland is responsible for the activation of T-cells, for example. The immune system is also circulatory in nature, as immune cells like macrophages and antibodies transverse the blood stream and lymphatic system. These channels render immediate pathways for transporting lymphocytes and the various byproducts of detoxification processes. This said, the ultimate source of the body's immune response is the programming features of the mind, which resonate to the 'self versus non-self' influence of the false ego.

This fourth *chakra* region resonates with the sense of touch. As we have experienced, the skin can sense minor changes in temperature, humidity, pressure, as well as electromagnetic radiation related to subtle and gross waveforms traveling within the atmosphere or local environment. The various tactile nerves can also receive slower waveforms vibrating through solids. This is why we can often feel the pounding of a drum beat on our skin. This is why many people like to go to loud concerts: The sensation of feeling the music on the skin can be quite appealing to music lovers.

Through this facility of touch, the inner self can channel emotions related to our dearest relationships. These would include intimate relationships with our partners or family members. For this reason, touching is considered a direct translation of our feelings for another person. We can thus see a relationship between this *chakra* region's connection with the heart and relationships. This *chakra* region translates the intentions of the inner self to love and be loved into the emotions and expressions of physical love and companionship.

Those intimate emotions are said to reflect through this center's hexagram shape. This center also reflects the frequencies of the green part of the spectrum. The skin is its organ of action while the hands are the predominating body part this center resonates with. This may be the reason why the hands tend to be so expressive: The translation of the intention to communicate with others is easily noticed by ones hand gestures. We might notice that when a person becomes frustrated with their ability to communicate their intentions to others, their hand gestures tend to increase. We are also especially attentive to the hand signals of others, and we are sensitive to positive signals and often hurt by negative signals. For this reason, most of us feel extremely offended should someone give us the 'finger.' This is because hand signals connect intimately with this intimate *chakra* region. We might add that probably one of the most precious expressions of our care for another person is expressed through the holding of hands.

The inner self resonates strongest through the fourth *chakra* region between the body's twenty-first and twenty-eighth years. During this time, the person typically begins to develop their conjugal relationships as well as reaches toward activities related to family life. During this time, a person will typically heal their relationship with their parents and siblings, get married, and possibly have children. We also see people developing issues related to social conscience during this phase of physical development. This is why we see many activists promoting human and animal rights during these years, then assuming more conservative in later years.

The shape of this *chakra* region is often described as a circle with twelve petals because this hexagonal shape expands in all directions and dimensions—between the physical, emotional, intellectual, spiritual, and transcendental aspects of ones being. Often this multi-dimensional aspect will put the inner self into a confused state, as our physical choices draw out into different results. The emotions typically channeled through this *chakra* region are love, duty, and devotion.

Within this twelve-petal *chakra* region also resides a still deeper access point or inner channel of spiritual devotion. This inner channel is said to connect with a broadcasting of the Almighty. Some might also refer to this feature as the "Lord within the Heart" or the "Holy Ghost." The intentions of the Supreme are said to vibrate through this *chakra* region to accompany and facilitate the inner self's process of growth and evolution.

The Purifier

The fifth *chakra* region is referred to by ancient Vedic texts as *vishuddha,* meaning *"pure."* This *chakra* region is located in the region of the throat. The fifth *chakra* region is associated with the plasma-aether-electromagnetic waveforms, translating through sound vibration. The connected sense organ is the ear (as it also converts sound to electromagnetic waves), and the mouth is the primary work organ activated through this *chakra* region. The fifth *chakra* region is been compared in *Ayurveda* to a sixteen-petal flower, with its rhythmic effects channeling out into sixteen directions and nerve plexes. This *chakra* region is most active during the body's twenty-eighth through thirty-fifth years.

As we analyze sound, we see it has a number of unique yet powerful characteristics. Through sound we can instantly communicate our intentions and desires. Immediately we can convey our thoughts through the vibration of our vocal cords. Sound itself is made up of air pressure waves. The process of vibrating the vocal cords from the mind's intentional messengers requires an electromagnetic translation, just as the conversion of sound back to electromagnetic waves does. Conveying intention through sound allows us to communicate our purpose, plan or philosophies immediately. We can instantly influence our surrounding environment with our feelings and emotions through sound. This immediate release of consciousness into sound also provides some purificatory and reflective tools, assuming our sounds are thoughtful and reflective. For this reason, psychologists have noticed those who do not communicate well or express themselves in sound tend also to bottle up their emotions, which can end up being expressed in unhealthy ways.

This *chakra* expresses through the plasma-aethereal elemental state, or *akasha* from the Sanskrit translation. Through the plasma-aethereal layer, thoughts and intentions can immediately be converted to physical attributes by using sound. Through sound a listener can be immediately affected by the thoughts of the sender. Through sound we reach a plane that is particularly more subtle than that reached through vision or touch. Through sound we can communicate the highest of thoughts, opinions, and intentions, along with our most intimate emotions. Through sound we can connect with each other precisely, as we share our most private goals and objectives. Through sound we also hear musical melodies and the gentle sounds of nature. Through sound we can express (and hear) the highest of spiritual aspirations. This can be done not only through conversation, but also through prayers, hymns, and devotional chants.

The fifth *chakra* region also resonates with the thyroid gland and the subtle connection between the conscious self's intention and the body's cells. This center translates intention to the production of the hormones that regulate the body's cellular activities. Thyroid hormones T3 and T4 are stimulated through the mediation of *thyroid stimulating hormone* (TSH), produced by the anterior pituitary gland. The waveform energies that regulate the process of converting TSH to T3 and T4 connect through the fifth *chakra* region.

Hence, the fifth *chakra* region is a channel of focus for those trying to grow and evolve personally and spiritually, or as an avenue for those who desire to help others. Aural reception is unique in that it allows us to receive knowledge and philosophical insight with ease—should we intend to. Thus aural reception has been the primary facility for transferring knowledge since ancient times. The passing of advanced information orally from wise teacher to receptive student allows subtle nuances and context to be conveyed. It also allows the teacher to develop an active rapport with the student, enabling the teacher to know immediately whether the student understands the concepts.

The Command Center

The sixth *chakra* region is located near the medulla plexus and pineal plexus, posterior to the axis between the eyebrows. This *chakra* region is referred to in the Sanskrit texts as *ajna,* meaning *'unlimited command.'* It is not the point on the forehead as one might imagine from some illustrations. Rather, its region lies beneath, reaching back towards the brainstem. It also encompasses the limbic system—the translating system between the various neural networks, emotions, the master endocrine system and executive control. It also amalgamates the frontal cortex and neocortex within its network. The frontal cortex is seen by brain researchers as the dispatching center for the broadcasting of the decisions and directions that stimulate the limbic system. The frontal cortex amplifies brainwaves and neuron transmissions that are converted to executable physical instructions. The deeper stimulus of the frontal cortex is of course the prefrontal cortex and the inner self.

A significant part of the command center is the harmonic synchronization between the body and the waveforms of the larger universe. This synchronization takes place among this *chakra* region, more specifically around the pineal gland and its innervations. Within the pineal gland is a network of SCN cells. Here the body's master clock and the pacing of time are orchestrated with the infusion of light. As these SCN cells respond to light, they also broadcast in waveforms to synchronize the other body clock systems around the body. Some of this process takes place with a hormone pathway between the pineal gland, the pituitary gland and the hypothalamus. This center also uses subtle waveform broadcasting mechanisms to stimulate the network of clockwork genes around the body. Our research has yet to catch up with this technology, just as our research has yet to fully understand and characterize the waveforms of the mind.

This sixth *chakra* region is positioned above and aloof of the first five *chakra* regions. These five 'gross physical' *chakra* centers directly convert and translate particular types of intentions to physical action. The first five *chakras* can also be programmed for response, and synchronized with each other to respond congruently. This ability of the self to organize and program the first five *chakras* all lies within the facility of the sixth *chakra* region.

Thus through this *chakra* region the subtle intentions of the inner self translate into the waveform web we refer to as the mind. As intentions are converted to the more significant brainwaves, they are further translated through the limbic system. The limbic system is composed of a number of devices that each translates these waveforms from the mind into physical activity. These include the thalamus, the hippocampus, the amygdale, the gyrus of cingulated and fornicate, the hypothalamus, the nucleus accumbens, the mammillary body, the orbitofrontal cortex, and the parahippocampal gyrus. These various centers negotiate the impulses between the mind and the sensory nerves, into activity stimulus and memory waveforms to be crystallized into storage neurons. This takes place through a constant sorting of the interference patterns of billions of back and forth response-feedback waveform impulses from around the body. These are also mixed with the waveform pulses emanating from the intentional inner self.

Many of the subtle energies of the mind are translated through the hypothalamus, which, after a waveform hand shaking with the pineal gland, stimulates master hormone release by the pituitary gland. Through this release, the pituitary gland stimulates the endocrine systems around the body. This is accomplished through the production of key neurochemical messengers, including growth hormone (GH) sent to the liver to encourage protein synthesis; thyroid stimulating hormone (TSH) to stimulate the thyroid gland secretions of T3 and T4; prolactin to stimulate breast milk production; ACTH to stimulate the adrenal glands; follicle stimulating hormone (FSH) to stimulate both the testes and ovarian follicles in their production of sperm, estrogen and others; luteinizing hormone (LH) to stimulate the production of progesterone and testosterone; ADH to stimulate blood vessel wall constriction; and oxytocin to stimulate the contraction of the uterus and stimulate breast milk release. All these secondary release mechanisms resonate with other specific *chakra* regions, and this resonation would be considered a cascading harmonic process, as these master waveforms synchronize with the various other *chakra* regions down through the spine.

The self utilizes these facilities of the sixth *chakra* region to also draw out a direction or process to implement our desires and intentions. We utilize the sixth *chakra*'s intuitive channeling to the inner self to design creative programming tools to orchestrate and harmonize the body's functions. The ultimate 'hologram' of the body is conceived in the sixth *chakra*, formed from the inner self's desires and consciousness. This holographic model allows the self to manipulate the command center of the sixth *chakra* to design methods to accomplish our desires through stimulating individual *chakras*. This might be similar to a person having a small-scale model of a building to formulate the various elements and rules by first arranging them on the small-scale model. Through the sixth *chakra* region, the self can also express our desires and objectives through the virtual hologram of dreaming. Typical dreams consist of the utilization of the various crystallized sensory inputs and memories gathered within the web of the mind and memory to play out an assortment of situations. These situations can be ridiculous as well as educational. This facility is thus used to work out problems or dilemmas. Sometimes the mind can even stretch this facility to extend dreams and thoughts into the physical environment. These abilities, together with the various other extrasensory mental abilities studied by parapsychologists, indicate that the mind is able to generate subtle magnetic field pulses that interfere with the geomagnetic field surrounding us.

The skin of the human body will easily fluctuate with temperature ranges of several degrees. However, the skin in front of the sixth *chakra* region (between the eyebrows) will register and respond to temperature changes of as little as one-sixtieth of one degree. Some researchers have proposed that the mysterious stimulation of the blind person's pineal-pituitary-hypothalamus complex and SCN cells is via these sensitive nerve endings located in the skin in front of this region. Perhaps these nerve impulses reciprocate with the special clock receptors in the eyes to communicate the light stimulation.

These characteristics are also expressed through the body's immune system via the sixth *chakra* region. Via the pathways of the various antibodies and macrophages, the self expresses our governance and judgment upon the "good" and "bad" elements within the body. Through this facility, these special cells electromagnetically scan each and every cell and every invader into the body. This scanning system requires an intricate broadcasting effort that carefully matches specific molecular information with a holographic mapping system of the body. This sets up a harmonic that allows each immune cell to activate specifically only against invading entities or existing cells that create risk for the organism as a whole. We could probably compare this process with cars utilizing GPS maps for directions. Each car only needs a section of the map, but it downloads that section or sections from a central database that contains the all the maps. The mapping system facilitated by the sixth *chakra* region provides the main database.

The sixth *chakra* region is said to reflect with white-bluish frequencies. It is thought to vibrate in the shape of a circle with two luminous petals. This *chakra* region also channels cognition, awareness, penance, clairvoyance, intuition, and brilliance. In addition, this *chakra* balances the conscious emotions of mercy, gentleness and compassion. The elemental layer of this *chakra* region is an amalgam of the other elemental states. Thus, this *chakra* region is often referred to as containing the three basic drivers of the three *gunas* of the organism, namely goodness, passion and ignorance.

The Bridge

In between the sixth *chakra* and the seventh *chakra* is a gateway that provides the bridge between the inner self and the mind. It is called the *soma chakra,* and located in a position referred to as the prefrontal cortex. *Soma* is usually referred to as 'nectar' or 'moon.' The moon signifies illumination, and nectar signifies desire. This gateway is often referred to as a 'minor *chakra'* because it does not provide the full conversion of consciousness to physical action, yet it does provide executive function. Rather, the *soma chakra* is a viewing station and steering module for the self and our desires. These arise from waveforms organized within the frontal cortex and neocortex. This viewing allows the self to ultimately access the body and mind, and steer the functions of the sixth *chakra,* which ultimately sets up the programs that orchestrate the five elemental *chakras* of physical action.

Often we hear references to "the third eye" and its ability to see into the future. Actually, this is a somewhat shallow version of this *chakra* region. Through this access region, the inner self channels intelligence and conscience, which balances the *yin* and *yang* of physical existence—the duality of life—together with intuitive concepts of good and bad, and happiness and sadness. Through conscience, the self is able to connect action to reaction, and consequences to learning. It is through this *chakra* center the guilty conscience is channeled, along our intuitive search for knowledge and fulfillment.

In other words, the *soma chakra* provides a window for the self to view and steer the grand programming designs. We might compare it with the window and dashboard instruments of an airplane. The self might be compared to the pilot, who constantly views the plane's speed, direction, altitude, fuel content and so on. The *soma chakra* provides the inner self a projection of the mind's images, input from the body, and programming dialog. With these, the self can steer according to our desires.

The self can thus watch from this perspective, and input our desires and objectives into prioritizing the processing that takes place in the sixth *chakra.* The sixth *chakra* is the command center, calculating the programming according to the intentions of the self as directed through the gateway of the *soma chakra.* Thus, the *soma chakra* provides the interface between the self and the mind, allowing the self to view not only the input and programming from the command center, but the ability to stimulate subtle changes.

Again we can compare this to driving an automobile. When a person is driving on the freeway and all the gears, motor and electrical systems are working, there is little need for large adjustments in the steering wheel. Just slight adjustments will keep the car in the lane. Even when ready to turn or stop, the driver actually does very little to stop the car. He may take the foot off the gas and press the brake a little, but the preprogramming among the car's gears, brakes, motor and wheels do the big work. The driver makes slight adjustments. This is analogous to the self's steering of the entire process of the mind and all the physical activity centers of the body. The self is on another platform, viewing the process through the instrumentation, and making slight adjustments to keep the body on the freeway of physical life.

The Doorway

The seventh *chakra* is complex because it is said to contain several different sub-features that, depending upon the spiritual development of the inner self, may or may not be developed. At the crown of the cranium, we typically find a slight indent at a spot called the *fontanel.* In babies, this spot is more pronounced, and it is typically soft, until the bones of the skull grow together. The takes place as the inner self becomes increasingly entrained into the physical body.

Sahasrara is the name of this *chakra* region. *Sahasrara* means *"thousand petalled."* Some also refer to this *chakra* as the *crown chakra.*

The seventh *chakra* region resonates with the activities of the higher intellectual abilities that govern logic, justice, and intelligence. Thus through this center the inner self can resonate with the higher Authority.

The seventh *chakra* region also channels our sense of direction from a deeper realm. This direction becomes evident should we mature in our spiritual evolution. Our sense of direction with regard to desires involving the more mundane elements of our existence are channeled through the *soma chakra* into the sixth *chakra.* Therefore, this seventh *chakra* region channels not only a deeper sense of direction, but also our ultimate sense of purpose.

The inner self thus draws our creative abilities through the doorway, from a greater Source of creativity. Our processes of intuition and intelligence are also drawn from within the doorway. We also draw from this deeper realm, understandings we might describe as 'coming from within.' The self is the driver that embellishes our desires through lower *chakra* function. The doorway provides access to a larger realm of consciousness.

Throughout the physical body's younger years, the seventh *chakra* region resonates with the relationship and guidance of the body's physical father. The father of our physical body represents our early guiding principles. Should our relationship with our father be abnormal, we may experience a shunting of this subtle *chakra* region, bringing about a state of isolation and irregular relationships. However, a normal relationship with ones earthly father—especially one who provides a guiding hand—produces a progressive evolution with this *chakra.* As this relationship naturally wanes during young adulthood, the intellect begins to develop and ones personal search for Truth expands. Along with this intellectual growth come rational thinking, logic and analysis. Progress in this opens the seventh *chakra* region further, helping to awaken greater realization.

A person consistently translating intentions at the level of this *chakra* region is considered working at the highest levels of productivity and growth as an individual. We often see this in evolved philosophers who tend to focus their energies upon the mysteries of life. Still reaching the doorway is a difficult step according to *Ayurveda.* On the inside of the doorway is the veil of false ego—concealing the doorway with the false sense of identity that we are our temporary physical bodies. Outside the doorway of course is the realm of the spiritual or transcendental. A process of detaching from the temporary desires associated with the physical world is required to gain entry through this doorway. For this reason, there are a number of advanced devotional practices described in the ancient Vedic texts to prepare one for gaining access to the "other side." The "other side" of this *chakra* doorway is considered spiritual perfection in *Ayurveda.* Most Vedic texts define this as the *Brahman.* Some define *Brahman* as an impersonal white light or effulgence; other texts have defined the ultimate *Brahman* more specifically as the Almighty.

The ancient practice of *kundalini* is described as the development of the ability to raise the life air through the chain of *chakras* and up through this seventh *chakra* region. This skill is considered quite rare during this era, although the Ayurvedic and TCM texts contain descriptions of yogis who accomplished this feat.

Incidentally, there is a basic misunderstanding regarding the Vedic term *"yoga."* It has largely been mistranslated and misinterpreted to mean a practice of twisting into various difficult postures, and/or particular breathing techniques. *Yoga* is more directly translated as "link up with the Supreme." Although one type of *yoga* called *hatha yoga* does include postures to prepare the body for meditation, this is considered a preparatory step on the path towards enlightenment. There are a number of other types of *yoga*—all outside the breadth of this discussion.

Channels of Nadi

A close translation of the word *nadi* is *'motion.'* This is because the *nadis* provide channels for the movement of conscious waveforms. The *nadis* provide the network of channels for the various waveforms that move through the body, originating from the intentions of the inner self and translated through the *chakra* regions. The *nadi* channel system is thus the network for communications between the inner self and the outer physical body.

The *nadi* channel networks each circulate unique waveforms that resonate within the mediums of the solid, liquid, gas, thermal and plasma-aether states. According to ancient Vedic texts, there are hundreds of thousands of these channels circulating the airs of the body, each originating from a particular *chakra*. Some sources have specifically named over 72,000 *nadis*. The basic types of channels connect the various organs, glands and tissue systems, linking them with a particular *chakra* region. Each type of *nadi* network will resonate with the waveforms related with its connected *chakra*. Thus, we achieve a branching of nerves, bloodstream, lymphatic system, alveoli, bones, organs and cells. From these major thoroughfares, branch more minute pathways, which circulate through each cell the nutrients, enzymes and information messengers like hormones and neurotransmitters. Also through some of these *nadi* channel networks circulate more subtle waveforms to communicate specific information. These include the ion channels, the brain waves, seismic waves (like peristalsis), air and water pressure waves, thermal pulses and various electromagnetic waveforms.

The *nadi* channels thus conduct conscious waveforms of various types and specification from the senses and every tissue within the body. Balancing and switching this information like the various gateways systems within the body. These shunt some information while broadcasting other information. The main control center for these switching functions is the sixth *chakra* region as we discussed. These large and small gateway facilities are balanced in mental and physical health, and imbalanced in either mental or physical disease. The major gateways include each nostril, each eye, each ear, the mouth, the genitals, the throat, the tongue, the fontanel, and the anus. Below are a few of the primary *nadi* channel networks of *Ayurveda*. It should be noted that they often have windy and complex pathways with various forks and inclusions. They rarely form a straight line from "entry" and "exit" points.

Like the other *nadi* networks, the ***sushumna channel*** has several *nadis*, including the famed *brahma* and *sarasvati nadis*. *Sushumna* also provides the main channeling for the gross and subtle waveform channels of the seventh *chakra* region. The *sushumna* originates at the foundation *chakra* region (first) at the pelvic plexus, and runs up the spinal column. From the base of the skull, the *sushumna* branches into two directions, one anterior (front) and one posterior (back) within the skull. The anterior branch pierces the palate and moves upward and around the skull where it meets the posterior branch—which branches through the posterior skull—and terminates at the cerebrospinal axis in the gap between the two brain hemispheres. This is located at the fontanel, known for its softness. The fontanel region is also the location of the seventh energy channel as we have discussed. This channel thus provides a constant gateway for the inner self to access while in the womb. The fontanel typically stays soft through the sixth month after birth, when it begins to harden. Through this *nadi* flow the waveform currents between the grounded earth elements and the intellectual and creative elements related to artistic development and intuition. This *nadi* is well utilized in artists and other creative people, as well as those involved in philosophy and devotional practices.

The ***ida channel*** flows through the gate of the left nostril, and through the left side of the body to the groin area. It is often referred to as the *left air* channel because it flows on the left side. It also is sometimes referred to as the *inner left eye* channel. This channel supports the expression of maternal and feminine emotion and is thus nourishing, potentially purifying, and spontaneous. Closing the right nostril and breathing through the left nostril can stimulate and increase relaxation, balance and greater alertness. This is because *ida* focus stimulates the endocrine glands and the emotional, intuitive energies of the conscious body. *Ida* has also been connected to the flow of lunar energy, and thus can affect the psyche functions of the more subtle mental waveforms.

The ***pingala channel*** flows through the gate of the right nostril and through the right side of the body, terminating at the right groin region. It is considered the *inner right eye* and the *right air* channel. This channel supports masculine energies, along with verbal and rational natures. Efficiency and power are traits of this channel. As it is energized with masculine consciousness, it increases vitality, stamina and vigor. This channel also conducts the logical activities of the neural network and physical responsiveness. To stimulate the *pingala* channel one can inhale through the right nostril while closing off the left nostril. This method can also be helpful to increase strength and endurance when challenged by physical or logical stress.

The ***gandhari channel*** flows from the lower left eye corner and terminates at the left big toe. The rhythmic energy of this *chakra* region supports *ida's* feminine, intuitive waveforms. This assists in the raising of consciousness. Grasping the left big toe with the right hand while abdominal breathing can increase the circulation of the airs flowing within this channel. Abdominal breathing is vital for the overall immune health of the body and its digestive functions.

The ***hastajihva channel*** also supports the flow of the *ida* waveforms, but crosses the body from the lower corner of the right eye, and terminates at the big toe of the right foot. This crossing allows a more balanced movement of the *ida* rhythmic flows. Grasping the right big toe with the left hand while abdominal breathing can increase the circulation of this channel.

The ***yashasvini channel*** supports and balances the flow of the masculine vitality of the *pingala* waveforms. It originates in the left ear and terminates at the big toe at the right foot. Again, grasping and holding this toe, but also holding the ear with the other will increase waveform circulation within this channel. Acupressure or acupuncture can also be used to stimulate the waveforms flowing within this channel.

The ***pusha channel*** also supports the flow of the *pingala* waveforms, and runs from the right ear to the big toe of the left foot. Again, these locations can be stimulated to increase its circulation.

The ***alambusha channel*** flows between the anus and the oral cavity. Its waveforms stimulate the assimilation of food and the evacuation of digested food. This channel incorporates the vagus nerve and the action of rhythmic peristalsis. Within this channel also flow creative waveforms for new thoughts and ideas.

The ***kuhu channel*** flows between the throat and the genitals. Its waveform flows stimulate or channel the release of seminal and vaginal fluids. Its flow can also channel conscious expressions of love. For this reason, the *kuhu* is extremely important to raising consciousness. Expressing love through this channel can override the expression of sexual lust. The expression of love also increases the expression of neural talents such as memory and concentration.

The ***shankhini channel*** begins at the throat and terminates at the anus, but it is positioned between the *sarasvati* and *gardhari* channels. Through this channel flow detoxification waveforms stimulated through the colon and anus. Enemas and colon hydrotherapy (otherwise known as the *colonic)* are powerful tools to stimulate this channel. Other ways to stimulate this channel include exercise and fasting.

The ***sarasvati channel*** flows through between the gates of the tongue and throat. Its path begins at the tongue and ends at the throat. Its waveform flow extends into speech and taste. The waveforms created by our vocal cords can have various effects upon ourselves and others. With kind words, we can add harmony to the environment. With words of insult and criticism, we can add discord to our environment. Therefore, this channel can be used to express both harmony and conflict.

The ***payasvini channel*** conducts waveforms between the right earlobe and the cranial nerves. Through this channel flow the messengers related to pleasures and addictions. Acupuncture also utilizes this location for needle insertion to assist in the curing of addictions. This channel also provides a gateway for ionic travel. The traditional use of earrings on the right ear had its original basis in the stimulation of this channel with particular minerals from metals like silver, gold and copper. These metals were chosen originally because of their various effects upon health and detoxification.

The ***varuni channel*** flows in the opposite direction, parallel with the alambusha channel. Together the two channels create a polar waveform current, which stimulates the release of waste within the body. This channel originates on the left side between the throat and ear, and terminates at the anus. This channel also synchronizes with the flows of the rhythmic airs of the lower intestine. It is thus a critical channel for the colon processing and defecation.

The ***vishvodara channel*** flows between the *kuhus* and *hastajihva* channels, and localizes around the navel area. This channel is the center of the flow of the emotional waveforms reflecting the consciousness of the self. The waveform flows through this channel stimulate the activities of the various organs, including the adrenal glands, the liver and the kidneys. This channel also creates heat in these various parts of the body. We can stimulate the circulation of this networked channel by exercising the *core muscles,* of which the primary is the *rectus abdominis.* The flows of this channel can be stimulated through properly executed breathing exercises and abdominal strengthening.

Meridian Flows

A clinically manipulative sub-network channel system within the *nadi* network was expanded upon in the TCM texts approximately 3,000 years ago. Here we will summarize the twelve basic *nadi* networks, which are now referred to in TCM as *meridians.* As described in these texts and promulgated over thousands of years of clinical experience, these *meridian* channels connect and flow *qi* waveforms through twelve organ and tissue systems. *Qi* and its Sanskrit version *prana* are considered synonyms for the thermal waveforms emanating from the self. The *meridian* channels have been described as a branched subset of the *vishvodara* channel. In this view, they would be considered thermal waveforms that flow between critical organs. Others note that some of the *meridian* channels have some crossover with some of the other *nadi* channels and may transduce other waveform types. This view takes the position that *meridians* are the clinically relevant portion of some of the other *nadi* channels.

Each science has its specific focus in terms of treatments, conditions and body types. As they developed in different cultures yet likely originated from the same source, their application over the centuries may have crossed over with each other in order to establish efficacy for particular issues. As mentioned, the *nadi* system has well over 72,000 channels, and there are billions of nerve endings within just the neural network—only one *nadi* network. Obviously, there are countless channel systems within the body, which ultimately accomplish every specific metabolic and sensory operation. We would venture to say that each different waveform vehicle also operates through its own, slightly different pathway. Each pathway, whether it is biochemical, nervous, genetic, peristaltic, or ionic, will conduct through the body in a unique manner. One pathway might conduct waveforms through a portion of the bloodstream from a particular organ using a particular hormone and receptor, while another may conduct waveforms through specific neurons and specific neurotransmitters. Yet another immune pathway may travel through part of the lymphatic system. Each type of waveform conducts through the body using a unique pathway. We can extrapolate this into the more subtle waveforms that motion through the body. Each should have a unique pathway and unique cascading process.

Though others have been described, twelve central *meridians* are generally accepted in TCM. Recent research has indicated that within the *meridians* flow waveforms in the microwave and infrared (Litscher 2006). These waveforms and *meridians* allow a practitioner to directly influence the health of the body through opening or modulating the gateways of these flows. These gateways are typically referred to as *acupuncture points.* An acupuncturist will, for example, diagnose a particular set of symptoms, and determine the connection between the flow of waveforms and the possible cause of the symptoms. In some situations, the waveform flow will be blocked or otherwise modulated. In other, the flows could be imbalanced between different *meridian* channels. For example, an acupuncturist might see a liver problem being caused by the liver not having enough heat. The acupuncturist will then penetrate or manipulate particular gateways along the liver channel to stimulate heat within the organ.

Over the past few decades, thousands of studies have been performed on the clinical effectiveness of acupuncture *meridian* therapy. Many of these have been controlled and double-blinded, and many have compared electronic manipulation as well as needle therapy. In studies too numerous to document here, acupuncture has proven to be effective for the treatment of hundreds of disorders related to the nervous system, the skeletal system, the digestive system, the cardio-pulmonary system, the brain, the liver, the kidneys and various endocrine systems. A recent review of the literature reveals over 12,000 research papers and studies have been published on the therapeutic effects of acupuncture over the past few decades. Some of the more recent research illustrates efficacious acupuncture treatment for herpes (Yu *et al.* 2007), autism (Yan *et al.* 2007), paralysis (Fu, 2007), hyperlipidemia (Chu, *et al.* 2007), diabetes and pancreatic disorders (Chu *et al.* 2007; Tian *et al.* 2007; Liao *et al.* 2007), kidney diseases and chronic pain (Grasmuller and Imich 2007), insomnia (Chen *et al.* 2007), myofascial pain (Shen and Goddard 2007), arthritis (Wang *et al.* 2007), chronic fatigue (Guo 2007), hormone balance (Bai *et al.* 2007), gastrointestinal discomfort (Wang *et al.* 2007), osteoarthritis (Brinkhaus *et al.* 2007), lipid metabolism (Kang *et al.* 2007), Sjogren's Syndrome (Bai *et al.* 2007), cancer pain (Cassileth *et al.* 2007), and many others.

In the early 1980s, the Shanghai Institute performed exhaustive research on the various physiological effects of acupuncture therapy. Their research concluded immune system stimulation, cardiovascular improvement, digestive function improvement and many other positive effects from acupuncture treatments. They also confirmed that acupuncture significantly increases or otherwise modulates the secretion of various hormones, including oxytocin, vasopressin, follicle stimulating hormone, corticosteroids, ACTH, and norepinephrine (O'Connor and Bensky 1981).

Today many western hospitals are using acupuncture for chronic pain, surgery, childbirth, and speeding the healing response. The quality of training and its long safety record give acupuncture therapy one of the best health records of any clinical and acute therapy. For this reason, a growing number of disorders are now being referred to acupuncturists.

The *meridians* are waveform vessels conducting particular frequencies that in essence circulate consciousness through the body. They are invisible to the naked eye and gross instruments. This is simply because these waveforms conduct with lower power and amplitude than we typically measure. Here are the main twelve utilized in acupuncture therapy. Each *meridian* channel is considered to be connected to a particular organ system, and each has either a *yin* or *yang* feature. Most also consist of two channels, one on the right side of the body and another on the left side. Here is a description of the twelve *meridians* and some of their characteristics:

Liver (Liv) is a paired set of channels also called the *lower yin meridian.* They run from inside the big toes up the inner (medial) legs and out to the hips, where they travel up through the rib cage on the side under the arm and towards the midline where they end under the breasts. The liver *meridian* resonates greatest between one a.m. and three a.m.

Lung (L) is another paired arm set also called the *upper yin meridian.* They travel from the nail-side of the thumbs up the medial (inside) arms to the front of the shoulder and then down the chest, ending above the breasts at the pectoral muscles. This *meridian* pair is most active between three a.m. and five a.m.

Large intestine (Li) is also a paired arm set also called the *upper yang meridian.* They start at the index fingernails and run directly up the top of the arms, over the shoulders and up the neck and jaw to the upper lip, where they split to end just outside the nostrils. They are most active between five and seven a.m.

Stomach (S) is a paired leg set also called the *lower yang meridian.* They start under the eyes on each side, circle down through the cheek and back, heading over the forehead and down next to the inside of the eyes near the nose bridge, and down the front side of the neck, down each breast, abdomen and legs, ending at the second toe. This *meridian* pair peaks in activity between seven and nine a.m.

Spleen-pancreas (S) is a paired leg set also called the *lower yin meridian.* They travel from the big toes up the inside of the legs, up the abdominal region to underneath the armpits and back down toward the outside of the ribcage. This *meridian* pair is typically most active between nine and eleven a.m.

Heart (H) is a paired arm set also called the *upper yin meridian.* They start at the inside of the pinkies and head up the inside of the arm to the arm-side of the armpits. They are most active between eleven a.m. and one p.m.

Small intestine (Si) is a paired arm set also called the *upper yang meridian.* They start at the outside of the pinkies and flow straight over the shoulder, down over the scapulae (shoulder blades) and then up the neck to the cheekbones, where they run back towards the ears. They are most active between one p.m. and three p.m.

Bladder (B) is a paired lower leg set also called the *lower yang meridian.* They start between the eyebrows and head up over the top of the head and then down the back of the head, neck and back, over the buttocks—

ending at the little toes on each side. They are most active between three p.m. and five p.m. everyday.

Kidney (K) is a paired lower leg set also called the *lower yin meridian.* They start at the bottom of the feet and head up the inside of the legs, up the midline of the abdomen and chest, ending at the sternum area. They are most active between five p.m. and seven p.m. each day.

Pericardium (P) set is also called the *heart constrictor meridian.* Some also call this the *circulation-sex meridian.* They travel up the outside of the breasts on each side up the armpits and up the arms ending at the middle fingers. They are most active between seven and nine p.m.

Triplewarmer (T) is a paired arm set also called the *upper yang meridian.* They start at the ring fingers and head up the outside of the arms, shoulders and neck and up around the ears—ending at the temples. They are most active between nine p.m. and eleven p.m.

Gallbladder (G) is a paired lower leg set also called the *lower yang meridian.* They start at the second toes, head up the outside of the legs, up the obliques, over the back shoulders up the neck over the crown and then back around the ears—ending at the temples. They are most active between eleven p.m. and one a.m.

Conception vessel (Cv) and ***Governor vessel (Gv)*** are both unpaired mid-body line *meridians.* They serve to balance the body from the front and back. The Cv starts at the pubic bone and travels up the midline of the abdomen, chest, neck and chin to just below the lower lip. The Gv starts at the tailbone and heads up the spine, neck and over the top of the head—ending at just above the upper lip.

The ***auricular channels*** are located around the ear. According to TCM, within the ear pinna anatomy exists a holographic image of the entire body. Therefore, the auricular points may be stimulated simultaneous to the stimulation of the main *meridian* points, or even alone to stimulate particular organs or channels.

The piercing of the acupuncture points with needles is not a physical necessity to modulate the waveform gateways. This is one strategy allowing the waveform energy of the practitioner to be transferred via the needle into the *meridian* vessel. This will typically increase the waveform flow through the vessel and open the gateways, although the treatment may also require a slowing of the flow. Contrary to popular belief, the needles do not accomplish this. The change is accomplished by the practitioner's own conductivity, interfering with the flow of the waveforms within that particular channel. The acupuncturist simply utilizes the needle as a transducer or conductor for the waveform flow.

This might be compared to splicing a wire into an electrical circuit. A dangling wire without any connection to anything else will not affect the flow of electricity within a circuit. However, as soon as that wire is connected to another circuit or electrical source, there is an immediate change to the circuit. In the same way, a needle in itself inserted into an acupuncture channel will have no effect. The focused intentional conductivity of the practitioner is being inserted into the channel. The needle is simply a carrier, as the wire is a carrier of electricity. Therefore, we must consider our acupuncturist's qualifications and patient reviews carefully before a treatment.

There are many other established means to stimulate or modulate *meridian* conduction, including trigger-point, *acupressure* (finger and thumb pressure), electronic impulse, and *moxibustion* (the burning of the mugwort herb and putting the smolder onto the points). One of the newer techniques to stimulate the *meridians* is through laser. As Sutherland pointed out in 2000, the term *meridian therapy* is a better description than acupuncture, because there are many efficacious alternatives to piercing the skin.

In other words, the same waveform modulating effects of needle acupuncture may be transmitted via the human hand, thumb, finger, burning herb, electromagnetic signal and now laser. The elbow, palm or foot can also be used. This method of applying pressure to *meridian* or acupuncture points within the context of massage is called *Shiatsu*. Again, it is the skill of the practitioner that translates to success in *meridian* therapy—not the device being utilized. The practitioner could theoretically conduct waveform modulation through almost any vehicle assuming the right skill level and healing intentions.

Acupressure technique may be attempted by oneself with guidance from literature or from professionals on the particular points of interaction. The safest way to apply pressure for someone not trained is to use the heel of the thumb. As the heel is applied to the point, it can be massaged in a deep, slow, circular manner *in the direction of the meridian flow.* Slowly and rhythmically massaging points along the *meridian* will serve to strengthen the organs and stimulate the waveform flow through those *meridian* channels. A number of good references published by professionals illustrate the specific points to massage. For best results, a skilled practitioner is recommended, however. Acupuncturists undergo rigorous training to not only learn the technique of needle insertion into the proper point with the correction intention and consciousness, but also learn other methods of modulating the *meridians*. They also practice five-element healing and herbalism. Visiting an acupuncturist remains about the best healing value in medicine today.

The TCM acupuncture system has located and mapped about 500 specific gateway points on the twelve *meridians*. Almost any deficiency of a particular organ or area intersected by a *meridian* channel can be energized by treating or even massaging the channel. Benefit may also be obtained by lightly massaging a channel over the entire *meridian* length; or even by *tracing* over it (Eden, 1998) without physically touching the skin.

Chapter Four

The Sentient Senses

According to the Ayurvedic sciences there are seven sense organs. Their inputs are organized by the mind's programming. After sensory nerves conduct sensory waveforms into their respective cortex, they are translated by the cortex neurons into waveforms that provide holographic reflections of the sensory images. As streams of these waveform reflections converge, they form holographic waveform interference patterns. These collective patterns create reflective images, and provide a viewing screen for the self. The mind's programming initially prioritizes and organizes these incoming images according to the self's goals and objectives, to filter the images before viewing. Once viewed by the self, the mind's programming orchestrates their prioritization for memory storage. According to *Ayurveda*, the seven senses and their sense organs are:

- The sense of sound: the ears
- The sense of touch: the skin
- The sense of vision: the eyes
- The sense of taste: the tongue
- The sense of smell: the nose
- The sense of defecation: the anus
- The sense of sex: the genitals

In *Ayurveda,* the seven senses are compared to seven horses drawing a chariot. The chariot's reins are compared to the mind, and in the chariot rides the self. This analogy is used because either the senses can be tamed by the intelligence (the reins) or the senses can run wild and carry the chariot out of control. In the same way, each of us has the ability to utilize the mind to control the senses for particular purposes.

The senses essentially import the raw data for the mind's view of the world around us. This naturally means that the mind is limited by the inputs given to it by the senses. The mind also receives input from the self as well. The mind's programming is created by the intentions of the self. The self in turn can draw from a deeper identity. This is often referred to as intuition, while some have called this the sub-conscious mind.

Many of us do not trust intuition because it is not physically recognizable. Intuition is real, however. There are many instances of people recognizing the need for action on an intuitive level and being right on the money. Therefore, some have described intuition as a sense: As in the *sense of intuition.* It should be clarified however, that this is not a physical sense organ, but a subset of intelligence. Like intelligence, intuition comes from a deeper source of information.

The body's sense organs coordinate their activity with the outside world through a process of waveform reception, conversion and projection. Reception is performed by groups of special neurons that collectively make up each sense organ. Each of these neurons is composed of specialized receptors. Each receptor is tuned to a particular type of waveform with a particular frequency and amplitude. The receptor and neural pathway then converts those waveforms to unique electromagnetic informational pulses. These informational pulses are conducted through specialized neural superhighways to the designated cortical center where they are projected onto the mind.

The Optical Reflection

Our eyes sense the world around us through the reception, conversion and transmission of waveforms that reflect the visible light portion of the electromagnetic spectrum. The eyes are cylindrical (sinusoidal) with an adjustable lens and shuttering mechanism to focus and limit the entry of light to specific waveforms. The cornea, the aqueous fluid, the iris, pupils, lens, and ciliary muscles all operate in a coordinated fashion to focus on a specific range of wavelengths, frequencies, and amplitudes. The eyes blink and the pupils contract to filter out waveforms, images, or debris that would otherwise disrupt the images we expect to see. These facilities of the eye are all pre-programmed to accomplish the intentions of the self to see the world in a particular light.

Once the lens mechanics do their work to narrow in on particular waveform ranges, inverted light is filtered through the cornea and lens and inversely reflected onto the retina. The retina is made up of specialized waveform-sensitive receptors. Some one hundred and twenty-five million narrow receptors called *rods* are sensitized to light and darkness. Another estimated seven million round photoreceptors called *cones* gauge color and depth. The underlying nerve cells use the rods and cones as waveform conversion devices. They effectively translate waveforms of visible light into bioelectromagnetic nerve pulses. These waveforms are conducted through neuron ion channels that provide a pathway through the millions of nerve fibers that make up the optic nerve.

The area where the optic nerve connects to the back of the retina has no rods or cones. This is referred to as the eye's *blind spot* or *optic disc.* To see our blind spot we can simply look at an image with one eye covered and move our perspective until the uncovered eye loses sight of a particular object.

As mentioned, the eyes are trained to pick up specific waveforms of reflected light and not others. They typically do not pick up wavelengths outside of 380 to 760 nanometers. Each type of retinal receptor is also limited in its scope. The rods are sensitive to brightness. They contain a light sensitive photo-pigment called *rhodopsin.* The rods thus respond to lightness or grayness—but not color. Their input is grayscale.

The cones are the color sensor photoreceptors. There are three types of cones: Red cones respond to primarily wavelengths in the red spectrum. Green cones respond primarily to green spectrum wavelengths. Blue cones respond primarily to blue spectrum wavelengths. As a painter's palette may combine these basic three colors to make up the various other colors, wavelengths with different color traits are blended to communicate a particular color.

In the center of the retina is a circular indentation filled with a greater density of cones used for focusing upon brightly lit objects. This is called the *macula.* The macula's cones have direct nerve pathways to the brain when compared to the more spread out rods and cones of the retina. Thus images received through the macular cones tend to be more distinctive and sharp than images received through the more spread out pigments among the retina. This design allows us to center and fix our eyes upon the visible zones directly in front of our eyes. This allows us to focus upon the views we are most interested in as we turn our heads. Conversely, this focal point allows us to unfocus waveforms of images in which we are not particularly interested.

Our vision is also limited by a number of other factors. Waveforms outside the wavelength range will typically not be converted into impulses. It is unlikely they will even register through the optic nerve mechanism. This is not to say waveforms outside of these wavelengths do not exist or are not visible using the right equipment. The concept of *visible spectrum* is based solely upon our visible range. The 'visible spectrum' for other organisms differ from that of humans. Human technology has also unveiled many other electromagnetic waveform spectra outside the visible spectrum. Even so, many physicists agree that we are still only aware of a tiny sliver of the entire electromagnetic spectrum.

During nerve transmission, visual waveforms also undergo filtration as they are translated through the neurotransmitters within the optic nerve. The chemistry of the neurotransmitter fluid is designed to filter and modulate waveforms, screening out incompatible or unwanted waveforms while leaving others emphasized. Drugs and alcohol can further affect the neurotransmitter content, causing a further alteration of waveforms as they pass through the optic nerve.

The intention of the self also affects neurotransmitter content and waveform filtration. The self's subtle programming of the mind also modulates the acuity mechanisms of the lens and pupils—as focus is centered upon the subjects that interest us the most.

The optic nerve provides the pathway for waveforms translated through the retinal cells to the *lateral geniculate nucleus* (or *LGN*) located within the thalamus. The LGN is made up of a series of bent neuron layers, which alternatively receive visual waveforms through the optic nerve while performing a sorting or integrating function. Each LGN layer also has a unique combination of cell types, and each cell type appears to process a different part of the information. For example, *parvocellular cells* integrate color and detail about the images, while *magnocellular cells* conduct a short-term integration of images without a lot of detail. *Koniocellular cells,* on the other hand, integrate other sensory information with the images, adding texture or *somato* information. Research has so far discovered six types of LGN cells, some of which integrate waveforms while others provide cancellation in order to spatially assemble and convert images (De Valois *et al.* 1966). Once sorted and converged through the LGN, the resulting waveforms are pulsed to the V1 portion of the visual cortex. Here they interfere with other projecting waveforms to create a mapped screen for the self to observe.

This last point is important to understand clearly. Individual waveforms reflecting through a specific rod or cone and relayed via the optic nerve have no meaning alone. Rather, it is the converging of multiple waveforms into an interference pattern that projects an image onto the mind. Without this convergence, there would be no information contained within the image. A single waveform would appear merely as a single band of color and light. We might compare this to looking at one pixel on a computer screen. That one pixel will convey no image in itself. Vision is not a singly pulse or view of a particular object. It is the confluence of waveforms that creates the total image.

Furthermore, the eyes are designed to receive waveforms from reflected light. These reflected images give shape and contour to vision. When we look directly at a light source, we generally only see a rounded image with rays bursting from all edges. We can look directly at some light sources, like fires and stars. Even still, their images are quite fuzzy.

If light does not reflect off an object at just the right angle, the eyes will not transmit an image of that object. The object will be invisible. Objects with different densities or molecular structures reflect light differently. This is why we cannot see air. An object with the wrong density or molecular structure will thus appear not to exist.

We cannot see in pitch-blackness because light is not being reflected off any objects. Even if we can see an object in partial darkness, we will still probably not see its color. The rods do not pick up color wavelengths well in dim light. The cones also need wavelengths with a minimum of light intensity. As a result, our eyes are almost useless in a dark closet. The little light that may seep under the door may allow us to see a few dark shadows. Without the right range of light reflection, however, there will be no visible perception. If we are smart, we will feel our way around the closet. The tactile sensory nerves also project waveforms for the self to observe.

Meanwhile, many animals—such as foxes, wolves, owls and rodents—can see quite clearly in the darkness. Their eyes have larger pupils to let in more light than ours can. They also have more of the photosensitive pigment *rhodopsin* within their rods. Many nocturnal animals also have a thick reflective membrane under the retina called the *tapetum lucidum* (the reason why these animals' eyes glow at night). The rhodopsin pigment lowers the threshold for light reflection. The tapetum reflects a second image onto the rods. This increases the nerve cells' ability to convert rod imagery into nerve pulses. Other organisms see colors differently. Ants do not see red. Deer and rabbits see primarily in grey shades. Prairie dogs cannot see red or green. Owls are altogether colorblind. Insects see the world in much greater curvature than humans do—much like looking through a thick crystal ball. Some insects like butterflies see in ultraviolet range. Other creatures can see infrared wavelengths.

Furthermore, if a fish were to look up into the air above the water, most likely he would see everything within a circular orb—much like an insect would. This is because of the refractive index of water. The fish's view would thus be circular, simply because the view of the eye is at one point, and the light bending in would have an angle of forty-nine degrees from zenith as opposed to the ninety degrees from zenith (according to our measurement) as the human eye perceives. The total difference or refraction then would approach forty-one degrees, inward toward the fish's point of perspective. Therefore, fish have the perception of the world outside of the water as circular. Trees, buildings, and other items are curved inward, with everything condensed within an orb.

Fish also pick up different ranges of waveforms. Many fish have the rhodopsin-based pigment *kyurenine* allowing absorption at the 370-nanometer range, *mycosporine*-like amino acids allowing absorption in the 300-360 nm range, and carotenoids allowing absorption in the 425-480 nm range. Many fish and amphibians also have *porphropsins,* rendering a range in the 625 nm region. This mix of photoreceptors among various species of fish—especially deep-water fish whose photoreception is geared to the dim-lights of the deep-water environment—make many fish blind outside the medium of water. A fish's photoreceptors are entrained to the refracted spectra within water and their sclera are conditioned for water. Thus, many images we see in our atmosphere above the surface of the water simply cannot be observed by the fish. For this reason, some fish are practically blind outside of water. This scenario is logically applicable to the limitations of human acuity. Evangelista Torricelli thus wrote in a 1644 letter, *"We live submerged at the bottom of an ocean of air."*

Invertebrates and vertebrates alike also have varying sorts of imaging photoreceptors lacking in humans. Reptiles for example have photoreceptors in the area between the eyes known as the *pineal zone.* Photoreceptor sites among other species include the *harderian gland* and *chromatophores*—light receptors on the skin of amphibians and fish. Most do not have the photoreception picked up by our rods. Many, however, do have visual and light reception ranges our eyes do not (Lithgoe 1984).

There are also forms of life around us that barely if at all reflect light. Certain jellyfish and bacteria varieties, for example, have only been discovered recently because they blend in to their environment. They reflect practically no light as a defense mechanism. Only through special instruments and staining techniques have we been able to see some of these organisms. Noting that light must be reflected for our vision, we can easily assume there are a number of other life forms we have yet to observe. Varying densities or molecular structures could very well eliminate the opportunity for visible light to reflect in a number of species.

The shape of our eyes is critical for vision. Should the cylindrical nature of the eyeball become distorted due to nutrient deficiency, free radical damage, aging or infection, our ability to see becomes further obstructed. Disorders such as *myopia* and its jealous cousin *hyperopia* can be the result. Myopia is typically considered being *near-sighted,* and hyperopia is considered being *far-sighted.* In near-sightedness, far-away objects will appear distorted and blurred. This is typically caused by a lengthening of the eyeball or steepness in the cornea. Once the circular nature of the eye is distorted, the image will fall onto the wrong area of the eyeball. The other problem—hyperopia—is caused by the opposite effect: A shortening of the eyeball or a flattening of the cornea. In other words, vision is a circular affair. Without our eyes' natural circular shape, our vision is disrupted. It is notable that the larger aspects of the universe around us appear for the most part circular. We must therefore ask ourselves how much of our rounded view of the outer world of planets and sun could be a result of this curvature combined with the refractive elements in the atmosphere? Could the curved shape of our eyeballs create a distortion just as we noticed for the fish viewing life outside the pond?

Just as the fish are limited to their water world of visual range, human eyes are limited by the atmosphere our senses perceive. For example, we cannot see through more dense matter such as rock or mercury. We can see through clear water, but visible light traveling through water renders fuzzy and non-distinct images for us, unless we dawn masks or other underwater screening equipment. Although water is an atmosphere familiar to us, waves of the visible spectrum will still travel substantially differently in water than they do within our oxygen-nitrogen-carbon atmosphere. Light will bend through water, distorting accuracy and dimension.

This phenomenon was described by Dutch astronomer Willebord Snell in the early seventeenth century, and now referred to as *Snell's Law of Refraction.* This law takes into account the refractive index differential between two mediums, and the resulting angle variance of a beam. Refractive index is a relative calculation: A comparison between the waveform transmissions through one medium compared with another medium.

Of course, the situation becomes exponentially more complicated when we extend this refractive quantification beyond a single beam of light and a comparison of water and air. Within an expansive environment of multiple mediums with different densities and radiation made up of different waveforms, relative refractive indices can alter a host of waveforms, translating to different shapes and colors among each medium.

Our exploration of outer space has confirmed to us that there are numerous atmospheres. Spectroscopy methods and in the case of Mars and the Moon, direct measurement tells us that each planet contains a unique type of atmosphere. For example, Mars appears to have an atmosphere composed primarily of methane. Saturn appears to have an atmosphere made primarily of sulphur. Under Snell's Law, in each of these different atmospheres, light should bend and refract differently. Could it be that the refractive and reflective differences of these atmospheres simply position objects and possibly even life forms outside of our sensory and instrumental ranges? Just as we see among insects, fish and other organisms when compared to humans, could our senses be specifically tuned to the atmosphere of nitrogen-oxygen and not capable of perceiving others?

Just as we consider water a denser atmosphere with different refractive and reflective characteristics, different planetary atmospheres should also refract and reflect light differently. Furthermore, just as in water, different atmospheres should be suitable only for specific types of molecular structures with particular densities and metabolic function. As a result, objects or living organisms within different atmospheres may simply not be visible to human eyes or those instruments designed for our atmosphere. We are reminded of the mystery of the unmistakable waterways lining Mars. Perhaps the type of water that circulates around Mars is simply not within the molecular scope of our range of vision. Perhaps many of our surrounding planets also have life outside of our molecular scope.

The unmistakable deception our physical eyes present to us is illustrated by the illusion of watching television or cinema. There in front of us, flashing on the screen, is a series of still photographs—each one slightly different from the previous. Each still picture is replaced by another still picture at a rate of some twenty-four frames per second. Meanwhile our eyes, LGN, visual cortex and mind can only process at a rate of about fifty or sixty images per second. As a result, while our eyes and minds are ambling through one photograph, another is flashed. This blurs the two images together, giving us the false impression of movement. We fail to see that about half the time we spend watching TV or a movie we are actually looking at a blank screen.

Seeing is not actually taking place within any of the anatomy anyway. The eyes, optic nerve and brain are simply transmitters—like an antenna and video terminal. All of these instruments merely receive, convert and relay informational waveforms of particular specification. Once the information waves pass through the optic nerve they are mapped through the visual cortex and reflected interactively among neurons that resonate with those waveforms. These interactive waveform reflections create a sort of mental mapping system. This mapping creates a holographic 'screen-shot' of the image onto the mind. This facsimile of the image might be compared to a scan or copy.

The act of seeing is quite different from this holographic screen shot. *Seeing* is what takes place by a *seer*. Seeing thus requires consciousness—someone who is aware—observing what the neurons are flashing upon the screen of the mind. Moreover, the equipment this conscious seer utilizes is not absolute. The seer thus can adjust the foci of the senses to perceive what is most beneficial to the objectives of the seer.

Because of this subjective ability, we can miss so much of existence simply because we do not want to become aware of it. We will often not recognize things even when they come into plain view. Just as two people attending the same event may recall two entirely different versions of the event, we each have distinctly different recognition levels due to our expectations of the world around us. It is when we communicate and intentionally compare those views that we gain a consensus view. Sometimes this occurs after the event. Other times it may occur instantly, as we look around us for other's responses. As most of us seek the love and acceptance of others, we tend to quickly inherit the collective view.

Meanwhile, research has concluded that particular colors affect cognition, moods and behavior. Brain imaging illustrates that color stimulates corresponding brainwave patterns—linked with particular moods and behaviors. *Ayurveda* also correlates colors with particular *chakras* and energy levels. The mechanism for this subtle electromagnetic bridge is explainable using wave resonance and interference models. Touching a piano key in a room full of pianos would cause the other pianos to vibrate in the same chord. With color resonance, we can associate particular waveforms with other waveform patterns occurring within the body. These waveforms stimulate internal waveform responses.

The longer wavelengths of red colors stimulate higher frequency beta waves in the brain at more than thirteen cycles per second and wavelengths of 630-700 nanometers. Red colors tend to stimulate autonomic systems, increasing heart rate and blood pressure. Red also stimulates circulation, hostility, violence, jealousy and competition. Red stimulates passion and sexual activity. Red resonates with the first root *chakra*. Red is stimulates healing in the areas of the anus, coccygeal areas, hips and feet. Red also stimulates movement and greater energy production. Therefore, it is useful when a burst of energy is needed.

Orange stimulates high alpha brainwaves between ten cycles and thirteen cycles per second at wavelengths of 590 to 630 nanometers. Orange also stimulates energy like red, but without some of the heat or intensity that red brings. Orange is warming. It tends to encourage enthusiasm, creativity, inquisitiveness, sincerity, thoughtfulness, and decongesting effects. Orange resonates with the second *chakra* according to *Ayurveda*. This is associated with the sacral area—the back and lower spine—and the lower abdominal area. Orange stimulates appetite and colon movement. Orange resonates with aspects of family, parenting, friendships and group organizations.

Yellow stimulates lower alpha brainwaves at eight or nine cycles per second with wavelengths of 560 to 590 nanometers. This color resonates with the third *chakra* region around the solar plexus. Yellow resonates with spontaneity, compassion, memory, learning, and appetite. It stimulates the stomach, upper intestines and the adrenal glands. Yellow can thus trigger stress in certain situations. Because yellow reflects light with a greater intensity, it can be tire the eyes and mind after some time. Activities associated with yellow include memorization, study, and focus. Yellow can be cheerful, but this can also lead to fatigue with an overload. Research has illustrated that babies tend to cry more and couples tend to argue more in yellow rooms.

Green stimulates higher theta region brainwaves at six to seven cycles per second with wavelengths of 490 to 560 nanometers. Green is calming, balancing, healing, soothing and invigorating. It stimulates growth, love and a sense of security. Green resonates with the fourth heart energy center, and is therefore connected to devotion and giving. Green stimulates healing, particularly related to the cardiovascular system and lungs. Green has been shown to stimulate the immune system. Increased T-cell levels have been observed. Green tends to suppress the body's endogenous melatonin, aiding the body to cool down, relax and sleep. Green also stimulates problem solving, negotiation and resolution.

Blue stimulates lower theta waves in the five to six cycles per second at wavelengths of 450 to 490 nanometers. Blue is cooling, calming and stable. Blue resonates at the fifth *chakra* region. Therefore blue is associated with the lungs, breathing, sound, and thyroid function. As the thyroid is part of the temperature regulating system, it helps stabilize core body temperature and the cellular metabolism rates. Blue stimulates creativity and communication. Blue also stimulates detoxification and purification systems within the body. Blue is a very good color for over-active children and stressed situations, because it tends to calm and relax the mind.

Indigo stimulates low delta waves around one cycle per second at wavelengths of 400 to 450 nanometers. It resonates with the sixth *chakra* located in the region of the eyebrows. It is thus considered the color of the 'third eye.' Indigo is associated with clarity, decision-making, leadership and intelligence. The sinuses, vision, and the immune system are stimulated by and resonate with indigo. Activities most associated with indigo would be highly intellectual activity, humanitarian behavior, medical research, and philosophical contemplation.

Violet stimulates higher delta waves from two to four cycles per second—slightly faster than indigo. Violet waves are associated with the seventh *chakra* region. Violet is associated with consciousness and intuition. It is a color linked with personal growth and learning. It is also associated with brain circulation, spinal fluid movement, and joint fluids.

Violet activities are associated with inspiration, prayer, and spiritual insight.

Certain blended colors have yet their own unique effects. Pink has been associated with tranquilizing, sedative and muscle-relaxing effects, for example. Notably, Dr. Alexander Schauss reported in his color research that these same effects occurred among colorblind patients.

Color pigments are also nutritional and therapeutic in foods. Lycopene, curcumin, carotenes, rhodospsin, lutein, canthaxanthin, zeaxanthins, sulforaphanes, isoiocyanates, anthocyanidins, pomeratrol, pycnogenol, and other polyphenols all contribute to giving botanicals color. These pigments also provide cancer prevention, antioxidant activity and various other nutritional benefits.

It thus appears that vision and color are not as simple as we might like to think. Vision provides a waveform bridge between the physical world and the conscious self. What we decide to look at and reflect upon truly affects our consciousness, just as our consciousness affects what we perceive and take away from what we look at. It is a cycle of awareness and perception steeped in consciousness.

The Pressure Transfer

The ears also convert waveform information to bioelectromagnetic pulses. Rather than translating electromagnetic waveforms from the visual spectrum as the retina does, the auditory physiology converts air pressure waves to neuron transmissions. Sound is transmitted at frequencies much lower than visible frequencies. Sound waveforms exert pressure upon the medium created by moving air molecules, and these pressure-waves beat the eardrums, initiating an almost comical Seuss-like chain response through the middle and inner ears.

The human ear will pick up air-pressure frequencies from 20 to 20,000 cycles per second, although sensitivity is most prevalent between 1000 and 4000 cycles per second. The higher the frequency, the higher the *pitch* the sound appears to our ears. Meanwhile, louder waves have greater amplitudes.

When these pressure waves enter the external ear and into the ear canal, they first oscillate the *tympanic membrane* (eardrum) at the same frequency of the sound. With this tympanic oscillation, the pressure waveforms are transferred through the middle ear to three fragile bones—the *malleus*, *incus* and *stapes*—in such a way as to amplify them into seismic pulse form. These tiny seismic pulses are reflected through the *oval window*. The oval window vibrates the inner ear fluids and basilar membranes. The waves of the liquid membrane travel through the *basilar fiber hairs,* which translate their waveforms into bioelectromagnetic pulses within the cochlear section of the *vestibulocochlear nerve.*

These tiny hairs are considered to be at the center of this translation effort, and damage to them from acoustic shock, inadequate nutrition or aging, create hearing loss. As these tiny hairs undulate with fluidic waveforms, they bump up against a stratified ceiling membrane called the *stereocillia.* When the stereocillia sections are bumped by the hairs, they open ion channel gates. These ion channel gates stimulate an electromagnetic pulse through the cochlear nerve system. The cerebral cortex of the temporal lobe is activated first with these pulses. It is believed that auditory waveforms move through neural pathways to trigger synapse responses within the *medulla*, the *midbrain colliculi,* and the *thalamus geniculate body* of the brain. Here the impulses are converted and intermingled with other waveforms to provide interference patterns.

Recognized synapse impulses are then flashed onto the mind, where they are sorted and prioritized for viewing by the conscious self within. The entire process supports several filtering mechanisms to remove atypical frequencies, unexpected sounds, or unwanted information. As a result, noises within range may or may not be perceived by the self, even though they indeed vibrate the eardrum. Even if they are not filtered out through the inner ear, they may still be filtered as they flashed onto the mind. They also may be immediately shuffled away into the memory mapping system, as we will discuss in detail later.

Like the eyes, the auditory system only allows specific waveforms with specific parameters to be converted to nerve impulses. Dogs can hear many frequencies and amplitudes we cannot, for example. Other species pick up higher or lower frequency wavelengths. Dolphins and orcas use a sonar system with an entirely different frequency system to "hear" and "see" as well as "scope" objects at great distances.

Furthermore, we must expect to recognize certain sounds as they interface with the mind. This is required in order to consciously identify and prioritize sounds as they translate through sound pathways. These waveform-filtering mechanisms screen and prioritize sounds. This can be seen in people living next to a freeway or in a noisy city. Initially they may become irritated by the noise. After some time, they become accustomed to it. Soon they may hardly notice it.

An electrophysiological encoding takes place as sound waves are converted to mental perception. This process has been called *cortical auditory evoked potentials.* Researchers have used EEG spectra modeling to images these visualize specialized sound transmission neuron channels—called corticothalamic pathways. These produce cortical projection.

Prior to its entry into the ear canal, sound is a longitudinal wave. These waveforms undulate through air molecules without moving the medium. Longitudinal sound waves move through a matrix of resonating waveforms by interaction and interference. Wave pulses are transduced through the air molecules. It is a sort of hand-off mechanism—a conduction from one molecule to another. This conductance can be measured through pressure gradients, because the waveform interference modulates the density of waveforms within each microenvironment. This modulation of air pressure is what physically vibrates the eardrum.

We can see a similar effect as we watch a boat moving through the water. The boat's movement creates waves, which interact and ripple through the existing ripples on the water. Just as the boat is identified by its effect upon the existing water surface and existing waves, the information within sound is determined through its effect upon the air surface and waveforms already existing within the air.

A natural balance of sound waveforms is critical to the well-being of the body. Research on sound and stress has demonstrated that practically any mechanical sound over the 90 decibels level stresses the body and mind. This type of stress can be just as harmful and dangerous as any other toxic burden or stressor. Sound vibration affects not only the tympanic membrane, ear bones, cilia and neural network, but also the entire body and mind.

Research has documented these effects. Automobile traffic noise levels are often sited as major threat to health, for example. Outdoor traffic noise levels between 55 and 65 dB(A) and considered stressful, and levels greater than 65 dB(A) are considered disruptive. The recommended exposure guidelines given by the *Occupational Health and Safety Association* defines a 90 dB(A) exposure for more than eight hours as hazardous to physical health and hearing. Consistent noise above these levels has been known to cause sleep disturbance and communication interference, create coordination problems, damage social behavior, and cause hearing loss. A number of studies have cited that sustained levels of 90-95 dB(A) will cause hearing loss and otherwise damage hearing, and 125 dB(A) levels will cause painful hearing. 140 dB(A) is considered the top painful threshold of human hearing. A typical conversation is 55 to 65 dB. A washing machine is about 75 dB(A), while close-in city traffic can get up to 85 dB(A). A subway will have a maximum level of 112 db(A) inside and around subway platforms. A lawn mower might run up to 95 to 110 dB(A), while an average household hums at about 40 dB(A). A power saw will easily push out 110 dB(A), while a pneumatic riveter will easily create

125 dB(A) sound levels. The sound of a jet engine can easily top 150 dB(A).

Interestingly, we have a much greater tolerance for decibel ranges in music than for machinery noise. The typical concert piano ranges from 60-100 dB(A), while most classical instruments range from 85 dB(A) to over 100 dB(A). The trombone, clarinet, cello and oboe for example, can each reach 110 dB(A). Meanwhile a symphony might peak out at over 130 decibels, while a rock concert may easily reach 150 decibels. A walkman headset at mid-volume range will push some 94 dB(A), while a headset and digital music player will easily reach the 105 decibel level, often peaking at 110 decibels. Harmonic distortion in headsets can add 10 dB(A) to these levels, so the equivalent of 120 dB has been measured with personal digital music players.

This all means our tolerance of harmonic or chromatic sounds is much greater than our tolerance of machinery-generated noises like automobiles, airplanes, or jackhammers. One is irritating and stressful, while the other is enlightening and relaxing. Mechanical sounds, made of repetitious bursts of forceful pounding, are *monotonous.* Although music also has repetition, it is not monotonous. This is illustrated by the breakdown of the word "monotonous:" *mono,* meaning "single," and *tonus,* meaning "tone." In other words, mechanical sounds are not only repetitious, but they have a singe tone range.

The prime distinction between music and mechanical noise is variable harmony. The beat and tempo of music is based upon a harmonic—meaning a particular rhythm is repeated or multiplied. In music, we find a changing of notes pacing with the beat and tempo. A machine noise might also establish a harmonic with its repeating beat, but there is no variance of notes with the beat, and there is little or no tonal change. Machinery noise is repetitious and monotonous because there is no variance.

Research by Garcia-Lazaro *et al.* (2006) at Oxford University's Laboratory of Physiology determined that nature's sounds exhibit primarily *1/f spectra.* The researchers also found that human subjects prefer melodies with 1/f distributions than 1/f0 (slower) or 1/f2 (faster) distributions of fluctuations in loudness and pitch. The researchers then tested the sound fluctuations with auditory cortex imaging, and found that the auditory cortex responded more positively to the 1/f distributions. The researchers concluded that a form of tuning existed between 1/f sounds and the auditory cortex pathways.

The variances in tone and tempo within music reflect the fact that music is informational. We consider the sounds of birds and crickets as *songs* because their noises are informational. These are conscious living beings communicating their territory or calling for a mate. This is why birds singing and crickets chirping are calming and soothing sounds, and the roaring of the city and highways is stressful. Conscious communication requires harmony.

Harmony can be heard among singers in a choir or musical instruments in a symphony because the composers originally were communicating their emotions within their compositions. Even a large crowd of fans in the stadium who are all shouting and cheering at different levels communicate harmony when they are heard as a whole from a distance. Individually each person's sound is spoken using a harmonic, and collectively many people speaking different harmonics still creates a larger harmonic. This might be compared to listening to a beehive. Each bee individually is buzzing differently, but the whole hive creates a harmonic hum.

Consciousness is inseparable from harmonic sound. Within each harmonic sound wave resides the imprint of its conscious source. This means that sound coming from a positive, uplifting consciousness will have a better effect upon us than sound originating from a hostile, angry consciousness. Humans, plants and animals all respond similarly to certain kinds of music. Australian psychologist Manfried Klein, for example, conducted research testing hand-muscle responses to music. He found that regardless of the language and cultural background—whether Japanese, Australian aboriginals, Americans or otherwise—the emotional response to the same music passages (indicated by hand-muscle tension) were identical. It mattered not that the music had not been heard before. The emotional response was the same regardless of whether or not that style of music was familiar (Ackerman 1990).

Every sound wave carries the consciousness of its origin. When we hear music or singing we like, our pupils will typically dilate and our endorphin levels will rise. As all of us have experienced, certain music enhances particular types of activities and invokes various emotions and feelings. Even a comatose person responds emotionally to music. Because sound waves carry consciousness, sound will connect the intentions of one conscious self to another conscious self.

Once sound vibration translates through the body, it interferes with existing waveforms, translating the information the self can perceive. The type of information created by the sound vibration depends upon the conscious source of the waveforms, and the conscious receiver. Should the sender's intentions be congruent with the receiving source's intentions, the waveforms will *resonate* with the receiver. This resonation creates the positive affects we relate to certain sounds. This means that we like the music we like because it resonates with the music already playing within us. Because the inner self is an intentional being with individual hopes, desires and personality, sound that reflects these intentions becomes attractive.

This feature is reflected in the expression that people tend to *'hear what they want to hear.'* This filtering mechanism sometimes creates the situation where we do not really hear the thoughts and considerations of others as we could. Sometimes, we may not be prepared for certain sounds. A sudden loud or unexpected noise can cause *acoustic shock injury.* This injury can cause pain around the ear, phonophobia, vertigo, and tinnitus.

On the other hand, we are almost always prepared to hear music. A musical octave—also referred to as the *perfect octave*—is the interval occurring between notes with a doubling or halving of frequency between them. Another perfect octave will occur when the frequency is doubled or halved again. This is referred to as *equivalency.* The *diminished* or *augmented* octave has a slight variance from a precise doubling, forming a flat or sharp note.

Absolute harmonic is accomplished when sound frequencies are whole integer multiples of a particular frequency. The first four harmonics of a 200-hertz frequency are 400 hertz, 600 hertz, 800 hertz, and 1000 hertz, for example. The whole integer multiple of a sound will harmonize with the first sound simply because its frequency is reflective. By reflective we mean the successive sound mirrors the waveform of the first sound. This reflective waveform is typically referred to as the *fundamental frequency* in a harmonic sequence. If we look at the concept of harmonic from a broader perspective, we can understand that each harmonic is actually a reflective fraction of a larger, expanded fundamental frequency.

The pitch of a sound may be related to its frequency, but frequency is not the only characteristic of pitch. The pitch of a sound is rather its perceived frequency. Frequency is a two-dimensional measurement related to cycles per second. A sound's pitch will still incorporate a variety of *overtones* into the total sound. These include changes in amplitude, tempo, and intonation. These qualities give the waveform informative variance. A sound may be *pitched* in such a way to appear very much like a note of a particular frequency, yet the sound waveform may not have that precise frequency. The pure note *A,* for example, should have a frequency of 440 hertz. Most concert tuning forks are set to the A-440 frequency for this reason.

Flat or sharp notes move the pitch or frequency adjustment into the *enharmonic genus,* which is based on the Greek *tetra chord.* The tetra chord concept calls for notes to be tuned in intervals of *perfect fourths.* The four-stringed lyre was its early basis, but later the tetra chord concept was expanded into other instruments. The *diatonic and chromatic* interval systems are also part of the enharmonic system.

Pitch variances are measured in *tones.* A shift to flat or sharp may become a variance in *semitones, quartertones, duotones,* or even *microtones.* These shifts may also be represented as fractions. For example, a *ditone*—or third major tone—may be 16/13 of a full note. The octave concept expressed in tetra chords would thus be a whole tone plus two tetra cords. The *chromatic scale* is a common scale used in music to denote the rise through a series of related notes. The chromatic scale is usually based upon the C note, but the B note and other notes may also be used as fundamental pitches as well. There are typically twelve total pitches in a tempered chromatic scale. Each of these pitches is a half step or semitone step from the prior pitch.

As music math has further developed, the perfect fourth led way to the disjunctive *perfect fifth.* Also called the *diapente,* this is a music interval providing harmonious latitude with surrounding tones. On the piano keyboard, perfect fifths are separated by exactly seven keys. The perfect fifth also provides the root of the major and minor chords and their extensions. The *just fifth* provides a 3:2 ratio. The *perfect fifth* has seven semitones—two less than the just fifth.

When notes harmonize, they resonate together. An A-440 tuning fork will resonate at the 440-hertz frequency, transferring this frequency through the air until it is interfered with by other waveforms. A concert tuning fork will typically be tuned to the violin's third string. As the violin is tuned, the tuning fork and the violin's third string will resonate together. This occurs because of a facility within the violin's construction to allow it to become an *acoustic resonator.* An acoustic resonator is a point on an instrument or body that carries the vibration of a note for a period of time. In other words, it vibrates at the same frequency. On a violin, for example, the string, the bridge, and the body of the violin all facilitate this resonating system. When the tuning fork is struck and the A note resonates through the concert hall, a violin tuned to the *A* note will resonate with the tuning fork, forming a harmonic to tune by. This is the same mechanism occurring within our bodies as we listen to the sounds we like.

Resonators and entrainers appear throughout nature. A canyon resonates with the sounds of the wind, birds, trees, and animals. An ocean beach or bay is a resonator of the waves marching in from distant storms. Nautilus shells and conch shells resonate wind in such a way that they sound like the ocean. Garcia-Lazaro *et al.*'s 1/f spectra research confirms that our bodies resonate with nature's sounds. This implies also that the sounds of nature originate from consciousness—from the largest to the smallest of microsounds.

Dr. Jacques Benveniste and his associates illustrated this directly when they found that biochemicals like hormones and neurotransmitters actually create tiny harmonic waveforms. They were able to digitally record these just as one might record a song. Like a song, the recorded frequencies could be played back in the presence of living tissue, and those frequencies stimulated effects identical to those stimulated by the biomolecules themselves.

For this reason, *sound therapy* has been remarkably successful for the treatment of a number of disorders. *Voice analysis therapy, Audio-Psycho-Phonology, Tomatis Method,* and various music therapies have all been observed to invoke healing responses. *Music therapy* has a long tradition. Pythagoras and his students explored the relationships between music, the universe, and health quite extensively. His *Music of the Spheres* treatise, handed down by Pythagoras' students, illustrated the harmony existing within the universe; and how this harmony related to music. The writings of Aristotle and Plato describe healing with music. Homer prescribed music to counteract mental anguish, and Asclepiades of Bithynia is said to have prescribed Phrygian music for sciatica and other illnesses. Democritus prescribed various flute melodies, and Pythagoras is said to have clinically applied music for nervousness. The respected Roman physician Galen applied music to his healing repertoire. Among other therapies, Galen prescribed a *"medical bath"* inclusive of flute song for nerve pain. The famous sixteenth century Swiss physician Paracelsus was a strong believer in sound therapy as well. His recommendations included not only herbal remedies, but colors and sound to achieve health. Classical composers like Bach, Beethoven and Brahms expanded these theories in their musical works, providing therapeutic music to millions of listeners.

Modern western medicine rediscovered music therapy during the twentieth century, after finding that world war vets healed faster with music. Today music therapy is an evidence-based healing modality. It is used in hospitals and therapy centers around the world. In the 1980s, the Certification Board for Music Therapists began to certify music therapists. Today this organization claims over 4,000 board certified music therapists.

Most researchers agree that a combination of harmony and tempo that gives music its soothing effect. Not only slow harmonious music provides this effect. Music with faster tempos and drumming beats can also provide therapeutic results. EEG testing has shown many relaxation tapes do not help as much as native music, Celtic music, and even certain rock and roll music can. Evidently, rhythmic beats provide a balancing effect between the left and right brainwaves. Flutes have also been shown to be particularly therapeutic. Research has also shown that live performances seem to provide more therapeutic results than do recordings. The right mix of therapeutic music increases deep breathing, lowers the heart rate, balances thermoregulation, and increases serotonin production.

Playing an instrument or percussion provides a special benefit. Playing music promotes not only the hearing of music, but allows an expression of creative personality. Most people can find at least one instrument they can play, even if it is just a makeshift drum of some sort. Listening to music while working lowers stress and increases productivity. Music with slower rhythms—slower than one's heart rate—increases relaxation in the research. Music with faster beats—faster than one's heart rate—tends to increase energy and stimulate activity. Familiar music from the past soothes anxiety and depression, especially among the elderly.

Studies in the 1960s by Dr. Georgi Lozanov demonstrated that learning and memorization increases with paced recitation. He found that if information was repeated either every eight seconds or every twelve seconds, its memorization was higher than repetition at other rhythms or randomly. This led to comparisons between combinations of beat (frequency) and intonation. This led to an investigation of various forms of music. He discovered that particular beats and melodies had greater effects upon the body than did others. In particular, he found music playing around sixty beats per minute—close to the average human resting pulse—substantially relaxed the body. This also had the effect of calming and synchronizing breathing rates. More importantly, music at this tempo consistently increased memory retention, recall, and learning. As Dr. Lozanov's research continued, it became apparent that Baroque-style music as composed by sixteenth, seventeenth, and eighteenth century composers such as Handel, Bach and Vivaldi had the greatest positive effects upon learning and memorization skills. These music forms seem to relax the body and focus the mind more than other types of music.

It is not simply the 60 beats-per-minute (or 3600 herz) frequency rate that encourages this high cognition state—enabling better memorization and physical relaxation. It is the 4/4 or 4/3 tempo along with the various tonal and pitch variances. Numerous beats and intonations have been tested in this research. Few, however, have the effect of increasing learning and relaxation to the degree certain music can (Ostrander 1979).

Geneticist Dr. Susumu Ohno of California's *Breckman Research Institute* underwrote this effect within the realm of DNA. Dr. Ohno's research indicated that that our gene expression rhythmically resonates with Fourier interference patterns. These interference patterns provide a repetitive sequencing common among all life forms (Holmquist 2000).

Plants also respond positively to the rhythmic effects of music. Researcher Dorothy Retallack published (1973) controlled research whereupon plants preferred certain types of music over others. Ms. Retallack discovered plants growing in rooms with Baroque-like music (such as Bach or Ravi Shankar) had robust growth with generous foliage and root systems. Meanwhile, plants grown in rooms inundated with rock music shriveled, died, or were generally weak. Her trials concluded that plants were impartial to country music, but positively responded with greater growth to Baroque style music and some types of jazz.

Dr. Jagadis Chandra Bose documented extensive experiments with plants in the early twentieth century. Dr. Bose utilized an instrument called the crescograph, which measured the responsiveness of plants. After numerous trials, Dr. Bose indicated that plants grew faster when exposed to traditional Indian music. Dr. T.C.N. Singh of a Madras music college continued this research. Between 1960 and 1963, Dr. Singh was able to increase crop yields by 25% to 60% when the crop fields were exposed to particular types of Indian and Baroque-like music. To this we add that Eugene Canby's Bach violin sonatas played to a plot of wheat resulted in heavier, larger wheat stalks with 66% greater yields (Newton 1971).

Canadian researchers Mary Measures and Pearl Weinberger at the University of Ottawa tested spring and winter wheat germination on 5,000 cycles per second (83.3 BPM) and 10,000 cycles per second (166 BPM). Both frequencies significantly stimulated germination. The largest germination increases, however, were achieved with 5,000 cycles per second (Weinberger and Measures 1968). Note that 83 beats per minute (5,000 cycles) is closer to the 60 beats per minute rate suggested in Dr. Lozanov's research on learning.

A few years' later, horticulturist and dentist Dr. George Milstein worked with a commercial sound engineer to test various frequencies on plant growth. Dr. Milstein determined the best growth rate to be 3,000 cycles per second (50 beats per minute). He later produced a record using what he found were the optimal sounds and tempos most encouraging to plant growth. He recorded this music onto a well-received L.P. album (Conely 1971).

In 1972, Dan Carlson, a student at the University of Minnesota, also conducted research into stimulating plant growth with sound. His research led him to a discovery that the tiny pores on the leaf's surface that absorb nutrients—called *stomata*—appear to open further around an environment of sounds with particular frequencies. The sound frequencies causing the greatest stomata opening ranged from 3,000 cycles to 5,000 cycles per second. As he investigated the frequency results further, Carlson discovered the sounds were remarkably similar to the sounds of common morning songbirds. The songs of swallows, martins, and warblers appeared to provide the closest match. The songs of these birds stimulated the opening of the stomata the greatest.

Most of us have experienced the calming and rejuvenating effect of listening to morning birds singing outside our window. Our own experiences and observations clearly indicate that natural melodies can induce a calming effect, together with a higher level of alertness and mental activity. Biofeedback research confirms that these moods are connected to a preponderance of alpha brainwaves.

These phenomena are all arising from consciousness. Research comparing human musicians and computer metronomes (music notation entered into a computer) has demonstrated that computerized sound facsimiles do not resonate with a listener in the same way a live musician playing the same song will. Converting a song to the precise computerized metronome simply does not precisely translate the consciousness of human musical sound.

Research has illustrated that our conversations have a tremendous effect upon our health. In a 35-year study completed at the Department of Psychology at the University of Arizona (Russek and Schwartz, 1996), Harvard University undergraduate men recorded their perception of the love and caring they received from their parents. Those using fewer positive words describing this had significantly more disease pathologies in mid-life than those who used more positive words.

In addition to focusing upon a particular sound itself, we can probe a bit deeper into the intention of the person creating that sound. Intentions that resonate with the goodness within us promote mental and physical wellness. Intentions resonating with our greedy side bring discord and illness to our bodies and the bodies of others. For this reason, serotonin, dopamine, and oxytocin neurotransmitters—all associated with wellness—are found more prevalent among those exchanging loving feelings (Esch and Stefano 2005).

Giving and caring for another, even if it is not returned, is the natural consciousness of the self. When we give and care for others without the need for return, we are doing what comes naturally. Words that express this natural inclination resonate with the self. Therefore, sounds from these intentions create harmony within and around us. This is why we all get a warm and fuzzy feeling when we hear of people caring for and helping others. Sounds expressing love are harmonic with the inner self.

Tactile Perception

The human body's membrane is only a couple of millimeters thick. This multi-layering of cell types has a complicated structure nonetheless. The epidermis cells, making up the outer membrane, have several functions. Their most obvious function is to protect the body from the environment. Epidermis cells produce and accumulate important substances like *keratin* and *melanin,* which help protect the body's membrane by creating thickness and natural sun block. Epidermis cells also help purge toxins out of the body. Underneath the epidermis lies the dermis, which houses the various functional systems like blood vessels and *sudoriferous* or sweat glands—along with *sebaceous* glands, which store and secrete *sebum.* These secretions provide the skin with an acidic surface, cooling lubrication and a convenient pathway for toxin release.

Sensing nerves located throughout skin cells are specifically designed to pick up a particular range of waveforms colliding with the skin's surface. These nerve cells contain touch receptors called *tactile corpuscles.* They are located primarily in the dermis, and are spread throughout the body. They are concentrated however, in areas we especially utilize for tactile sensations: Hands and fingertips, for example, have more tactile corpuscles than do many other skin regions.

Pain receptors are not enclosed like the tactile corpuscles. They are considered *free nerve endings.* Thus pain receptors are contained within nerve fiber branching. More importantly, these pain receptors are not exclusively located in the skin. They are located throughout the body, receiving waveforms from muscles, joints, internal organs and other tissue systems.

Pain receptors convert the waveforms within a particular range into bioelectromagnetic signals. The types of waveforms that affect the different sensory nerves include temperature variation (cold, heat), touch (surface sensitivity), pressure (weight, mass and force), or injury. Each type of waveform is sensed by a specialized nerve receptor. Each of these receptor types has a distinct pathway through the nervous system. For example, branched neuron skin-pain receptors extend closest to the skin's surface and spread out like a tree. Both touch and pressure receptors are more bulb-like and positioned deeper under the skin.

Heat and cold receptors are altogether different structures from the other skin receptors. Heat receptors are also distinctly different from cold receptors in structure. Heat temperature-sensing nerve cells pick up thermal waveforms. Cold-sensing receptors only quantify cold temperatures. The cold-sensing nerve endings are in the first one-fiftieth inch of skin deep. The heat-sensing nerve-endings lie somewhat deeper. There are also significantly more cold-sensing receptors than heat-sensing receptors. The skin contains about 150,000 cold-sensing nerve receptors and only about 16,000 heat-sensing receptors. Each type of waveform signal also travels a different pathway through the nervous system.

Pressure or puncture skin sensations are also waveform transported. The frequency of these types of waveforms may be quite low, with typically long wavelengths. An accidental blow to the leg, for example, might consist of one large waveform with a rather large amplitude. An infrared waveform on the other hand, is much smaller, with a shorter frequency and smaller amplitude. Cellular damage affects nerve endings quite differently. Neuron responses signaling damage to cell membranes or contents are designed to stimulate an immune system response. Pain sensitivity appears to be integrated with temperature-sensing receptors, as the body assimilates and compares the three types of sensitivity responses. Apparently, there is an interaction between the sensory paths for pain and temperature responses (Defrin *et al.* 2002).

This illustrates that like the other sensory stimuli processes, multiple waveform interactions with multiple sensory nerves are required before a full impression or response can be made. Different waveforms give reference to each other. In a body with trillions of nerve endings, it is not hard to get a confirmation among nerve endings of a particular sensation. Whether it is a sharp, soft, hot or cold sensation, many different waveforms from the source have to stimulate many different nerve endings in order to accumulate the necessary convergence of waveforms and their interference patterns required to create a complete sensation translated through the nervous system. In most cases, an object or contact will stimulate several types of sensory nerves with differing waveforms. These will all be sent through the central nervous system to converge first within the local *chakra*. As they converge, an interference pattern will be formed, which will, assuming the programming, cause a sympathetic nerve response. This will initiate the pre-programmed response, such as pulling our hand out of the fire. Alongside the automatic response, the waveform convergence simultaneously relays up the spinal cord to the sixth *chakra* region. Here it will reflect upon the mind the temperature, size and shape of the fire for the self to see and consider if further response is required.

A good way of visualizing tactile pain responses is to follow the circuitry involved in sensing a burning sensation from an electric oven. Alternating electromagnetic waveforms are piped into the house wiring from the grid and power generation facility. The oven circuitry converts the alternating electromagnetic waveforms into thermal waves, which radiates through the stove element. Should we touch the element, the element pulses intense thermal waveforms into our dermal layers, which interrupt the electromagnetic bonds within the molecules making up the skin cells and basal fluids. This will initiate molecular damage to the cells, which sets off a communication relay from these cells to local pain receptors. An informational broadcast of damage stimulates the pain receptors, which stimulate an informational waveform pathway (cascade) through their nerve channels to the local *chakra* region.

Simultaneously, the thermal waves stimulate the ionic-electromagnetic gateways of the thermoreceptor neurons. A switching of these neuron gateways initiates a waveform pathway, sending the sensory information to the local *chakra* and *vertebral internuncial neurons*. The pathway between these thermoreceptors and pain receptors located around the skin and the internuncial neurons in the *chakra* region create the autonomic *spinal reflex arc* response. This reflex arc stimulates the immediate response of pulling the skin off the burner before our skin melts away.

The thermoreceptors are nerve endings that convert and translate particular waveforms into nerve impulses. These impulses initiate and open neurotransmitter and ion gateways between the nerves, stimulating not only the spinal reflex arc, but also a conscious interpretation of the burning sensation as painful. The signals are relayed through the peripheral nervous system towards the brain centers. This neural pathway channels waveforms to neurons in the limbic system (within the sixth *chakra* region) consisting of the thalamus, cerebral cortex and/or reticular formation, where their impressions will be converted and imprinted onto the mind's screen. Here the conscious self can view these sensations, prompting physical responses to prevent a recurrence of the pain. The conscious response(s) will complement the sympathetic system's responses of the spinal reflex arc. Reactions such as calling for help or applying first aid may be appropriate, for example.

In the same way, the alternating grid-born electromagnetic current completes a house circuit as it converts to thermal waves in the appliance and back to electromagnetic waves. In the body, the circuit is completed through the body's nervous system when the pain and sympathetic nerve response are fed back.

Pain signals can sometimes refer to other locations not directly in touch with the pain: This is a pre-programmed mechanism for resolving pain. For example, a waveform relay from the liver when the liver's cells are being damaged or insulted might be felt somewhere else in the body. This is often termed as *referred pain*. This stimulates a signaling process for indicating a problem somewhere in the body—signaling to the self that an investigation must be done to fix the problem.

Sometimes waveform relays of pain information stimulate brain neurons when there is no obvious cause for the pain. Doctors may refer to this as *psychogenic* or *nociceptic pain*. Conventional medicine classifies this sort of pain relay as either a neurological disorder or a psychological disorder. We will discuss this further as we explore pain in more detail later.

The skin typically does not have a tactile response from sound rhythms, unless they occur at the lower frequencies known for vibrating the skin's molecular structures or structural surroundings. These are seismic waves. Waves in the seismic range will be sensed by the human skin through its tactile corpuscles. Seismic waves are a recognizable form of information communication. Any prisoner of war will testify that Morse code tapped upon walls or pipes can be an effective vehicle to communicate even the most intimate feelings.

The tactile sensory nerves and the skin provide an even more intimate form of communication device in the form of touching. Through intention, the self creates subtle pathways of communication via tactile sensory perception. When touching another person for example, a waveform pathway for emotion and consciousness can be created, assuming the intention is there. We can certainly sense the heat and surface area of another person's touch with our skin's thermoreceptor relays. However, the deeper waveform pathway for emotional intention may or may not be perceivable. Typically, this "loop" of intention can be closed with the other party's intention, creating an open channel for emotional exchange. Regardless, we know through empirical studies that touch is important to healing and a healthy physical existence.

In the fifties and sixties, psychologist Dr. Harry Harlow conducted a series of studies related to touch at the University of Wisconsin at Madison. The studies focused upon the necessity of contact between rhesus monkeys and their mothers—or in many cases surrogate or façade mothers. Some baby monkeys were pulled away from their mothers at birth and put in isolated cages. These monkeys quickly became hostile, depressed, and unstable compared to caged monkeys united with their mothers. Some of the baby monkeys were left alone with wire-built frames or cloth-covered frames made to look like the shape of a monkey. Some of these frames were even built with milk bottle-breasts so the monkey could feed from a pair of fake nipples. Although the baby monkeys would try to hug the fake monkeys and suck milk from the fake breasts, they also became hostile, depressed, and unstable compared with monkeys caged with living mothers. Some of the monkeys previously isolated with wire surrogates were introduced to live monkey surrogates who were not their mothers. These monkeys immediately began to hug the surrogates, and these stressed and hostile monkeys gradually became "normal" (for being imprisoned in cages) (Harlow *et al.* 1965; Harlow *et al.* 1962; Harlow 1964).

Other studies, such as those of Dr. James Prescott (1979 and 1996), have confirmed that human sensory deprivation during the formative years causes the incomplete development of the neural network associated with the limbic system. Dr. Prescott's work connected these effects with violent and antisocial behavior later on in life.

Studies with infants and pre-term preemies (infants born prematurely) have also confirmed the importance of human touch to the well-being of the body and self. Preemie babies who were held more often and stroked or massaged more grew faster, had shorter hospitalizations, were significantly more alert, and were more responsive to the world around them than preemies who were more isolated during incubation. The touched babies were also calmer and better adjusted later in their childhood than babies who were not touched as often (Ackerman 1990, Browne 2000; Klaus 1998; Rapley 2002).

Experienced "touchers"—such as masseuses—understand this technology first hand. Trained in the art of vibrating and stroking the skin to relax muscles, increase blood circulation and speed up lymph flow, masseuses see immediate response among their clients every day. Medical massage has been practiced for thousands of years with great clinical success. This type of rhythmic stroking also can have tremendous effects upon a person's psyche and mood. Research has confirmed that higher levels of neurotransmitters such as serotonin and dopamine are released in response to massage.

We can see a direct correlation between sensory nerves and a radio picking up a broadcast. Tactile and thermoreceptor nerves are generally thought of as requiring physical touch. However, they also sense other types of waveforms. A cool breeze or some exposure to the hot sun will stimulate significant response. The skin's nerve receptors respond to air currents, thermal waves, electromagnetic waves, and liquid motion. If we add to this the ability to sense emotion through touching, we arrive at a conclusion that touching is intimately connected with consciousness.

Savory Sensation

Like dotted islands and atolls of the South Pacific Ocean, thousands of taste buds lie on the surface of the tongue. They also even lie sporadically on the roof of the mouth, pharynx, and larynx. These receptor 'islands' have small surface pores that reach up to sit above the saliva 'shores.' Connected to these receptor pores are thin nerve fibers, ready to sense the waveforms being released from the food slurry being churned inside the mouth. These nerve fibers will bundle together, connecting different pores in a network of channels—communicating converted electromagnetic taste pulses to the brain stem and eventually to the thalamus. From here, the transmissions are conveyed to the *somatosensory cortex* in the *postcentral gyrus* in the parietal lobe of the brain, where they can be converted and projected onto the mind's screen for the self to observe and interface with.

There are four basic types of taste buds strategically placed around the tongue. Sweet taste buds are aggregated around the tip of the tongue while salty taste buds lie on each side of the tip. Sour taste buds lie along the sides of the tongue. Bitter taste buds lie primarily at the back of the tongue top. These taste receptor cells have some crossover ability, but they are designed to resonate with certain waveforms and polarities.

The odor sense works in much the same way. Olfactory bulbs are positioned mostly at the top of the sinus cavity on either side of the nasal septum. Olfactory bulbs lie at the epithelium mucosa surface, where nerve fibers connect to the bulbs. These nerve fibers sense the waveform and polarity of odorous molecules traveling in the air as they interface with the mucosa of the nasal cavity. This electromagnetic waveform and polarity means odor is an oscillation—it is a waveform. So we are in effect sensing pulsating 'odor-packets' traveling within and around gas and air molecules. Upon reception, these pulses are converted through nerve fiber synapses within olfactory nerves, and relayed to the cerebral cortex. Here these waveform pulses are converted through the hypothalamus for imprinting onto the screen of the mind.

Special olfactory nerve bulbs, collectively called the *vomeronasal organ* (VNO), or *Jacobson's organ,* may be stimulated on a more subtle level by *pheromone* waveforms. Pheromones carry subtle informational waveforms through the environment to the limbic system. Pheromones tend to stimulate sexual responses among animals, plants and insects. Some debate has continued as to whether humans exchange pheromones.

Though humans have anatomical VNOs—known for pheromone exchanging in animals—significant nerve conduction has yet to be observed on a gross basis. The assumption has been that without obvious VNO nerve pathways, there would be little chance of conduction to the endocrine mechanisms such as the pituitary gland. This is countered by the fact that biocommunication signaling does not always require nerve pathways.

Consideration might be given to the work of a well-respected rhinologist Dr. Maurice Cottle. Dr. Cottle, known for his contribution towards the development of the electrocardiogram, invented a diagnostic machine in the mid-twentieth century called the *rhinomanometer*. Dr. Cottle wrote two books on the subject of rhinomanometry, and was a professor and head of Otolaryngology at the Chicago Medical School. Dr. Cottle was able to diagnose a number of ailments in other parts of the body simply by measuring the swelling or shrinking of the tissues and the airflow through this region during breathing. The turbinates throughout the mucous membrane house subtle waveform channels connecting to various organ systems and processes. The delicate turbinate membranes are more than mucous membranes: They are erectile, with thousands of tiny receptors. They respond to stimulation just as do erectile regions such as the penis, clitoris, and nipples. The turbinate erectile receptors respond to and coordinate airflow with the rest of the body. Clinical evidence demonstrated that Dr. Cottle's machine could accurately diagnose coronary heart disease and depression, for example (Cottle 1968).

Dr. Wilhelm Fleiss was also an otolaryngologist. He and Dr. Freud also worked with the turbinate membranes of nasal tissues. They found associations between various physiological processes in the body and the turbinates just as Dr. Cottle did later. For example, they found a swelling in one part of the turbinates indicated an ulcer. Apparently, an extensive mapping of the turbinates with respect to particular organs and disorders was in development prior to World War I. This work unfortunately came to a halt when the war started.

After reviewing this research, it seems plausible that since the turbinates can be considered a part of the VNO organ, the ability to receive and send pheromones is not such a radical concept.

The process of sensing odor and taste is extremely complex, and has perplexed physicists for many years. Particle physics proponents described olfactory and organoleptic sensory stimuli as being the product of molecular contact. This is unlikely, however, when considering the sheer dilution factors involved in these sensory organs. Humans can detect sourness in one part in 130,000, and bitterness in one part in 2,000,000.

Odors can be communicated instantly from miles away. Using the same logic used by the scientists that reject homeopathy because these dilutions defy the chance of a molecule being present in any random sample, no molecule is logically active at these levels. This means the communication of taste and odor could not be wholly molecular-based.

Dilution factors are enormous in most olfactory sense perception scenarios. An olfactory event might initially be driven by molecular reaction. However, gas pressure tests have concluded in many cases little or no presence of the gas molecules of the reaction. Still, the odor is pervasive. Some have concluded that subtle molecular reactions must be occurring in the air between the source of the odor and the nasal passages. Such a model, however, would require every odor to create molecular changes within the air, affecting the air's toxicity and the availability of oxygen.

Many physicists have linked odor perception to particle adsorption within the context of weak *van der Waals forces:* These are the attractive or repulsive forces between molecules and atoms. Their electrostatic properties carry odor particles through the air to stimulate the olfactory bulbs, according to the theory. This attempt to insist upon a particle theory of odor sense perception is commendable. In reality, however, these van der Walls forces between the molecules are also waveform agents. Van de Walls forces are magnetic field-related waveform forces, and they are observed in context with anisotropic matter dispersion. *Anisotropy* is the dispersion of matter outward in orientation to respective magnetic fields. Some describe these as dipole moments, but this technology is little understood, primarily because our knowledge of magnetic fields is still in its infancy.

Because we have yet to observe these "olfactory particles" attached to other molecules or particles, and because there is no change to the molecular composition of the air in many cases of olfactory reception, we must accept the possibility of waveform transmission. In rare cases, odorous gases can dramatically change the atmosphere content, but this is due to the particular gas not the odor. In a majority of cases, as we have all experienced, we can get a sniff of something far away instantly without any recognized dispersion of gas.

Informational scents have been connected with mood, energy level and social behavior. An ancient science—now called *aromatherapy*—has been practiced for thousands of years, revolving around the scents certain natural extracts create. These scents have been shown to evoke significant mood and activity responses. In a controlled, double-blinded study done by Ohio State University scientists (Kiecoit-Glaser *et al.* 2008), fifty-six healthy men and women underwent exposure to odors of lemon, lavender and water during three different visits. Expectations were additionally subjected to controls. Lemon oil caused a "robust" rise in positive moods as compared with the other odors, accompanied by an elevated rise in norepinephrine levels. In another controlled double-blind study (Kim *et al.* 2007) on fifty-four post-operative anesthesia patients, significantly fewer analgesic medications were required in the lavender aromatherapy group.

As we analyze the waveform model for the sense of smell, we might consider a series of studies that emerged from Britain (McCulloch *et al.* 2006) on the ability of dogs' olfactory senses predicting—more accurately diagnosing—instances of cancer in human subjects. This exciting research—much of it double-blinded and controlled—illustrated that dogs were able to sense the growth of lung and breast cancer among humans by smelling their exhaled breath or by sniffing their skin. As this research has progressed, a number of volatile waveform biomarkers have been identified in cancer patients. These appear to stimulate subtle olfactory receptors in dogs (Machado *et al.* 2005; Phillips *et al.* 2003).

If we consider the ramifications of this research, we see three waveform mechanisms revealed: 1) The ability of certain diseases to produce unique waveform transmissions; 2) the release of the waveform transmissions through the skin and/or lungs; and 3) the ability of the dog's olfactory receptors to receive and translate that information into the conscious perception of a problem. The key operators here are the information, and the circuit. The circuit loop began with the disease and closed with its recognition by the self within the body of the animal. Because there are obvious gaps in biocommunication using a biochemical/particle theory of transmission, we are left with the conclusion that olfactory sense perception is a waveform biocommunication, and pathways between conscious beings can be opened with intention.

Another important mechanism was demonstrated by this research: Like humans and all other living organisms, dogs have an ability to empathize.

Sexual Sensitivity

Sexuality is due to the sensory reception of the erectile cells lying within and around the genitals. The genitals are equipped with extremely sensitive regions, consistent with the proliferation of these sensitive neurons. On the male, the head of the penis contains a dense population of these sensory nerve endings. On the female, the clitoris is most populated with these sensory cells.

In the male, spermatogenesis—the production of semen—occurs in the testes in a relay circuit stimulated by the signaling of the biomolecular messenger *follicle-stimulating hormone* from the adenohypophysis gland.. The testes are small round organs divided into segments filled with twisted channels called *seminferous tubules.* Within these tubules spermatozoa form through a special type of cell division called *meiosis.* Here 46 chromosome (44 plus an X and Y) *spermatogonia* divide to form the basis for the spermatozoa. This process is staged through a primary and secondary process of spermatocyte production. During the last step, the cytoplasm of the new cell is thrown off and a tail is formed.

Some believe life begins at as professed by a number of theologies. The Ayurvedic science details that the living being enters the sperm while in the testes. This observation is consistent with spermatozoa suddenly becoming motile within the testes. *In vitro* testing has demonstrated that spermatozoa motility is negatively affected by a number of mechanisms. Sperm are thus challenged by oxidative radicals, incorrect pH, or the wrong scrotal temperature.

The female vaginal discharge further discourages sperm entry. Yet even in these sorts of hostile surroundings, a determined sperm will seek out survival and continue to advance towards the ovum. As they travel up the vagina into the cervix, they seek continued survival in the same way we strive to keep this body alive. The nature of a living being is to pursue survival against sometimes challenging and hostile surroundings.

Another perspective comes from the thousands of hypnotherapy regressions by Dr. Newton and other doctors who have documented findings that the soul may join with the fetus at a much later stage.

According to this research, this joining can range from between immediately after conception to after the first trimester. In such hypnotherapy regressions, the person or patient recalls directly when they entered their current body and when they entered previous bodies.

This of course brings to matter our definition of "life." If "life" means a physical organism having physical activity, then we can safely assume the Ayurvedic and most other religious doctrines' premise that the life of the physical body begins at conception and there is at least a part of life that is present in sperm.

But if we insist that "life" requires the presence of the living soul joining the physical body, this would mean "life" as we know it will begin sometime when the baby is in the womb and the incarnating soul joins with the fetus inside the womb.

Certainly, the view that sperm becomes a host to the living self during the spermatogenesis would present some problems. This would mean that millions of living sperm with souls would die with every ejaculation. If lucky, one will survive. Are all of these entities with souls dying off with every ejaculation?

Sperm have a life cycle similar to many bacteria. Millions can be born in one moment and die a moment later with exposure to sunlight or any other environmental challenge.

Two milliliters of sperm can contain 300 million spermatozoa in a healthy person. Only one is required for fertilization upon entry into the ovum. Should a sperm contain a soul, it would drive the development of the fetus body with a combination of genetic and spiritual expression.

Such an expression would change the nature of the fetus immediately after conception, fueling a distinct development of the DNA hapmap. The seeds for the hapmap are expressed from the mother's and father's genes. Would the entry of the soul at this stage harm the careful combination of genes that develop the fetal brain tissue?

The research indicated through hypnotherapy regression indicates that the soul or self waits until this process is completed and the fetal body and brain has developed to a certain point at a later stage. At that time the soul can arrive and project its changes onto the developing fetus.

Because our topic relates to consciousness, it is fair to say that anytime there is a soul joined with a body there is consciousness. But does this mean that a fetus without a soul doesn't have consciousness? Certainly we can assume that at the very least, that fetal consciousness would be connected to the consciousness of the mother.

Once the soul does enter the fetus is must begin to setup shop so to speak.

We might compare this process with how an office worker might customize a work cubicle. The design and parts of the cubicle are dictated by and supplied by the company. The employee will customize the workspace with his or her own belongings, posters, and so on. Should we walk through an office of 'cubes' we will see an array of various colors, ornaments, wall-hangings and desk arrangements that sufficiently express the employee occupant. We can see from the lives of twins that duplicate base genes do not dictate duplicate body features in entirety, and certainly do not determine personality and lifestyle preferences.

The ovum provides a genetic host to this process. As the ovum is entered by the sperm, it becomes charged with the self. Until then, it is simply one of many cells within the female body—albeit designed for the possibility of being entered by a new life form. A process called *oogenesis* occurs in the ovum, with a special pathway of cellular division that involves oogonia with 44+XX chromosomes dividing to form oocytes, which divide twice to eventually become the 22X chromosome ovum.

The only way a sperm can find an ovum is if it bursts through the uterine wall where it is assembled. For this purpose, follicles grow on the surface of the uterus. When a follicle bursts, it can release its underlying ovum. This follicle growth is stimulated by the well-known waveform biochemical messenger known as follicle-stimulating hormone. Once it bursts out the uterine wall, the ovum will await penetration by the sperm.

For most humans and animals, sexuality consumes a major portion of our life's focus. Why is this? Many also point at the evolutionary-rooted drive of the body to procreate: As if we were evolutionary machines and there is no one inside who might have any intention or purpose.

This indicates that sexuality combines the intentions of woman and the man as they conceive together. These drives include pleasure and that is expressed towards the creative process of producing a host for an incarnating soul to occupy.

Why is the feedback response from sexual activity more powerful than that of the other senses? This relates to design, reflecting the importance of procreation. Without a significant incentive to mate and have offspring, the challenges presented by carrying offspring would likely prevent procreation. By design during and following the orgasm, the sexual organs are feeding back to the nervous system a series of endorphins, serotonin, dopamine, and pleasure-feedback electromagnetic waveforms to encourage the inner self to complete the task.

There is another incentive for sexual activity, however. This incentive relates to the innate need of the inner self to exchange love, service and affection with another living being. In this case, sexuality is a tool or resource the inner self uses in to exchange a relationship with another soul. This however is often frustrated, as the desire to obtain pleasure can have negative consequences if there is no love involved, which the inner self needs.

The assumption and subsequent problem with these attempts for fulfillment through sexual activity is that the inner self is ultimately not fulfilled by being sexually pleasured alone. This is because the inner self has an identity separate from the physical body.

It is like a car driver having their car washed and waxed. The driver does not feel the car getting scrubbed and rubbed. The driver has no means to obtain any physical satisfaction from it, because his body is separate from the car's metal exterior. The driver will certainly get feedback that the car is clean and shiny, however.

Such a driver will see the reflection on the car surface and have some feedback that the car is now clean. The driver identifying with the car's image might obtain a positive mental feedback response—but this is not the same as direct fulfillment. These indirect feedback responses are not the same as *feeling* the effects of the car's surface being rubbed.

In the same way, the inner self, misidentifying the body as the self, is not actually touched by sex—sex touches the physical body only. Once the body feeds back positive nerve sensations and positive biochemical messengers, the inner self may have some sense of positive feedback following the organism. Still, the orgasm does not specifically affect the inner self—so it does not bring any true satisfaction.

It is for this reason that we find couples anticipating becoming satisfied by having sex—and displaying excitement in anticipation—only to find afterward that they are not fulfilled by the sex act. For this reason, we find so many marriages and relationships that were founded upon sexuality end, due to a mutual letdown from the expectation of sexual fulfillment.

Defecation Senses

Most of us think of defecation as an action of the body rather than a sensory activity. However, the colon and the anus are both receiving sensory information in the form of peristalsis waves stimulated by the vagus nerve and propelled through the intestinal tract. This sensory motion is coupled with the propulsion of waste materials through the digestion process.

The process of defecation is a sensory process because we must have significant incentive to perform this activity. Much like sex, we must firstly be attracted to defecate, even though the actual physical act is somewhat disgusting and smelly. Still, most of us look forward to defecating, not just because we want to drop our waste off, but also because our bodies transmit a positive feedback sensation during and following the process of dumping our waste.

This positive sensation is driven by special nerve endings located around the *anal sphincters*. These nerve endings reciprocate a number of cascading informational waves that stem from the vagus nerve. A parasympathetic reflex is stimulated when the contents of the colon increase the pressure at the rectum to about 50 mm Hg. This reflex then stimulates contractions of abdominal muscles, which drive up the pressure at the rectum to 200 mm Hg and higher, providing the propulsion necessary to eject the waste. Peristalsis waves also offer a feedback-response mechanism that signals to the sphincter that it is time to open up and allow waste from the colon to escape. As researchers have traced this feedback and response mechanism through the nerves, they have located a bundle of nerve endings at the lower spine called the *defecation center*. The location of this center is consistent with the location of the first *chakra* according to Ayurvedic science.

While this is happening, the biofeedback signals through the central nervous system (and *chakra* linkage) that the colon will be relieved with the opening of the internal anal sphincter. This positive feedback response also stimulates the voluntary sphincter muscles to relax and open the external anal sphincter, which allows the contents of the colon to proceed. At this point, the mind and self are fed back positive response waveforms signaling that the body is positively relieving waste materials. Like the sexual feedback messengers, these positive sensory signals motivate the body to overlook our stool's strong smell and awful appearance and feel good about this activity.

We conclude this discussion on the senses with a comment made by fifteenth-century physician Paracelsus:

> *"The power to see does not come from the eye, the power to hear does not come from the ear, nor the power to feel from the nerves; but it is the spirit of man that sees through the eye, hears with the ear, and feels by means of the nerves. Wisdom and reason and thought are not contained in the brain, but belong to the invisible spirit which feels through the heart and thinks by means of the brain."*

Chapter Five

Metabolic Awareness

The body contains a variety of processing systems, each centered around a particular function, a specific elemental state, and a particular range of waveform biocommunications. Each organ provides the body with a practical purpose. The anatomical parts and physical processes of each organ can be referenced in any modern anatomy textbook. Here, however, we will briefly touch on how each organ system functions within the matrix of the body's intentional biocommunication systems.

Digestion

Digestion is probably the most misunderstood process the body undertakes. Amazingly, nutrition and digestion are only briefly discussed in medical schools today. As a result, doctors rarely understand the process, and as a result, western society is increasingly succumbing to a variety of digestive disorders such as irritable bowel syndrome, ulcers, polyps, acid reflux and many others. These disorders are typically treated for their symptoms but not for their causes. This in itself is a symptom of a bigger problem: A lack of understanding of digestion.

Ayurveda has recognized that each part of the digestive process draws upon different elements and different states of consciousness. The upper digestive tract, made up of the esophagus, throat, mouth and nasal cavity are all classified as *kapha* oriented, as they draw from solid and liquid elements. The stomach, liver, gall bladder, pancreas, and upper intestines are classified as *pitta,* as they are oriented toward the thermal element. They are driven by the fires of digestive enzymes and other heat-producing molecular reactions. The lower intestines and the colon are considered *vata* oriented, as they tend to accumulate the elements of gas and plasma-aether. These three *doshas* tend to reflect our consciousness through each part of the digestive process.

The Stomach

Most of us assume digestion takes place in the stomach. Not true. A few carbohydrates and proteins might be broken down in the mouth and stomach, and water is absorbed through the walls of the stomach along with a few minerals. Most of the nutrients from food are broken down and absorbed through the upper intestinal tract.

One of the most important parts of the stomach is actually the mouth. This is where the body masticates our food, liquefies it, and breaks down many starches. Under the tongue are *salivary glands.* They produce amylase. Amylase is an enzyme that breaks down starches into simple sugars. This is one reason the body is driven to eat starches. As the body chews them, the tongue tastes the sugar. This feeds back to the mind that this food is good for the body. The mind has programmed the body to see sugar as positive because the cells use sugar in the form of glucose to produce energy. Particular molecular bonding waveforms between carbon and hydrogen in glucose provide the cell with energy when released. What are these waveforms? These are the waveforms converted from the sun's rays through photosynthesis by plants into carbohydrates. The tongue is programmed to sense these waveforms and feed back to the mind that this is good for the body and the body should get more of it. This particular feedback mechanism is often misconstrued by the self as a possible solution to the self's search for fulfillment, however. This is the cause for addictive eating and depressive eating disorders.

Because of this feedback mechanism, most of us hastily jam our faces with consecutive mouthfuls as if our food were under threat of capture. We also tend to hold our breath as we eat. This habit encourages hasty chewing and swallowing, forcing unprepared food into an unprepared digestive system. Little do we realize that it is the intentional act of focusing on food that predicates the biochemical processes involved in digestion.

Taking our time and chewing a little more liquefies our foods and mixes them with important mucus and enzymes. Chewing well also works our jaw and face muscles. The mouth contains several *parotid glands,* located in the jaw behind the ears. As we chew, the parotid glands are stimulated, releasing T-cells into the blood, mucous and lymphatic pathways. This stimulates the immune system to guard against any invaders obtained by eating. It also stimulates the immune system in general.

The trick to better mastication is to take some slow easy breaths while chewing. It is also important to not to wash our food down with fluids. Better digestion can be accomplished if we let our saliva and amylase liquefy our food thoroughly while in our mouth prior to swallowing. We can swallow when it feels like runny mashed potatoes. In this form, the food will be prepared for the stomach. Drinking too many liquids while we eat dilutes all the enzymes required to break down the molecular structure of the food. When our enzymes become diluted, the stomach must work harder. By diluting important enzymes, we slow down their action potential. This leads to less nutrient absorption and longer digestive times. A sip now and again to rinse the palate is sufficient.

The esophagus is the staging area for food. If the mouth masticates the food well enough, the food will pass through the esophagus to the stomach within ten seconds. At the bottom of the esophagus is a valve called the esophageal sphincter. This valve lets food into the main stomach while keeping acid and food from backing up into the esophagus. An unhealthy sphincter does not close tightly enough—causing heartburn as acids and food irritate the sensitive mucous membranes of the esophagus. If the food delivered to the sphincter comes in too fast and rough, the *cricopharyngeus* muscle, which controls the sphincter, will weaken. When this muscle loses tone, the valve weakens, and the stomach's acids can leak back.

This is not the only cause for what is called heartburn. As food is dropped into the stomach, it undergoes intense churning and breakdown by the stomach's digestive juices. Special glands called *gastric cells* secrete a mixture of biochemicals within the stomach. This blend is composed primarily of hydrochloric acid, pepsin, rennin and special mucus made primarily of mucopolysaccharides. Depending upon the health of the stomach, these cells also secrete lipase, a fat-splitting enzyme. The enzymes pepsin and rennin break down proteins, preparing them for intestinal assimilation.

Gastric juice must have a particular pH to be effective. The pH is the action potential of its waveforms to break apart the waveform bonds that hold together the food molecules. This means the ionic waveforms within the gastric juice will interfere with the bonding waveforms of the food molecules just enough to break apart those molecules into essential portions. If the waveforms broke apart all the bonds like a nuclear explosion, there would be no nutrition potential left. Rather, we are talking about a precise breaking apart of long fatty acid chains to shorter fatty acid chains, and a breaking apart of complex carbohydrates into simple glucose molecules, for example.

In order to affect this, the acidity of gastric juice must be precise. In a healthy body, this ranges from a pH of one to three. Hydrochloric acid (HCL) is the central molecular component to reach this pH range. An acidic pH is critical to sterilize our food as well. Without enough HCL, the body runs the risk of allowing unwanted bacteria to grow in the stomach and intestines. One of these is *Helicobacter pylori*. Recent research has linked a majority of ulcers to *H. pylori* overgrowth in the stomach.

The common premise is that heartburn means too much acid in the stomach. Western medicine's solutions are antacids and acid-blockers. These will only provide a short fix for some—those with leaking esophagus sphincters. For others, antacids may not help the pain at all. Here the sphincter is not the problem. In these cases, antacids may even make matters worse, because they will push the pH too high. When the pH is too high, our food will not be broken down correctly, leaving the intestines with food too raw for absorption. This will also open up the stomach to invading organisms such as bacteria.

Acid-blocking medications may further exasperate the problem in many cases. These may be helpful for temporarily easing pain and removing the symptoms. They also can create the reduction of the very digestive juices needed to break down foods for intestinal absorption. They also cut back HCL production, allowing bacteria to possibly expand.

Research has been indicating that possibly more than three-quarters of ulcers involve an *H. pylori* infection. This seems to provide evidence showing that *H. pylori* might cause ulcers. However, it would be interesting to see how many *H. pylori* infections occurred after a heartburn sufferer self-medicated with antacids and/or acid-blockers for a while. How could the bacterial infection overgrowth occur if the acidic environment was maintained? Could it be that the infection was the result of blocking or neutralizing the body's natural flow of antiseptic acids into the stomach? This could only be proved with a long-term study of heartburn patients before their digestive issues developed into an ulcer, and before they began antacids or acid-blocks to reduce stomach acidity. However, it does seem likely. Clinical observation illustrates that many heartburn cases develop into ulcer cases. In a majority of these cases, the heartburn sufferer begins self-medicating with various acid blocking and acid neutralizing medications.

Meanwhile, traditional healing modalities such as *Ayurveda,* TCM, and western herbalism have been promoting the use of various herbs and barks that that balance and even increase the stomach's HCL production for heartburn and ulcer patients. There are a number of pungent and bitter botanicals that balance gastric juices; including cabbage juice, fresh ginger juice, black pepper and dandelion flowers. These all promote the correct pH and stimulate gastric acid production. How? Because these are botanicals containing biochemical messengers that coherently and constructively stimulate similar activity within the botanical plant body.

Along with gastric acids, special glands in the stomach called *pyloric mucous glands* produce and secrete a thick mucus which will provide a lining and covering for the stomach *fundus,* protecting it from the heat within the enzymes and acids released by the gastric pits. These mucous glands are stimulated by the vagus nerve as we begin to eat. This mucus lines the stomach cells, buffering them from the harsh gastric juices. Sometimes heartburn is the result of too little mucus lining within the stomach and the lower esophagus. This is often the case for those who do not drink enough liquids, or those who are under stress. When the body is stressed, the programming of the mind focuses its energies upon muscle and nervous activity, depleting the resources of the mucous glands.

Antacids may temporarily neutralize the acids that may be damaging the stomach's cells. The obvious question is why the stomach's own acids should damage its cells. The answer lies within the health of the stomach's lining—its mucosal membrane. This relates to whether the diet is healthy and whether there is enough water consumption. This is because hydration and nutrition are directly related to mucus secretion.

Drinking water on an empty stomach improves absorption. One of the best times to drink water is first thing in the morning before we eat and before we brush our teeth. Drinking on any empty stomach will not only hydrate the body faster—as the stomach directly assimilates water into the bloodstream. It also delivers mucus from the mouth and esophagus into the stomach. To increase our stomach mucus, we might consider sucking on a little sour fruit or pressing our tongue around the mouth to produce more saliva. Then we can swallow that with or without water. Doing this prior to a meal will increase our stomach mucus. Note that water should precede the meal by at least 15-20 minutes to allow for absorption. It also helps to relax and breathe prior to and during a meal. This relaxes the vagus nerve, stimulating more mucus formation. When the body is stressed, the body's activities will be drawn away from the digestive activities, leaving the stomach with too little mucus. It is for this reason that people with too much stress will often also have heartburn.

Several herbs are known to increase the production of mucus in the stomach. They include slippery elm bark, marshmallow root, ginger root, and licorice root. Taking a daily tea with these on an empty stomach can do wonders for the health of our intestinal lining. They will also help a sore throat. Why? Because the throat and esophagus is also lined with mucous membranes, which can become raw when too little mucus is being produced. This is often the case in rhinovirus or rotavirus infections; the body's fluid and immune resources are often drawn away from the mucous membranes in order to fight the infection.

Imbalances in stomach acids typically reflect issues related to either taking on too much responsibility or taking our responsibilities too seriously. These scenarios can create stress without a relief valve, leading to frustration or even anger. The balance in our stomach acidity therefore reflects the balance among our work, family and other responsibilities. This is tied closely to our ability to express ourselves, and be honest about what we can and cannot do. Often those with stomach imbalances tend to 'hold things in,' trying to make believe that they can handle the load when in fact they need help. Part of this issue is not expressing ourselves when we have taken on too great a burden. We might assume that others will notice the burden we are taking on and come to our aid. Often this does not happen, simply because others are mostly focused upon their own burdens. After taking on the burden for some time without aid, the self may become frustrated and even angry for having to carry the load alone. If we need help from others, we simply need to express it.

We may also need the advice of others. Asking for advice does not diminish our standing, as many of us believe. Asking for advice in a situation where we feel burdened will only add to our base of knowledge from which we can draw. In addition, the people around us will respect the fact that we are open to their opinion. Too many of us go around thinking that we know all the answers and that our perspective is shared by everyone. In reality, we have one tiny perspective and others may have a completely different one. It is important that we understand where others are coming from at least. This simply takes open communication.

Expressing ourselves is not the same as blowing up at people. It actually means the opposite. It requires that we explain the problem calmly and clearly (not just to anyone, but the key person in the problem) with a humble approach—not feeling as if we are owed anything. Communicating clearly without an attitude, and admitting that we cannot handle something alone can relieve us of our burden, or at least make others aware of it so their expectations are reasonable. This can also stimulate a resolution to the issue, nipping the bud on any possibility of internal anger or resentments. This in turn should also result in a balanced flow of *pitta*, as too much *pitta* is a reflection of frustration. If we are suffering from either heartburn, indigestion or an ulcer, managing the issue with nature's botanical agents is important. For resolution and future prevention, however, we need to address the emotional issues of our inner self.

The Intestines

The small intestines are made of three parts: the duodenum, the jejunum, and the ileum. The duodenum is only about 30 centimeters long, but the jejunum runs about two meters and the ileum is another three meters in length. The intestine is a contorted tube about two to three centimeters in diameter. Throughout the inside of the intestines are finger-like protrusions called villi. These villi are filled with blood and lymph vessels to absorb and circulate nutrients.

We have been taught that nutrition is the sum of little parts called vitamins, minerals, proteins and fats. This 'parting' out of the elements of nutrition masks the real process. Most people figure that as long as the food (or pill) contains these nutrients we will have adequate nutrition.

This is simply not true. There are a number of studies reporting people supplementing with synthetic or isolated vitamins continuing to show the symptoms of deficiency in some of those vitamins.

Nutrients must be in a particular molecular bonding structure to be absorbed and do the body any good. It is also essential that these nutrients have the appropriate cofactors for assimilation. Minerals, for example are best chelated to particular proteins or fatty acids in order to be assimilated. Fat-soluble vitamins are best attached to sterols or lipids for digestion. Many other cofactors are also required. Vitamin C, for example, must be accompanied by cofactors such as bioflavonoids for proper absorption and utilization by the body. We might ask how we can obtain the right cofactors. Quite simply, they are obtainable from nature's molecular bonding combinations. The body is precisely tuned to the types of cofactors that exist among nature's plant kingdom. The nutrient combinations occurring within fruits, vegetables, nuts, roots, grains, grasses, seaweeds, and beans are presented in precisely the right combinations our body requires. This is because the physical body is permanently linked to the bonding waveforms transformed through nature's elements.

Botanicals provide all of the human body's nutritional needs. Many believe that meat is necessary to get complete nutrition. This, however, is not as efficient as obtaining nutrients from plant sources. Meat must also be cooked under intense heat to make it palatable, which destroys many heat-sensitive nutrients. Our bodies simply are not designed to eat raw meat. Our intestines are too long and narrow. If we compare the intestinal tracts of meat-eating animals with botanical eating animals, humans clearly have intestinal tracts more suitable to eating vegetables, fruits, nuts, beans and roots. Our intestinal tracts have a particular shape, length, enzymes and anatomy best suited to break apart high-fiber foods and convert them into nutrients. Meats have very little fiber. For this reason, meat-eaters predominantly suffer from colon cancer, irritable bowel syndrome, polyps, and a variety of other intestinal tract disorders. A plethora of studies have documented that these disorders are significantly related to a lack of fiber in the diet.

The intestines, bile, enzymes and villa must also exist within a particular environment to enable the proper breakdown and assimilation of nutrients. There is a sensitive balance required between the ionic state of the food and the intestinal tract environment. This environment is dictated primarily by the various mucous membranes, the liver, the pancreas, and the vagus nerve, which all work conjunctively to orchestrate the supply of various enzymes, pH and liquefaction into the intestinal tract.

In between the villi are glands that secrete bile from the liver via the gallbladder, and various enzymes from the pancreas. The vagus nerve stimulates the intelligent release of these substances. How does this happen? The vagus nerve responds to relayed waveform interference patterns that originate from a combination of sensory perception and the biofeedback messengers from around the body. Thus, the sensations of taste, smell, vision, satiety, metabolism, blood glucose levels and more are converged to display an immediate combined projection onto the *chakra* region. The *chakra's* programming imparts specific responses such as the mucus and gastrin production and peristalsis motion.

The various biochemicals expressed by a healthy stomach wall and a healthy diet will maintain a particular pH within the food and mucus mix—or *chyme*. This enables enzymes to adequately reach and break down the food contents into nutrient-combinations the body can recognize and utilize. Proteins are broken down to polypeptides (amino acids) by protease. Fats are broken down to glycerol and fatty acids by lipase. Lactose is broken down into glucose and galactose by lactase—just to name a few of the many enzymes the body uses to break down foods for assimilation.

How does the body know how to break these molecules down? Long protein or fatty acid chains could be theoretically broken down into a variety of combinations. For example, particular polypeptides are produced when long proteins are broken down by protease enzymes. The body performs this process through waveform scanning processes. Molecules are intelligently scanned by immune system cells like IgA and IgE antibodies, along with T-cells and B-cells. Food molecules are also scanned as they enter the gaps between the intestine's microvilli.

The intestinal *brush barrier* is a complex mucosal layer of enzymes, probiotics and ionic fluid. It forms a protective film over the intestinal epithelium. It also provides an active nutrient transport mechanism. This mucosal layer is stabilized by the grooves of the intestinal microvillus. It contains glycoproteins and other ionic transporters that attach to nutrient molecules, carrying them across intestinal membranes. Meanwhile the transport medium requires a delicately pH-balanced mix of ionic chemistry able to facilitate this transport of amino acids, minerals, vitamins, glucose and fatty acids. The mucosal layer is policed by billions of probiotic colonies that help process incoming food molecules, excrete various nutrients, and control pathogens.

Typically, intestinal barriers let only smaller molecules access to the liver and bloodstream—usually beneficial nutrients. Should larger, undigested food molecules enter the bloodstream—even if from a food consumed for decades—the body's immune system will not recognize them. This can lead to IgA and/or IgE responses, with associated histamine conversion causing skin and/or sinus inflammatory response. This can thus result in the double-edged eventuality that a food, formerly a source of nutrition, can suddenly be identified by the immune system as toxic, resulting not only in an autoimmune allergic response, but also in nutritional deficiencies because of the lack of absorption.

The epithelium of the intestinal tract functions is a triple-filter barrier that screens for molecule size, ionic nature and nutrition quality. Much of this is performed via three mechanisms existing between the intestinal microvilli: *tight junctions, adherens junctions* and *desmosomes.* The tight functions form a bilayer interface between cells, controlling permeability. Desmosomes are points of interface between the tight junctions, and adherens junctions keep the cell membranes adhesive enough to stabilize the junctions. These junction mechanisms together regulate permeability at the intestinal wall.

The mucosal brush barrier and the microvilli junctions together form the boundary between intestinal contents and our bloodstream. Should the mucosal layer chemistry become altered, its protective and ionic transport mechanisms will become weakened, allowing toxic or larger molecules to be presented to the microvilli junctions. This contact can irritate the microvilli, causing a subsequent inflammatory response. Such a response will also weaken the microvilli junctions, allowing the larger molecules immediate access to the bloodstream.

Alteration of the intestinal mucosal layer and the subsequent weakening of the microvilli junctions can be caused by a number of factors. Alcohol is one of the most irritating substances to the mucosal lining and junctions. In addition, many pharmaceutical drugs, notably NSAIDs, have been identified as damaging to the mucosal chemistry and junction strength. Foods with high arachidonic fatty acid capability (such as trans-fats and cooked animal meats), low-fiber, high-glucose foods, and high nitrite-forming foods have all been suspected for their ability to compromise the intestinal lining. Toxic substances such as plasticizers, pesticides, herbicides and food dyes are also suspected. In general, substances which increase PGE-2 response are suspected to increase unhealthy permeability. In addition, the overuse of antibiotics can kill-off the all-important resident probiotic colonies. With intestinal probiotic colonies decreased, pathogenic bacteria and yeasts can outgrow probiotic colonies. This pathogenic bacteria growth invades the brush barrier, introducing an influx of endotoxins (the waste matter of these microorganisms) to the bloodstream together with some of the microorganisms themselves. Lack of hydration and stress are also suspected as contributing factors to irritable bowel issues.

Inflammatory responses resulting from intestinal disorders have increasingly been attributed to cases of sinusitis, allergies, psoriasis, asthma, arthritis, fibromyalgia and more by holistic doctors aware of these mechanisms. Overgrowth of *Candida albicans,* a typical fungal inhabitant of the digestive system at minimal numbers, has also been attributed to increased intestinal permeability. It has been proposed that systemic *Candida* infections have a route of translocation via increased intestinal permeability. Research further confirms a correlation between increased permeability and liver damage.

Should our pancreas be burdened or stressed, it will not produce enough enzymes. When the body is in stress mode, hormones and blood go elsewhere, leaving the pancreas in low metabolic gear. For this reason, it is important to relax when we eat. Otherwise, our food might end up significantly undigested.

Enzyme production can decrease with age. For example, lactase production can slow down as our bodies get older. For this reason, people have more difficulties drinking milk after many years of milk drinking. However, this does not necessarily mean we are lactose intolerant. Recent studies have showed that most people claiming to be lactose-intolerant could still drink at least a glass of milk a day without any problems. Prevailing opinion is that many suspect lactose intolerance simply because lactase production slows down a bit.

The research indicates the reality is that many adults lose some of the important probiotics that help our bodies digest dairy. Eating cheese and yogurt can in turn supply the probiotics that can help us digest lactose. These probiotics produce lactase to help ou bodies break down the lactose in milk.

For conditions related to cramping and indigestion, we can consider not drinking fluids with meals. This will better concentrate the enzymes. Beyond that, enzymes and probiotic supplementation should be considered. Enzyme supplements are readily available in broad mixes, and should be taken with meals. Probiotics are microorganisms that live in between our villi and elsewhere. This will be discussed in more depth later.

Intestinal issues like irritable bowel, polyps, and intestinal permeability relate to the self's issues regarding boundaries and giving up of oneself.

Often we give of ourselves to a person or people who may take advantage of that giving. As this activity continues we may begin to feel that we are giving too much, yet we are feeling too deep. We do not feel that we can withdraw without bad consequences. We feel therefore obligated to continue being a caregiver, regardless of the effects this may have upon our health. As this situation worsens, we begin to feel the knots within our intestines. The stress we are expressing physically (yet withholding externally) restricts the flow of bile into our intestines, and changes the pH of the intestinal tract, which changes the mucosal lining, probiotic colonies, and eventually the intestinal wall. As the intestinal wall changes, it begins to become damaged and diseased, and the body's immune system begins to attack the intestine's cells to get rid of them. The body begins attacking itself. This is an expression of the self needing something to give. We are feeling that we are giving too much and we need something to change. We need to rearrange the boundaries. This manifests into intestinal issues, as our feeling of giving too much manifests in a sub-conscious self-annihilation of our body. This does not indicate any sort of mental defect, however. It is simply the self needing to reconcile our sacrifices to others with our own needs.

The solution here is to be honest with ourselves and others. We need to draw our boundaries clearly and tell those we are caring for that we can only do so much. That we can only give so much. We need to also take care of ourselves. This lack of boundary can be immediately dealt with once we express our situation honestly within ourselves, and then humbly with those we are giving too much to. They will understand.

Intestinal health requires that sufficient bile with the right chemistry is released from our gallbladder . Without enough bile, our ability to digest fats, proteins and so many other nutrients will be altered. Undigested fats, proteins, sugars and carbohydrates in turn create gas, bloating, irritable bowels, and constipation among other things. Our gallbladder stages and times the release of bile and salts from the liver into the intestines as needed—timed intelligently to our intake of foods. Without the gallbladder, bile infusion does not time with our meals. We may still have enough bile, but the timing may be off. Therefore, a person who has their gallbladder removed is well advised to eat smaller and more consistent meals throughout the day.

The liver produces bile as it recycles its filtered components from the blood and lymph. In cases where the body has imbalances in calcium, cholesterol and other minerals, the gallbladder may crystallize the excessive components into gallstones. This can be worsened by a meat diet, as excess amino acids, uric acids and arachidonic acids result, precipitating more calcium from the bones to balance these acids in the bloodstream. (This is also a cause of osteoporosis, as the bones leach calcium for this same reason.) The best way to prevent gallstones is to eat a well-balanced plant-based diet with plenty of fiber, minerals, and sufficient water between meals.

As mentioned, fiber is also extremely critical for proper digestion. This is because fiber regulates the absorption process. It does this by absorbing excess water, allowing enzymes to be more concentrated, while softening indigestibles headed for stool. Without both soluble and insoluble fiber, starches will be broken down, assimilated and converted too quickly into glucose. As this glucose hits the bloodstream, it stimulates insulin production from the pancreas. This avalanche of glucose stresses the pancreas and the cells. As this forces an imbalance in the pathway, this in turn can create insulin insensitivity and glucose insensitivity among the glucose receptors and insulin receptors at the cell membranes. This insensitivity encourages obesity and type II diabetes because the cells are not utilizing the glucose, leaving blood sugar too high.

Our level of fiber intake relates directly to our trust in nature. Professional consensus suggests 25 grams of fiber a day is a bare minimum, and 40-50 grams per day is recommended by holistic nutritionists with at least 50-75% being soluble. The average American diet contains no more than about 12-15 grams of fiber. Nature presents us with whole foods with ideal fiber ratios designed to pace with the body's natural rhythms. Great fiber choices include whole fruits like apples, whole grains like oats, vegetables like celery and roots like carrots and potatoes. Every meal can have 5-15 grams of fiber. Low fiber meals stress the body's resources, and increase the likelihood of obesity, heart disease, and blood sugar problems.

Healthy fats from nuts and seeds are also helpful in balancing glucose absorption. Seeds, nuts and beans have lignans and phytoestrogens that also help balance our hormone secretions, which help normalize inflammatory response. Because fatty acids from these fats are complexed with various nutrients like vitamin E, they are broken down slowly. A meal with healthy fats will time-release absorption, giving us a steady stream of energy instead of the roller-coaster insulin-glucose ride.

Research has illustrated that the healthiest mix of fats is about 10% saturated; 10% gamma linoleic acid (GLA); about 40% long chain omega-3 fatty acids such as alpha linolenic acid (ALA), eicosapentaenoic acid (EPA) and docosahexaenoic acid (DHA); and 40% healthy omega-6 unrefined oils from nuts, sesame and sunflower seeds, olives and canola. GLA is found in green leafy vegetables, spirulina, borage and primrose oil.

ALA found in walnuts, pumpkin seeds, flax, chia seed, salba seed and canola will convert to the longer DHA and EPA chains using an enzyme called desaturase. For unhealthy people this conversion proves difficult, however, requiring the need to obtain DHA from other sources like fish, or even better, golden microalgae. The DHA from microalgae grown in tanks does have the risk of mercury, saturated fat and toxins seen in both farmed and wild fish. In addition, microalgae are not subject to extinction as many fish are.

Fortunately, most of the epithelial cells of the small intestine are replaced within about a week. With probiotic supplementation, good intentions, a high-fiber, nutritious diet with plenty of fresh foods, intestinal health can be regained in most cases. Botanicals helpful for healing and stimulating intestinal digestion include papayas, pineapples, fennel, peppermint, licorice, black pepper, ginger, and anise. A light, circular abdominal self-massage is also helpful after a large meal.

The Liver

The liver is a workhorse and the body's lifeline to useable blood, nutrients and detoxification. The liver sits just below the lungs on the right side under the diaphragm. Partially protected by the ribs, it attaches to the abdominal wall with the *falciform ligament.* The *ligamentum teres* within the falciform is the remnant of the umbilical cord that once brought us blood from mama's placenta. As the body develops, the liver continues its function to filter, purify and enrich the blood that courses through our blood vessels. Should the liver shut down, our body would be dead within hours.

The liver is the body's scrubbing mechanism. This takes place on a number of levels, but primarily through a process where particular cells attach and break apart foreign chemicals. Into the liver drains the nutrition-rich venous blood following its coming in from the intestines through the hepatic portal vein. This is blended with oxygenated blood through the hepatic artery. A healthy liver will process about 1500 ml (about 50 ounces) of blood per minute. The blended blood is commingled within well cavities called sinusoids, where blood is staged through stacked sheets of the liver's primary cells—called hepatocytes. Here blood is also met by interspersed macrophage immune cells called *kupffer cells.* These kupffer cells attack and break apart bacteria and toxins. Hepatocytes further filter and purify the blood. Nutrients coming in from the digestive tract are converted to biomolecular structures the body's cells can utilize. The liver also converts old red blood cells to bilirubin. The filtered, purified and metabolized blood is jettisoned through hepatic veins out the inferior vena cava, where it is then pumped through the heart, oxygenated by the lungs, and then pumped into circulation.

The liver's filtration/purification mechanisms protect our body from various infectious diseases and chemical toxins. After hepatocytes and kupffer cells break down toxins, the waste products are disposed through the gall bladder and kidneys.

The gall bladder channels bile from the liver to the intestines. Bile is made up of bile acids, combined with bilirubin, phospholipids, bicarbonate ions, and cholesterol. The bile acids thus act as an efficient carrier for waste materials. The gall bladder will concentrate and save bile until it is stimulated by eating. Once stimulated, the gall bladder pumps the bile into the duodenum, just in time for food being dumped into the intestines from the stomach. Here the bile acids such as taurcholic acid and deoxycholic acid help to break down large fatty acid molecular chains by electromagnetically attaching to certain fatty acid chains. This essentially breaks apart some of the larger fatty acid chains, allowing the body to absorb the shorter fatty acids. This process also helps make fat-soluble vitamins resonate with our body's biochemical needs, thereby increasing their assimilation.

Bile acids will make more than thirty roundtrips between the liver, gall bladder, intestines, colon and back to the liver. This cycling is part of the body's rhythmic process of escorting toxins out and nutrients in.

The liver assembles over a thousand biochemicals the body requires for various functions. The liver maintains blood sugar balance by monitoring glucose levels and assembling glucose metabolites. It assembles albumin to maintain plasma pressure. It assembles cholesterol, urea, inflammatory biochemicals, blood-clotting molecules, and many others critical to metabolism.

The assembly of metabolites within the liver is a highly advanced waveform process. Hepatocytes contain complex scanning and matching mechanisms within their ion channel gateways. Here waveform bonds with particular specificities are matched with other waveform bonds to form bioactive, intelligent molecules. What makes the liver so intelligent? There are no brain cells within the liver, are there? The liver is pre-programmed in the same way other organs are. The liver is innervated by a complex branching from the vagus nerve along with a plexus from the phrenic nerves, which tie together within the third *chakra* region. The programming drives both sympathetic and parasympathetic activities, giving the liver direct and autonomic control from the mind. The liver is also supplied with thermal heat converted through the third energy center or *chakra* system, which is pumped in through the *vishvodara nadi* channel and distributed through the body through the paired liver acupuncture *meridians*.

Interspersed within the liver are functional fat factories called *stellates*. These cells store and process lipids, fat-soluble vitamins such as vitamin A, and secrete structural biomolecules like collagen, laminin and glycans. These are used to build some of the body's toughest tissue systems.

Research on infectious diseases such as Ebola, SARS, *Salmonella, E. coli*, hepatitis, HIV, influenza and MRSA indicate that infection rates over the past decade are increasing. Meanwhile, toxicity-related and autoimmune diseases such as arthritis, allergies, irritable bowel syndrome and many others are also on the rise. Why are these illnesses rising in the face of increased availability of pharmaceuticals and antibiotics?

This is a complex question. Most researchers agree that our livers are weakening under the attack from an avalanche of toxins pelting our bodies, however. Today our diets, water and air are full of plasticizers, formaldehyde, heavy metals, hydrocarbons, DDT, dioxine, VOCs, asbestos, preservatives, artificial flavors, food dyes, propellants, synthetic fragrances and more. Every single foreign chemical requires the liver to work harder. Why? Because the liver's hepatocytes must be more focused and its immune cells must be deployed in greater numbers to scan, surround, snag, break apart and dispose of greater volumes of foreign molecules.

Frankly, most livers are now overloaded and beyond their natural capacity. Why is this bad? First, the hepatocytes can collapse from over-toxification, causing genetic mutation, cell death, and liver exhaustion. Secondly, a weak liver condition opens hepatocytes to diseases from infectious agents such as viral hepatitis.

Liver disease—where one or more lobes begin to malfunction—can result in a life-threatening emergency. Cirrhosis is a common diagnosis for liver disease. A malfunctioning liver can also result in fatty liver, jaundice, high cholesterol, gallstones, encephalopathy, kidney disease, clotting problems, heart conditions, hormone imbalances and many others. Cirrhosis can occur concurrently, resulting in massive hepatocyte die-off and subsequent scarring, causing the liver to begin to shutdown.

Most of us have heard about the damage alcohol can have on the liver. Many do not realize that pharmaceuticals and even some supplements can also be extremely toxic to the liver. The liver must find a way to break down these foreign chemicals. Many pharmaceuticals require a Herculean effort simply because the liver's various purification processes were not designed for these foreign molecules. As liver cells weaken and die their enzymes leak into the bloodstream. For this reason, blood tests for AST and ALT enzymes can reveal this weakening of the liver.

We must therefore closely monitor the quantity and types of chemicals we put into our body. Eliminating preservatives, food dyes and pesticides in our foods can be done easily by eating whole organic foods. We can eliminate exposures to many environmental toxins mentioned above by simply replacing them with natural alternatives. Phosphate-based soaps and other cleaners can be replaced with glycerin-based soaps, vinegar and baking soda. Synthetic fragrances can be replaced with natural essences and aromatherapeutic agents. Pesticides can be replaced with various oils like castor bean oil, elements like sulphur and lime, and other natural agents like sodium borate—also known as borax.

Reviewing our prescription medications closely with our doctor and questioning the necessity of each is also critical to the health of our liver. Today physicians often prescribe multiple medications without reviewing their combined effect upon the liver. Prescriptions should never be changed without our doctor's consent. Still, there is no reason why we cannot carefully question our physician or even seek a second or third opinion before medication use. We can also request a liver enzyme test, and we can request a referral to an herbalist or naturopath who can work conjunctively to offer herbal alternatives that do not endanger our liver.

A number of herbs help detoxify and strengthen the liver. These include golden seal, dandelion, milk thistle, garlic, cayenne pepper, black pepper and others. Dandelion and milk thistle are common "weeds" that can also be harvested locally and added to the diet as general tonics. A healthy liver also requires plenty of water to replenish itself and process its various metabolites. ½ ounce of water per pound of body weight is a good guide for an active person, less about 20% for the water in food. A healthy liver is critical for healthy cellular performance, mental acuity and skin health. Without a healthy liver, our body is destined for less than sub-performance.

Generally, an unhealthy liver reflects a problem with over-consumption. When the self is feeling empty and depressed because we are unfulfilled, we will be tempted to consume more than we should. This stresses the liver because too much consumption means the liver has to work harder to produce all the enzymes and biochemicals needed to process these foods.

A damaged liver may also reflect a self needing to escape. If we do not want to face our situation and do not want to grow from it, we may be tempted to try to escape the situation with alcoholism or drugs. These do not solve the problem, we later find out. They merely allow us to temporarily forget our issues. We soon have to face them in addition to a physiological addiction. So our problems only worsen. There are plenty of healthy ways to escape. Sports and exercise provide useful escape mechanisms if needed. Better to face our situations head-on and grow from them. Figure out why we are in the situation we are in, and solve the problem. Solving the problem is often easier than escaping from it. The weakened liver is feeding back to the body that it is time to solve our problems and not try to escape from them.

The Colon

Most of us think of the colon—often referred to as the large intestine—as no more than a pipe: Like an air duct or water main. Although the colon transports partially digested food-waste though a bending tube-like structure, it functions more like an organ than a pipe. In fact, a malfunctioning colon will disease the entire body, increase fatigue, lower athletic performance and cause various infections.

The gateway between the small intestine and the colon is the *ileocecal* valve. The ileocecal valve sits in a chamber called the *cecum.* The cecum is a drain-trap—similar to the bend plumbers build into pipes to trap sediment. To clean out the trap, the cecum is connected to the immune system via the appendix. The appendix is a part of the lymphatic network and immune system, which supplies antibodies and macrophages to remove toxins and bacteria before they can enter the colon. A healthy cecum is also colonized by probiotics that battle pathogenic bacteria.

A cecum chamber full of pathogenic bacteria can overwhelm the appendix. This can cause the appendix to swell, causing the well-known appendicitis attack. Why is it so important to for the body to keep pathogenic bacteria out of the colon?

The colon is typically about three to six feet long with three bendy sections. The first section ascends the right side of the abdomen. The second section transverses the abdomen. The third section descends the left side of the abdomen to the rectum. A healthy colon houses trillions of probiotic bacteria colonies. These bacteria, primarily of the *bifidobacterium* family, work to ferment and convert the residual fibers, nutrients and fatty acids left in our foods to short-chain fatty acids (butyric, acetic, valerate and propionic acids) and vitamins K, A and B. The colon also releases water and potassium into the bloodstream. Without these important nutrients, the body can become malnourished. For example, a lack of butyric acid has been linked to colitis and colon cancer.

The colon is an important detoxification organ. The liver dumps various waste metabolites into the colon and, assuming an unclogged colon—which many of us have—these are dumped out the rectum within hours. One of the more important metabolites the colon absorbs is cholesterol. A healthy colon with plenty of fiber in the diet will thus reduce cholesterol levels—especially the low-density lipoproteins (LDL) considered the primary cause for atherosclerosis.

If the colon is stagnant and not moving fast enough, it will release various waste products back into the bloodstream. A slow moving colon will release ammonia, histamines, skatoles, indoles, putrescine, cadaverine, hydrogen sulfide, tyramine, phenols, neurone and a number of endotoxins produced by pathogenic bacteria into the bloodstream.

The famous Harvey Kellogg, M.D., an early twentieth century physician and champion of colon cleansing, performed thousands of colon surgeries for colitis, cancer or other intestinal diseases. Dr. Kellog once said, *"Of the 22,000 operations that I have personally performed, I have never found a single normal colon, and of the 100,000 that were performed under my jurisdiction, not over 6% were normal."*

A toxic and slow-moving colon is a destructive source of pollution and acids into the bloodstream. These toxins can produce a number of unhealthy symptoms. These include sinusitis, asthma, rheumatoid arthritis, chronic fatigue, allergies, food sensitivities, fibromyalgia, acidosis, and general toxemia. Histamine, for example, increases the body's inflammatory activities, often accelerating the pathway of inflammation and swelling. This burdens the weaker areas of our bodies, driving the inflammatory cascade as the body works to remove these toxins.

The health of the colon is directly related to movement. Movement directly relates to the amount of toxins in the body. Toxins slow cells' metabolic performance because the cells also must work to detoxify. This diverts their functions from their primary tasks. Cellular toxicity also slows oxygenation and the removal of lactic acid. Lactic acid removal is critical in reducing muscle fatigue.

A slow colon diseases itself by putrefying various bacteria and waste materials. For this reason, colon cancer is one of the leading forms of cancer. Colitis has reached epidemic levels, and constipation is a common experience for a majority of Americans. Simply increasing the speed of movement and increasing probiotic colonies will slow toxin release into the blood and reduce the number of pathogenic bacteria in the colon.

The clearing of the colon is made difficult by a pervasive *mucoid plaque* layer build up in the colon. Years of overeating foods that move slowly through the colon and putrefy—low-fiber processed foods, red meats and fried foods—creates a thick layer of plaque along the walls of the colon. This plaque might be compared to the artery plaque of atherosclerosis. As it builds, it narrows the opening (lumen) of the colon, clogging and slowing movement.

Imagine a three-inch pipe, lined with sediment to the point where the opening is only one-half inch. This is the case for many who eat a modern western diet. Rather than sediment, colon plaque is a thick layer of gooey, bacteria-laden crud: A living layer of gunk. This layer of plaque can weigh up to ten pounds. Pathogenic bacteria thrive within this layer of mucoid plaque.

Clearing the colon is easier than we might think. Many supplement manufacturers offer various (and sometimes expensive) colon cleanse products, but these typically require many months of use to even make a dent in the mucoid plaque. These are certainly better than nothing. By far the easiest method of safely removing our mucoid plaque layer, however, is through colon hydrotherapy. This is a process where a colon hydrotherapist inserts a hose hooked to a hydrotherapy machine that gently circulates water through the colon and extracts the plaque and built-up waste. A few treatments of this "flushing" will remove most plaque immediately. Additionally, most colon hydrotherapists now provide a "probiotic insert," which delivers critical *bifidus* probiotic bacteria directly into the colon. This "insert" virtually guarantees the colon's immediate re-colonization of probiotic. Colon hydrotherapy centers exist in most cities, and they are typically very reasonably priced—especially when compared to expensive colon surgery or even colon cancer medical treatment.

Clearing out the plaque can turn around a bad case of constipation as well: Especially if we are eating right, and training our colon to eliminate regularly. Some of us wait to defecate when the urge comes on. The best approach, however, is to train the bowels by sitting on the toilet everyday at about the same time—a time when we have a few minutes to relax and preferably in the privacy of our home. This intentionally trains our peristalsis movement to defecate at certain times. Once in the morning and once in the evening is ideal. Still we may also need to answer the call outside of these times. For many, once a day may be enough. Less than once a day should be considered constipation.

Diet is key to colon speed. By reducing red meat and fried foods and increasing high fiber foods and plant-based foods, we can effectively speed things up. While a fiber- and plant-rich meal might take 24-30 hours from meal to defecation, red meat and fried meals will typically take about 48-72 hours. Our diet should consist of at least 40 grams of fiber per day. Increasing roughage will also keep the colon cleaner, and reduce mucoid plaque build-up. Most western meat-heavy diets barely contain 10-15 grams. For this reason, westerners have the highest rates of colon cancers in the world. Good sources of supplemental fiber are psyllium husks, flax, salba and greenfoods. Healthy laxatives include magnesium, rhubarb, aloe, and of course prune juice.

An unhealthy colon typically reflects a problem with the self's goals and objectives. The self needs to have clear goals and objectives. Without those, the body expressing the self moves aimlessly, without determination or discipline. The lack of discipline also tends to show itself in the form of our diet. If we do not have a goal or objective, we often do not care that an unhealthy diet can cause colon cancer, diabetes and various other pathologies. We do not make a determination to eat right. While developing nutritional goals and objectives may not heal an immediate bout with constipation, a change in our diet and eating habits will certainly achieve a long-term solution to the problem.

The best strategy to create goals and objectives in life is to first start with a lifetime goal: What do we want to accomplish with our life? After determining this major goal (or goals), we then draw those out into a twenty year plan (depending upon our age), a ten year plan, a five year plan, then a one year plan. The closer the date, the more specific the detail should be, so that we can define how we get from the point we are at now to the lifetime goal. As we develop our shorter-term goals, we will find that our life begins to take on new meaning. Our goals become a foundation upon which we prioritize our activities. We find that our body's health then becomes a vehicle for arriving at our goals. At this point, we will see the need for a good diet, without being too wrapped up in it.

The Heart and Cardiovascular System

The heart is not only an organ. It is also one of the most celebrated parts of the anatomy from a conscious perspective. The heart has been referred to allegorically for centuries, with expressions such as *"he broke my heart," "I gave him my heart," "that was heartless," "I put my heart into it,"* and so on. It seems that these references actually have a concrete basis. The heart lies within the fourth *chakra* region, which expresses and translates emotions of the self related to love, compassion, relationships, and giving. It is no accident that this region virtually controls all aspects of circulation and nutrition. The heart's connection with love and relationships simply reflects the importance of these aspects to the inner self. Without loving relationships, the inner self loses the purpose for living.

This is evident when widowers die shortly after their wife dies. Two decades ago, the U.S. National Institute of Mental Health found that within the six months of a wife's death, a widower over 55 has a 40%

greater likelihood of dying than other men of the same age (Hope 1989). The term "died of a broken heart," comes into context here.

Using some of this logic, Hippocrates proposed that the seat of the mind and the self was within the heart. This was challenged two centuries later by Erasistratus of Alexandria, Egypt, who found that sensory and motor nerves seemed to more closely relate to the functions of the mind. Erasistratus contended that the living self or vital force within the body was contained in a subtle vapor, which he referred to as *pneuma*. Modern medicine has of course dismissed any existence of a vital force within the body, whether in the heart or brain. The heart is considered simply a pump, and the brain simply a conglomeration of neurons. Nevertheless, the importance of the heart's health to remaining alive is irrefutable.

Without nourishment brought by the cardiovascular system, the cells will die immediately. Therefore the heart's beat has been accepted for centuries as the indication that the body is dead. Today physicians judge death by the cessation of brainwaves. Whether dead at the moment of the heart stopping or not, however, prior to the expanded use of the cardiopulmonary bypass (also known as the heart-lung machine) once the heart stopped, the rest of the body would soon fall. The heart therefore lies at the center of the body's existence just as love lies at the center of the inner self's existence.

The beating of the heart is probably the body's most obvious and famous waveform cycle. The rhythms of the cardiovascular system consist of more than a couple of thumps. The heart and cardiovascular system beats with a complex waveform interference pattern. The heart's valves beat to a particular rhythm as they pump blood from the veins to the lungs and from the lungs out to the rest of the body. The arteries dilate and constrict rhythmically to accommodate this pumping system, while priming the circulation network for blood pumping.

The veins have their own rhythmic pumping system. The veins return blood to the liver, lungs and heart utilizing a pressurization differential driven by the pumping of the skeletal muscles around the body. This system helps maintain a critical low pressure to collapse the veins until they are pumped. As they are pumped, *venous valves* open and close, to help pump and effectively stop any backflow of venous blood. This process lifts blood from the lower part of the body toward the liver, heart and lungs.

The human heart has four chambers. The right and left atria are the upper chambers. They each connect to a ventricle on each side by means of valves. There are four valves. The right *atrioventricular* valve (or *tricuspid*) and the left atrioventricular valve (or *mitral*) each connect the atriums to the ventricle spaces. Deoxygenated blood will flow into the right atrium from the vena cava. Once in the atrium it will flow into the right ventricle through the tricuspid, whereupon it is pumped to the lungs through the pulmonary valve and pulmonary artery. Once rich with oxygen from the lungs, blood re-enters the heart though the pulmonary veins and into the left atrium, where it is channeled into the ventricle and pumped out to the rest of the body via the aortic valve and aorta.

This valve and pumping operation between the right and left sides of the heart is orchestrated with precise harmonics. Each of these steps coincides with muscle contractions of the heart divided between two phases, coordinated with the opening and closing of the valves. The heartbeat moves into the *systole* phase as the atria cardiac muscles flex to draw in blood into each side. Once this phase is complete and the blood is channeled through to each of the ventricles, the atria cardiac muscles relax and the ventricle muscles contract, forming the diastole phase. Each cycle takes about .8 seconds to complete.

The cardiac muscles are precisely arranged so that stimulation for the entire muscle range can be initiated from single points. The heart's beating is said to be a system of nerve *conduction.* Two key nerve nodes stimulate the heartbeat. This produces a type of impulse wave that maintains the beat rhythm. The first node is called the *sinoatrial node.* This is considered the heart's pacemaker, although the *atrioventricular node* is also a critical stimulating component, which not only provides for a pacing of contractions, but also can substitute for the sinusoidal node should this first node fail.

Between and during the waveform stimuli that occur through these nodes is an impulse wave that travels through a nerve bundle called the *bundle of his,* and then through nerve fibers called *purkinje.* These three nerve groupings are part of the fourth *chakra* region, programmed to impart a rhythmic stimulation that keeps every heartbeat synchronized and buffered.

Harmonizing with these waves is so-called blood pressure, which is actually a combination of cellular rhythms driving blood vessel wall contraction and blood circulation volume. The heart's pace and output is only one of the major components determining the blood pressure. Cardiac output tends to be about five or six liters per minute. Meanwhile, *vasoconstriction* occurs primarily in the arterioles—the blood vessels running between the larger arteries and the smaller capillaries. Because blood—like water—tends to flow from higher-pressured regions to lower-pressured regions, the blood's circulatory pulse resonates to form pressure waves.

Blood pressure is directly related to blood volume. The greater the amount of blood, the higher the pressure will be. Fluid volume and speed are the critical elements of blood pressure. Managing fluid intake and output is a factor of the kidneys, the lungs, the skin, the digestive tract, and the signaling of neurotransmitters and hormones partially regulated by minerals such as sodium and potassium. Then of course, there is the conscious effort required to keep the body and bloodstream properly hydrated.

The subtle orchestration of neurotransmitter and hormone biocommunication keeps all of these processes informed of the various requirements of the body along with the various programmed instructions from the mind and *chakras.* Within the brain is a vasomotor center, firing sympathetic information pulses to coordinate the appropriate level of blood vessel dilation or contraction, fluid levels, heartbeat pacing, energy utilization, oxygen levels, and all the other synchronized pulses that flow within the blood. The receptors for this signaling system are found within various glands. Secreted signaling chemicals originate primarily from the endocrine system and stimulate activity through biocommunication to receptors found in the cells of the lungs, the intestines, the eyes, the heart, the liver, the artery walls, and various other tissue systems. The basic receptor types have been tagged *alpha-1, alpha-2, beta-1* and *beta-2 receptors*—named to distinguish physiological response.

To regulate artery flexibility, messenger neurotransmitters and hormones stimulate alpha-1 receptors on blood vessel wall cells to initiate either the expansion or constriction of blood vessels (*vasodilation* or *vasoconstriction,* respectively). There are a number of biochemicals that have been observed complicit in stimulating the alpha receptors, depending upon the circumstance. Norepinephrine is one of the most effective. Norepinephrine initiates an urgent all-out physical response. Other signaling biochemicals include ADH, renin, angiotensin, and aldosterone, which modulate various functions such as fluid levels, liver activity and kidney functions. These biochemical waveform messengers can also stimulate beta-1 receptors on heart muscle cells to increase both stroke volume and heart rate. Beta-1 receptors also exist on the kidney's glomerular cells to govern fluid loss and retention. Epinephrine is another vasoconstrictor messenger, but epinephrine tends to stimulate alpha-1 receptors as well as more specialized beta-2 receptors. Beta-2 receptors stimulate skeletal muscle arteriole cell walls to dilate. Epinephrine is thus more selective in its stimulation, allowing for a precise flight-or-fight response. Blood volume levels ebb and flow with the waves of cardiac output levels, artery wall flexibility and lumen (the opening size of the artery) size. Because these levels all are balanced with the body's mineral chemistry, sodium levels and hydration levels also relate to ADH release. In all, the orchestration of waves, tidal ebbs and flows, and fluctuating artery walls might be compared to the synchronous motion of waves and water working the beach and tidal zones.

This interplay of rhythms regulates and maintains blood pressure using a check and balance system throughout the cells that make up the blood vessel walls, the various nerves, and the biochemical messenger system. Larger arteries and the aorta might have an average pressure of 100 mm Hg. Arteriole pressure, however, will be less—ranging from 35-80 mm Hg. At this pressure, capillaries will be at only about 10-35 mm Hg. Venous pressure will be even less. Venules will only range from 5-10 mm Hg, and the vena cava will be close to zero most of the time. At the brachial artery—where most blood pressure is measured, a systolic pressure of 120 mm Hg and a diastolic pressure of 80 mm Hg are considered normal.

A number of other factors also affect blood pressure. These include circadian rhythms, body core temperature, hydration, external atmospheric pressure, outside humidity and temperature, and of course our emotions, moods and stress-levels. Sleep quality greatly affects the condition of the cardiovascular system as well. Fluid intake and environmental humidity affect the condition and volume of the blood. The diet certainly affects the condition of the heart muscle, blood content, and blood vessel walls. Thyroid hormones, vasopressin, dopamine, serotonin, cortisone, insulin, leptin, epinephrine and just about every other hormone and neurotransmitter all affect the cardiovascular system in one way or another.

The rhythms of the heart can be easily listened to by a trained doctor. This is called *auscultation.* The listening process practiced by western allopathic medicine focuses on the two systolic beats, called S1 and S2. The first sound during the pulse is the S1 and the second sound when the pulse disappears is the S2. The S1 and S2 are both created by the almost-simultaneous closing of the right and left corresponding valves. The S1, typically sharper, indicates the ventricle-atrium pressure differential, causing the AV valves (mitral and tricuspid) to close. After allowing blood to flow out of the heart, this pressure differential changes again as the ventricles relax. The out flowing semilunar valves snap shut from the backpressure of the blood, creating the S2 sound. There is usually a longer delay between S2 and S1 than between S1 and S2—allowing the physician to differentiate between the two heart sounds.

The allopathic physician will listen to the speed and timing of these two heart sounds, particularly noting the sharpness of their snapping sounds. When the snapping is not as sharp, heart congestion or valve problems are suspected. When a whirring or turbulence sound is heard between or around the sounds, a heart murmur is suspected. Further review of the sounds will usually indicate whether the murmur is critical, or perhaps not clinically significant. In addition to the S1 and S2 sounds, a physician may hear two other sounds: These are called the S3 and S4 heart sounds. S4 is often related to hypertension, but S3 can be more problematic. Should the S3 make a sloshing sound, this might indicate a regurgitation of blood moving through the ventricles. It is considered somewhat normal for a child or young adult with lots of energy to have an S3 sound. However, an S3 sound will often be problematic for the adult because it may indicate a valvular deficiency.

Heart arrhythmias are also sometimes heard during auscultation. Most commonly associated with heart disease or valve dysfunction, they may also indicate no immediate concern. When arrhythmias are serious, they can produce light-headedness, dizziness, or fainting, requiring immediate medical attention.

Heart palpitations are often the result of stress or fear. It is not well understood why a person will suddenly be aware of their heart's beat, however. Our heartbeat autonomically speeds up and slows down throughout the day as a matter of course. A heart palpitation means that a direct biocommunication channel between the self and the heartbeat has been opened up. This ability is also often seen in biofeedback. The normal feedback process is modulated by the self's becoming determined to directly link to the physiological system. The ability of the self to make this determination and the net result *is* a conscious awareness and possibly even some control over a normally autonomic function is proof positive of the intentional nature of the body's biocommunication functions. As to why the self accidentally gains such awareness: This would suggest a messaging process indicating there is something wrong with the heart or cardiovascular system. The message may be as simple as *if we do not let it [the stressor] go and relax, we are likely to have a heart attack.*

Traditional Ayurvedic and TCM physicians measure the heart's rhythms quite differently than do allopathic physicians. The Ayurvedic physician will feel the heart's pulse on both wrists at three positions. The physician will position the first three fingers along the radial artery towards the hand about a half-inch apart. The subtle waveforms felt at these positions indicate to the Ayurvedic physician the relative and subtle balance between the person's *chakras* and *doshas,* relating to imbalances of *vata, kapha* or *pitta* within the body. Each point on each wrist is pressed both deeply and superficially to reveal different specific aspects. This means that each wrist has six possible combinations. This renders twelve possible physiological systems for the Ayurvedic physician to assess with the patient.

The experienced TCM physician will also feel twelve pulses on the two wrists. Like *Ayurveda*, there are three positions on each wrist, each corresponding to a different *meridian* and organ system. Again, each position may be felt with either a superficial pressure or a deeper pressure by the practitioner. The deeper pressure will indicate the waveform flow through one set of channels and the superficial pressure at the same point will reveal the waveform flow through another set of channels. For example, the medial point on the left hand might indicate problems with the waveform flows through the kidneys when pressure is applied deeply. Issues with the bladder will be indicated with the more superficial pressure at the same point. Both the Ayurvedic and TCM pulse readings require substantial clinical training and mentorship.

The rhythm of the heartbeat can vary greatly between people. Research has indicated the average resting pulse for an American male is 70 beats per minute (or 4200 hertz), while the average American woman is 75-80 beats per minute (or 4500-4800 Hz). A resting pulse of 60-70 is considered normal. However, healthy people who exercise regularly often register resting pulses of 50-60. One study showed that only three months of exercise reduced the heart rates of formerly sedentary middle-aged men (45-55 years old) from an average of 72 BPM to 55 BPM. Meanwhile highly conditioned athletes can have resting pulses far lower than these can. In comparison, competitive distance runners have average resting pulses of 45 BPM while some marathon runners have rates as low as the mid-30s (Cooper, 1982).

The heart rate can rise significantly during stress. In a study of fourth-grade teachers, their heart rates would rise from 75 BPM to 110 BPM when they rose from their desks to speak to the children (Cooper 1982).

The connection between pain, fear, stress and the heart has been made repeatedly through study and observation. Most of us have heard of stories of deaths by heart attack during a fearful moment. This is illustrated by firefighter death statistics. One might think the vast majority of firefighter deaths come from being burned in fires. The statistics, however, consistently show that significant numbers die from cardiovascular events. The Federal Emergency Management Agency released a 2005 report on 2004 deaths among firefighters, for example. Of 107 firefighter deaths nationwide in 2004, 49 resulted from either stroke or heart attack. Most of us know that fear can lead to heart attack. Most, however, do not realize that anger also leads to many heart attacks. About 36,000 people experience heart attacks each year in the United States as a result of being angry.

Television can also be a source of dramatic heart rate rise. This is because television programs can be stressful. Dramas and sporting events can be especially stressful on television. Studies have shown that the chance of having a heart attack is significantly higher while watching a sporting event on television.

Studies have also confirmed that the dramatic rise in heart rate during anxious moments experienced by sedentary people is nearly non-existent in those who exercise regularly. Why is this? Exercise purposely puts the heart through the stress cycles, building its tolerance. This dampens the effect of an unnecessary fight-or-flight response. The mechanism of adrenal stimulation is muted because there has already been a recent stimulation—dampening the effect of an unintended response. Some experts feel that the amount of the biochemical has been used up, and this exhausts the adrenals somewhat. Others feel that the production of endorphin during exercise serves to slow the response cycle.

Exercise seems to put a type of 'governor' on the heart rate. This stems from the flow of biocommunication messengers from the adrenal gland, which include epinephrine, norepinephrine, cortisol and endorphins. The biocommunication pathways feed back to the self that the 'tough part' is over. The body no longer over-reacts to a stressor. After all, running five miles is painful (and so are most vigorous workouts). After receiving an hour or pain feedback from the body, the self becomes more tolerant. The self mellows for the time being. The flow of endorphins stimulates a reduction of physiological stress as the body works to recover. It is the self who ultimately 'views' this feedback, and intends to rest from the pain. Without the self mellowing, the body would continue its stress responses even after a workout.

This illustrates that the body is built for periodic fight-or-flight responses. This is because the body is a rhythmic machine—it is designed to increase stress levels periodically, alternating with a reduction of stress levels and a calm homeostasis. Should we not stress the body regularly with exercise, we find the body stores pent-up biochemical messengers. This, combined with an over-anxious self and mind (a self and mind not challenged by pain) over-responds with fight-or-flight responses to non-critical situations.

The body was ultimately designed to have periodic physical responses—to run away or fight for example. This is because the stress response was designed to get us out of danger in our natural environment—out of doors. Today we live in indoor environments, and no longer need to run away from or fight an animal. As a result, we stimulate these same stress responses when we fear losing our job or money. We might end up having a fight-or-flight stress response while driving home from the office. Instead of the physical activity, we might express our stress in our driving. Most of us have experienced the 'uptight driver' with pent-up job stress. All the adrenaline, glucocorticoids and other stress metabolites are built up in the blood stream. Like coiled springs, the cells are standing by for activity.

Often a person suspected of cardiovascular disease is given a cardiogram stress test. This utilizes a monitored ECG during stressful exercise. The resulting graph is printed and the physician looks for any abnormalities with the graphical representation of the heartbeat. Heart pulses monitored using an electrocardiogram will measure the electrical current moving through the heart during a heartbeat. The first *P wave* illustrates the atria activation, while the *QRS complex* graphs the ventricle movement. Finally, the *T wave* illustrates the recovery portion of the heartbeat, while the current spreads back through the ventricles in the opposite direction. The graphical representation of each heartbeat is probably familiar to most of us. The P and T waves are mild, while the QRS wave is renders a sharp and steep spike. Problems become evident should the P or T wave become steeper or pause when lower. Should the QRS waveform change in frequency, spike with more or less frequency, or be rounder in its shape or amplitude, this would also indicate cardiovascular issues.

A regular exercise program that brings the heart beat levels up to about 80-85% of the maximum heart rate for the age of the person has been recommended by various physicians. A twenty-year old body might have a maximum heart rate of close to 200 BPM, while a forty-year old body might have a range of 180-186. A fifty-year old body will typically have a range of 168-180, a sixty-year old 158-175 and a seventy-year old 147-170. These levels depend greatly upon the fitness level of the person, yet these were developed for the average adult. Thus for a forty-year old, getting the heart rate up to about 144 in a twenty minute workout would stress the heart just enough to work through all of the adrenal and nerve stimulation needed for a good fight-or-flight response.

Cardiovascular disease is serious business. CVD is the results in more deaths than any one disease in the United States and the leading cause of worker disability. The World Health Organization estimates some 17 million people die worldwide each year from CVD, about one-third of all deaths. Stroke alone disables more than a million Americans per year. CVD kills people in their prime of life and causes more than half of all deaths among women. Cardiovascular drugs are widely prescribed and prevention information has been widely available through efforts by groups like the American Heart Association. Still, this disease continues to ravage our society. Chemical solutions are typically applied too late and are complicated by side effects or interactions to be fully effective in thwarting this epidemic.

Although the heart is the cardiovascular command center, cardiovascular health is directly related to the elasticity and strength of the blood vessel walls and the health of the blood and liver. CVD conditions typically include:

- coronary artery disease: diseased or weakened arteries that feed the heart;
- hyperlipidemia/hypercholesterolemia: high levels of cholesterol, low- and very-low-density lipoprotein and/or triglycerides and/or low levels of high-density lipoproteins;
- ischemic heart disease: restricted blood flow to the heart, causing angina or myocardial infarction;
- hypertension: high blood pressure;
- atherosclerosis: artery wall lesions that result in a thickening of lumen and restricted blood flow;
- thrombosis/embolism: circulating aggregations that obstruct blood vessels;
- stroke: obstruction in cerebral blood vessels
- cor pulmonale heart disease: hypertensive obstruction of lung-heart blood vessels

The most common heart disease is ischemia, with causes purported to include elevated cholesterol, hypertension, and atherosclerosis. Current theory on atherosclerosis is that it is a narrowing of artery walls due to oxidative LDL and other free radicals, which inflict damage upon the arteries, stimulating an inflammatory response. This inflammatory response results in plaque build-up, fibrin and thickened lumen. Obvious signs are metabolic disorders such as obesity or diabetes, a sedentary lifestyle, and/or a diet high in saturated fats and/or fried foods. High blood pressure and fast or irregular heart rate, especially in persons over 40 years old should be considered CVD risk factors. Higher levels of total cholesterol, low-density and very low-density lipoprotein cholesterol and total triglycerides have been assumed to indicate high risk.

Although early research indicated that low cholesterol was a mortality risk factor among the elderly, these studies have not confirmed this. In fact, the cholesterol-mortality link has been refuted by subsequent studies such as Onder *et al.* (2003) and Miller (2004). These studies illustrated that higher cholesterol, especially among the elderly, is not associated with cardiovascular disease mortality. Small LDL particle size remains associated with higher risk of atherosclerosis (Gardner *et al.* 1996). A recent study of 1371 subjects (Goff *et al.* 2005) has connected insulin resistance with small LDL particle size. Additional diagnostic factors for CVD appear to include homocysteine, fibrinogen and C-reactive protein levels (Kullo and Ballantyne 2005). Higher CRP levels indicate the possibility of inflammation relating to atherosclerosis. Higher fibrinogen levels can indicate the potential of clotting events, which can result in thrombosis. Higher homocysteine levels may indicate a problem with trans-methylation—the liver-regulated glutathione process of exchanging methyl groups to reduce oxidative stress. Methylation problems can be the result of a lack of bio-available methyl groups such as B vitamins.

Cardiovascular conditions primarily reflect the intentional lifestyle choices the self makes. They reflect the relationships the self chooses. The cardiovascular system resonates with our relationships, commitments, and choices regarding the people we surround ourselves with. Relationships that are not working will likely cause high blood pressure and malfunctioning valves. Heart murmurs are often the result of inconsistent relationships. Pacemaker irregularities and weakened valves are likely related to weakened relationships that have lost their boundaries. Weak heart muscle and circulation problems tend to stem from inactive or poor relationships in general.

Modern science emphasizes genetic predispositions toward CVD. These are also directly related to the choices we make with the people we surround ourselves with. Research has shown that the primary reason CVD issues travel in families relates directly to the shared dietary habits and lifestyle choices passed down through families (Jensen 2002; Vauthier 2002). Poor choices predisposing one to CVD include smoking, faulty foods, a sedentary lifestyle, stress and alcohol consumption. Many of these habits are shared with friends and relationships. They are intentional activities shared with those people with whom we feel compatible. Is this a coincidence?

This begs the chicken-and-egg DNA question: Did the genes cause the habits or did the habits cause the genes? Many researchers like to assume the former. The later, however, is not only more logical, but agrees with the rest of the empirical evidence. The fact is, people make choices. Those choices become activities. Those activities affect the body in particular ways. The body in effect will become adapted to those activities. This changes the body's metabolism in slight ways. As the body changes, our gene sequences change.

The propensity for a particular activity may indeed be illustrated by certain gene sequences. Still this propensity in no way removes the freedom the self has to control that activity, and grow and evolve beyond it. As the saying goes, *"follow your heart."* Does this mean we let an organ or our genes govern our lives? Certainly not. This means the self should be in charge. The body is directed by the purpose of our inner being. We can decide to direct our physical lives before our physical lives direct us.

The Immune System

When a heart is removed from a dead body and put into another body, the body's immune system begins to immediately reject it. This is because the body's immune system recognizes this heart as not part of the natural body.

The immune system is located throughout the body. We find immune cells on the skin, in the blood, in the lungs, in the bones and in every organ system.

The immune system has a number of amazingly intelligent abilities. The first is *recognition.* The immune system has the facility to recognize molecules that endanger the body's welfare. The immune system also maintains *memory.* The immune system can remember the molecular structure of a toxin or pathogen by virtue of recognizing their *antigens* (byproducts or molecular structures). This is also the function of a vaccination—exposing the body to a small amount of a particular antigen so the immune system will develop the tools and the memory to respond appropriately the next time it is exposed to it.

The immune system is incredible in its ability to maintain *specificity* and *diversity.* These characteristics allow the immune system to respond to literally millions, if not billions of different antigens. Moreover, each particular antigen requires a completely different response.

The immune system is an intelligent scanning and review system intended to gauge whether a particular molecule belongs in the body. This is determined through a complex waveform processing system. We might compare this system to an iris scan, often used as a password entry system. Utilizing a database of waveform structures, the immune system checks current waveform interference patterns against this database. If the waveform combination matches a known invader, the immune system launches an attack. This is typically called an immune response or an inflammatory response.

Despite advances in vaccination and antibiotics, modern medical science is perplexed with the immune system. This symptomized by the lack of understanding of *autoimmune syndrome.* Most empirical data agree that autoimmune disorders were not as prevalent historically, and have been increasing substantially in recent years. A massive list of degenerative diseases are considered autoimmune, including irritable bowel syndrome, asthma, allergies, arthritis, urinary tract disorders and many others. Meanwhile many other pathologies such as cardiovascular disease, diabetes, liver disorders and many others have become linked in some way to autoimmunity. The rates of most of these diseases are increasing as well. This growing instance of the immune system rejecting its own cells is the topic of much debate among medical scientists. There is no debate among traditional medical disciplines such as *Ayurveda*, TCM and naturopathy, however.

Understanding that the body is precisely programmed to nature's elements and pulses is critical to our understanding of immunity. We must clearly understand what the immune system is. A better understanding does not necessarily require an electron microscope and *in vitro* research. A better understanding means knowing how and why the immune system can recognize and tell the difference between foreign invaders and inputs designed for the body or the body's own cells. This is the crux of the issue. Many scientists have yet to understand this mystery despite a wealth of empirical biochemical and genetic data. The fact is, the answer does not lie within the genetic sequencing or the tabulation of every ligand and receptor.

Harmful bacteria and funguses invade the body via either the digestive tract, the sinuses, the vagina, the lungs, the skin or even the ears and eyes. Bacterial or fungal infection can also be caused by normal residents of the body growing beyond their typical populations—such as *H. pylori, E. coli* and *Candida albicans.* There are four general processes the conscious body uses to prevent infection.

The first is called the *non-specific* immune response. This utilizes a network of intelligent barriers that work synergistically to prevent infectious agents from getting into the body. The barrier structures include the ability of the body to shut down its orifices. We can close our eyes, mouths, noses and ears to prevent invaders or toxins from entering the body. Inside of most of these orifices exist further defensive strategies. Nose hairs, eyelashes, lips, tonsils, ear hair, pubic hair and hair in general are all designed to help screen out and filter invaders. The layer of skin within most of the body's orifices is also covered with a mucous membrane. This thin liquid membrane film keeps many invaders from penetrating the body. Most of the body's passageways are also equipped with tiny cilia, which assist the body to evacuate invaders by snagging them. These cilia move rhythmically, sweeping back and forth, working the invaders that are snagged outward with their undulations. The mucous membranes lining the passageways are also lined with immune cells and antibodies (like IgA) that identify and stimulate a particular type of response. The objective and ultimate response is to remove the invading toxins before they encounter any tissue cells or the blood stream.

The digestive tract is equipped with another type of sophisticated defense technology. Should any foreigners get through the lips, teeth, tongue, hairs, mucous membranes, and cilia and sneak down the esophagus, they then must contend with the digestive fire of the stomach. The gastrin, peptic acid and hydrochloric acid within a healthy stomach keep the pH of a healthy stomach at around two. This is typically enough to or disrupt many bacteria. If the person is mistakenly weakens this protective acid by taking antacids or acid-blockers, the body's ability to neutralize invaders will be handicapped. In addition, a number of microorganisms are accustomed to acidic environments, and then some can tuck away into clumps of food—especially food that has not been chewed well enough.

The next wave of immune response takes place among the body's *probiotics*. The human body can house more than 32 billion beneficial and harmful bacteria and funguses at any particular time. Beneficial bacteria are in the majority in a healthy body. A healthy immune system requires the help of these probiotics, which quickly identify harmful bacteria or fungal overgrowths and work to eradicate them. Most probiotics produce biochemicals that can damage or kill certain pathogenic bacteria. These form the body's own natural antibiotic system.

The body's third form of immune response involves a highly technical strategic attack that first identifies the invader's weaknesses, followed by a precise and immediate offensive attack to exploit those weaknesses. There are more than a billion different types of antibodies, macrophages and other lymphocytes the immune system utilizes to mobilize and execute specific attack plans. As an immune cell scans a particular invader, it will analyze and recognize a particular biomolecular or behavioral weakness within the toxin or pathogen. Upon recognizing this weakness, the immune system will devise a unique plan to exploit this weakness.

This intelligent and specific immune response system centers around particular cells produced in the bone marrow and the thymus gland, *T* and *B-cells, NK cells, Kupffer cells,* and the various *antibodies.* These cells and specialized proteins work together to strategically damage and remove invaders. Both B-cells and T-cells are assembled by stem cells in the bone marrow. T-cells undergo further differentiation and expansion in the thymus gland while B-cells undergo a similar process of maturity before release from the spleen. Both T and B-cells circulate via lymph nodes, blood stream and tissue fluids. Both also have a number of special types, including memory cells and helper cells to identify and memorize invaders. These cells are assisted by scanning antibodies and various types of macrophages to analyze, program and attack different types of invading organisms and toxins.

Every particular toxin or pathogen has its own unique weakness for the body to exploit. For some toxins, a phagocyte might simply engulf it and break it apart with specific chemicals. For others, a macrophage might secrete a particular chemical that poisons the antigen. When a cell is infected, an immune cell may just directly kill the entire cell. One specialized lymphocyte that does this is called a *natural killer cell* or NK cell. Some cells actually contain NK cells—sort of like having a self-destruct mechanism aboard. Macrophages may also cut off the blood supply to an invaded cell so the pathogen dies as the cell dies. The healthy human immune system might be compared to a specialized hit squad. What makes it so smart?

The immune system is launched from several platforms. A primary launch pad is the endocrine system. This includes the adrenal gland, the ovaries, the thyroid, the parathyroid and the pituitary glands. This network of glandular systems intelligently drive and balance the immune response with a variety of messaging hormones and protein ligands that will either turn on a mechanism or switch it off. Receptors positioned strategically around the body receive these relayed communications. These include cortisol, plasmin activator, various basophils and many others.

These pathways begin with the immune system's initial ability to electromagnetically scan and assess waveforms within molecular bonding patterns. Following such scans, the system may embark on one of two basic immune pathways: the *cell-mediated response* or the *humoral response.* A cell-mediated response will typically be directed toward invasions into our body's cells. The humoral response will attack any invaders or toxins entering or circulating through the blood, lymphatic system, intercellular fluids or mucosal membranes.

A humoral response utilizes specialized B-cells (or *B-lymphocytes*) in conjunction with specialized antibodies. Cruising through the blood and lymph systems, the antibodies and/or B-cells can quickly sense and size up viruses, toxins or bacteria. Often this will mean the antibody will lock onto or bind to the invader to extract critical genetic information. This process will electromagnetically scan the potential invader's genetic makeup, biomolecular makeup and potential vulnerabilities. This type of scan could be compared to a CT scan or MRI scan. Their specific vulnerability arrived revealed by the nature of their antigen. Each invader will have its own type of antigen, though similar invaders might have similar vulnerabilities. The B-cell then reproduces the specific *antibody* designed to sense and communicate that specific vulnerability through the body's satellite transceivers. This antibody signals the precise information on how to damage or take apart the invader.

The cell-mediated response utilizes T-cells (or *Thymus-cells)*, which work through a complex system of *cytokines* to relay and command instructions to various killer cells. The killer cells include *macrophages, natural killer cells* and *cytotoxic T-cells.* The initial scanning of an infected cell by a T-cell utilizes electromagnetic means just as the B-cells do. This scan surveys an entire cell for bacterial infection or some sort of genetic mutation due to a virus or toxin. These strategies are most useful in invasions of protozoa, worms, fungi, bacteria and even viruses that intrude upon the cells. The T-cell immediately communicates the situation by releasing cytokines—tiny coded proteins, along with subtle waveforms that broadcast the information to coordinate macrophage response.

As to the form of these waveforms, we should recall the research on immunoglobulin IgE done by Dr. Benveniste and associates over several years, finding that molecular communication took place without chemical binding. Furthermore, remember that his (and confirming) research isolated specific frequencies among waveforms emitted from biochemicals like heparin and acetylcholine. These waveforms were recorded and played back at a remote location. Their recorded waveforms stimulated the same response the biochemicals could induce, yet without any molecules of the substance available. With this sort of evidence, combined with the impracticality of cytokines needing to chemically bond with each and every phagocyte around the body in order to instigate a full body response to the invader, it seems only logical to assume the immune system uses subtle waveform broadcasting technologies. When we consider the abilities humans have to send and receive subtle waveform communications using sound and electromagnetic radiation—utilizing waveform reception technologies—and the fact that stars are seen from billions of miles away through waveform technologies: Why would it be such a stretch to assume our extraordinary immune systems can at least utilize these technologies?

B-cells also conduct and receive technical information via waveforms. B-cells release antibodies and attack invading bacteria and viruses outside the cell using smart information. NK cells on the other hand, break apart cancerous cells or cells infected with viruses from inside of cells. How do the NK cells know there is a virus or cancerous growth among the cell? In a cell-mediated cytotoxicity study done at St. Luke Medical Center's Department of General Surgery, Chong *et al.* (1994) described their results: *"Since the transfected huICAM-1 interacts with NK cells at sites spatially separate from the NK cell-target cell interactions, our data suggest that LFA-1-ICAM-1 or MAC-1-ICAM-1 interactions can provide remote costimulation, via signaling events, to induce cytotoxic activity in NK cells."*

Furthermore, research has suggested that cytotoxic T-cells attack infected cells from outside the cell. It is assumed that the T-cell could somehow gain physical access to every cell, and insert a cytotoxic material into the cell. This however, appears illogical in the face of other immune cell communication research. It would be more logical to assume that the T-cell broadcasts a toxic command that stimulates NK or other self-destruct mechanisms within the cell, and/or stimulate the shutting down of circulation to that cell or tumor region. The T-cell's support network includes *helper-T-cells* and *delta-gamma T-cells.* These cells are known to share information between them. Should every piece of complex information require a chemical binding?

Delta-gamma T-cells, for example, are stimulated by specific molecular receptors on cell membranes. Somehow, in the signaling process, delta-gamma T-cells are able to understand that a particular cell has been invaded by a foreign bacterium, virus or other pathogenic structures. Upon receiving this signal, these T-cells initiate a particular response to that particular pathogen. We must wonder how the T-cells get this information. Do they go around and touch one of these receptors on the cell surface of each and every cell? Remember there are trillions of cells within the body. Many have compared this to a lock and key process, as if the molecular structure of the cell receptor takes on the role of the ligand and turns a key inside the T-cell.

Again, the only logical mechanism is a signaling process through informational waveforms, similar to what we might see in a radio broadcast. A cell under attack sends to the cell's surface a beacon protein, which initiates distress waveforms that are in turn received by delta-gamma T-cells. The question this leaves is how the delta-gamma T-cell can locate the signaling cell. Just as a radio will pick up a closer station clearer than a station located further away, T-cell reception from local cells can relay a dispatch of the signal, providing a location homing. This same technology is used by mariners as they use beacon signals to navigate. This immune system molecule signaling was first revealed to Dr. Benvienste accidentally as he and his associate were studying immune cell activity. As he and his colleagues confirmed the results from various angles, and eliminated the alternatives, it became obvious the immune system uses this technology. Dr. Benveniste and associates were so convinced of the results that they sacrificed their reputations (Dr. Benveniste was one of the most respected medical researchers in France) to continue this research for the next fifteen years with little acclaim or acceptance by the scientific media.

The T-cell system also has a memory protocol, wherein cytokines help store waveform information inside of T-helper cells. This allows the immune system to catalog and later access the specific genetic, molecular and physiological makeup of an invader scanned even decades earlier. This allows the T-cell to immediately mount a defense against viruses and cancers. Our bodies are under constant attack, and most invading organisms are broken up and disposed of within seconds of contact with the body. Unless of course the body is burdened with too many toxins to remove at once—stressing the body to its breaking point. In this state, the immune system can exhaust its supporting players—the liver, the adrenals, the kidneys and so on, slowing down the entire biocommunication relay and response mechanism.

Most immune cells (lymphocyte) have been assigned a particular *cluster of differentiation* (abbreviated as CD) classification by researchers. This classification is based upon the molecular arrangement of the particular protein—particularly the outer bonding formation. The molecular arrangement allows researchers to categorize how that particular protein might respond in the presence of other molecules, substances or invaders. Often a CD number will be used to define a molecular bonding arrangement. A particular CD number will also match to a specific type of receptor at the molecule. A CD2 molecule has an E-rosette receptor for example. The CD number also defines the waveform interference arrangement, which is often referred to as *adhesion* with another molecule. Because we understand waveform transmission, we know that adherence allows the waveforms of one element to begin resonating with another element in a particular array. The CD322 cluster has a *junctional adhesion* for example. Other CDs may define a particular *ligand* function.

Again, a ligand is the signaling end of a type of biocommunication while a receptor is the receiving end of the biocommunication signal. Currently there are about 339 known CD ligand numbers, although this database is quickly expanding. In addition, within many of the CD numbers there are sub-units called *variants*. For example, there are six CD49 variants, numbered CD49a through CD49f.

Each type of CD might describe a particular type of binding between ligand and receptor. The question, once again, is just how close do the ligand and receptor need to be in order to stimulate the receptor with the ligand's information? We know from physics that atoms never actually touch in a molecule. Their waveform bonds and polarities electromagnetically interact in some way. We know the ligand and receptor cannot physically touch. They electromagnetically interact.

Unlike bacteria, viruses are not living organisms. Viruses can gain access to the body's cells through a number of means, including airborne droplets, contact exchange through hands, arms or handles, sexual contact, and blood-to-blood contact. Viruses are genetic spores. They infect other cells by altering their DNA or RNA with destructive interference. This in essence forces a genetic mutation within the cell. Once a virus has disrupted normal DNA sequencing, the DNA's transcription to RNA becomes altered. This mutation then translates to altered activity. Furthermore, the DNA sequence alteration secures the virus' ability to spread. Many feel that this survival intention indicates a virus is alive. However, a virus is actually a messaging system—like a ligand. It delivers a particular and often destructive genetic message.

We might compare a virus to a computer email worm virus. The typical computer worm virus first invades certain files inside the computer, and uses the computer's own software to replicate itself. The initial virus program might have been originally written by a devious computer programmer. Once the programmer's emails are sent out, however, the coding within the worm's file does the damage automatically. The original programmer may be long gone by then—perhaps on vacation—while the worm could still be destroying software all over the world.

There are two basic kinds of viruses: DNA viruses and RNA viruses. DNA viruses damage the cell's DNA, changing the master instructions for that cell. An RNA virus will damage the cell's ability to replicate its DNA instructions, sometimes even replacing those instructions with the viral instructions.

Once the virus has changed the cell's DNA or RNA, that cell begins to function differently. Some super-viruses are incredibly resilient, using damaged cells to pass the virus on to other organisms. Some viruses, despite an immune response from the body to attempt to eradicate them, may remain dormant inside of certain cells. These viruses may become active when triggered, typically when the body is stressed and/or the immune system is compromised. The herpes simplex virus is such a latent virus. It typically becomes dormant within cells of the nervous system, intermittently becoming active. Once active, it causes its characteristic open wounds outside the mouth or in the case of HSV2, around the genitals (although HSV2 can also invade facial tissues as well).

Other viruses can also become latent, even common viruses such as rhinoviruses (including the common cold), various types of influenza, shingles, mononucleosis, cytomegalovirus, and a host of other viruses. If a weakened immune system does not completely eradicate the viral cells immediately following an infection, the virus may gain entry and remain dormant and unnoticed in some less-traveled space in the body, awaiting the opportune time to re-emerge. This opportune time is usually when the body is hit with a trauma or other cause to functionally reduce the immune system.

Noting that viruses are programmed messages, and most messages ultimately are programmed by consciousness, what are the messages being sent by viruses? We might consider a virus a pretty awful message—quite comparable to a landmine.

To understand the message each virus contains we must have a perspective upon the structure of the physical universe in general. It is a dimension of learning. We are each temporarily occupying physical bodies primarily because of our desires and past behavior, but once in these bodies, they become subject to the various learning experiences that result from our attitudes, decisions and the consequences of our prior actions. The facilities of this universe are tuned specifically so that each action and reaction teaches us particular lessons regarding how we treat others and how we conduct ourselves.

Lessons transmitted through programs such as viruses might seem cruel or hurtful. Still, we have to remember again that our bodies are not *us*. They are simply temporary vehicles we run that will wear out soon. Like any automobile, we will soon have to step out of our body. Hopefully as we step out, we will have grown from its lessons.

This is the only logical rationale that can explain why only some people contract a virus that is currently "going around." (Certainly, a 'lottery' perspective makes no sense.) During flu season, some will get the influenza bug while others will not. Even during devastating epidemics like the Spanish flu epidemic of 1918, many of those exposed did not contract the flu. Even unhealthy people do not contract flu viruses when exposed. Furthermore, despite attempts to immunize for flu season, new strains are always developing that outsmart the vaccines. Today there are a number of viruses that are resistant to most if not all the previous vaccines. Why are viruses so difficult to eradicate and prevent? Why does everyone exposed not contract the disease?

The answer lies within consciousness. We each must learn particular lessons at particular times. The virus represents a seed for a particular lesson. If we are due the lesson, we will get the infection.

For the most part, those who have stronger immune systems also happen to take better care of their bodies. Just about anyone will contract the flu—healthy or not. Still, a weakened immune system will more likely contract it, gauged by epidemiological research over the past decade. Any sort of crisis, whether stress-related, diet-related, or environment-related, will weaken the immune system. Most medical researchers agree that this *immunosuppressive* state tends to open the door to optimistic viruses.

If we analyze each of these stressors that lead to immunosuppression, most are related to decisions of the inner self. Job-stress is usually an expression of unrealistic expectations for over-achievement, and a distrust that things will work out in the long run. Therefore, a reduction of immunity due to job-related stress, and a subsequent virus is a lesson to teach us that our job accomplishments are really not all that important. The lesson becomes clear when we discover we cannot work due to the illness. This forces us to slow down and rest our bodies. We are focused upon our aches and pains, which communicate the triviality of who is getting more recognition at work. It might even stimulate an inspiration to consider the higher realms of existence.

There are so many lessons illnesses present to us. This is only one—albeit a quite common one that most people can relate to. Other lessons include an illness caused by a reduction of immunity due to over-consumption. By over-consuming, we are mistaking our need for inner happiness with food, alcohol or drugs. Because the livers are overloaded, this over-consumption weakens the immune system; leaving our body open to increased chance of illness—and a lesson that over-consumption comes with a price.

In some cases, we might be hard pressed to understand the lesson of a particular illness. We might ask why such a good person would be infected with a virus while another meaner person is not. We might first realize that the meaner person will also receive his due of lessons. We all do. In addition, the nicer person still has to learn lessons. Furthermore, sometimes a tough lesson is a blessing. The nicer person may well learn more from a tough lesson—giving that nicer person more wisdom. The bottom line is that we simply cannot compare our lessons with the lessons of others. We each get exactly what we need and deserve. Those who do not waste their time being angry that they have it worse than others will in the end gain the wisdom intended for us to receive.

Cancer is a gathering of genetically damaged cells that begin to thrive under a mandate contrary to the healthy body's homuncular objectives. There is often no clear agent of infection in cancer. The genetic damage can come as a result of the immune system trying to adapt to a new toxin, a free radical or a new stressor. Unfortunately, as are normal cells, genetically damaged cancerous cells are programmed to multiply. Thus, we are faced with an expanding network of mutated cells, which we refer to as a *tumor*. A tumor that has already expanded outside its original tissue region is referred to as a *malignant* tumor, while one which 'stays put' within its tissue region is referred to as *benign*. A tumor currently expanding outside of its tissue region is also said to be *metastasizing*.

This malignant behavior has many theories of mechanism. Though some research indicates it may be caused by an inactivation of tumor suppressor genes, no one understands how this mechanism is initiated. Some research indicates cell growth factors are involved. Although researchers are trying to pinpoint genes that increase the likelihood of cancer susceptibility, there is a growing consensus that over-exposure to environmental toxins called carcinogens are a likely culprit.

Environmental or food toxins can become potent free radicals once inside the body, damaging cell membranes, organelles and nuclei. A damaged cell membrane may cause genetic damage in itself as the cell adjusts to the damage, but often a toxin will intrude into a cell and then begin to damage the cell's internal organelles and genetic material. Studies have demonstrated some cancer cells are actually genetically damaged immune system cells. Once genetic damage takes place, the cell's activities become altered. This begins the process of *apoptosis*, or cell death. Genetically damaged cells can quickly multiply and take over a tissue region. They infect surrounding cells and move outside the construct of the body's instructional guidance systems. An accumulation of these maligned cells often functions as a well-organized unit, working to interfere with the actions of the body's metabolism in specific ways.

Quite simply, cancer is an expression of the body's self-destruct mechanism. We might compare this to a self-destruct mechanism that might accompany an ejection system in an advanced fighter jet. Because it is time to eject for whatever reasons, the body begins to dispose of itself with a programming feature that begins to shut down the vital organs and cells that keep the body alive.

Research has confirmed that the average healthy person has cancerous cells throughout the body on a daily basis. Only a few begin to flame out into a raging tumor. For most, it simply results in the cell collapsing and being eliminated from the fold. A simple overloading of stressors at a particular time and place will usually bear upon a few cells, which collapse as they attempt to adapt to the stressors. Why do some of these occasions result in a runaway of cancerous cells?

The whole process is a subtle biowave process. Not only do all the processes of the body—including the immune system—run on inter-related mechanisms, but each molecule—including DNA and RNA—is bound together through standing wave crystallography driven by an intentional self.

As we ponder this, we might consider how effective particular types of radiation therapy are in eliminating cancer cells. Anticancer radiation consists typically of high-voltage gamma-ray waveforms. Gamma rays are created using a cobalt-60, radium-226 or similar radioactive substance to provide a source of electromagnetic waves, shot through accelerators. As the beam is focused specifically onto a tumor grouping, those cells become obliterated, dying on the vine so to speak. Unfortunately, many other cells—healthy ones—that come into contact with these destructive waveforms also can be damaged. Thus, radiation therapy can be very dangerous. The treatment is just shy of being lethal for the patient, yet hopefully more lethal to the cancer cells.

Radiation therapy illustrates the waveform nature of every cell, including a cancerous one. When radiation at a particular frequency enters the cell, it interferes with the standing and radiating waveform structures making up the molecules of the cell. One of the primary structures of the cell is certainly its DNA. When DNA and RNA molecules of the cell are damaged, cell death or adaptation/mutation are the likely options.

As for weaker radiation coming into contact with the cells—say ionizing radiation such as gamma rays—the genes might be damaged enough to produce an adaptation—a slight genetic mutation to adjust to the new waveform environment. However, even ionizing radiation can be quite lethal—indicated by the massive cancer deaths seen in Japan in the decades following the dropping of the atomic bombs. Researchers have also seen this same radiation effect among many experiments with rats and other animals as they have been subjected to various radiation doses in the name of science.

What is it about DNA that makes the cell so sensitive to unnatural forms (or forms unintended by nature) of radiation? DNA itself is a transceiver molecule. It receives and transmits information. The information relates to the strategies for survival originating from an intentional self. Some of these strategies are programmed by the self through the mind, while other programs are inherited from the body's parents. Still even these inherited programs still have to be authorized for use by the inner self. This authorization is the subtle exchange of feedback and intention between the body and the self. Using this feedback system, the self adjusts to the given limitations of the body, and seeks to improve upon them utilizing creative problem solving. This might be compared to the housing industry. Each generation of humans has inherited from their ancestors' construction methods and architectural designs for building houses and other buildings. Each generation picks up what the previous generation has done, and first acknowledges this by learning it and even emulating those methods. Then gradually the new generation will also creatively improve upon those methods, adding its own methodology and design techniques. The next generation then repeats the cycle, inheriting those improved methods.

In the same way, the inner self assumes the genetic designs offered by the mother and father. It first accepts them, and begins to learn how to utilize the various tools and resources of the body, including its immune system strategies. Gradually, however, the child will build upon those strategies by trying to make improvements. The immune system will attempt to learn how to more efficiently cleanse the system of existing toxins, while learning how to eliminate new toxins. The child's DNA begins to adapt to the world with new creative strategies as well. Slight genetic changes will be made in order to adapt to new environmental exposures. Gradually, the new generation becomes on one hand more equipped to handle the new environmental exposures; and on the other hand becomes less tolerant, as it becomes more efficient at detoxification.

We are seeing the latter part of this process in the case of autoimmune syndrome today. Our DNA and immune systems have created new strategies for detoxifying the cells. One such strategy is logical: *Kill off the cell before they mutate and begin to spread the mutation around the body in the form of cancer.*

Yes. We are proposing that autoimmune syndrome is actually our body creating a new strategy to prevent more metastasizing cancerous tumors from spreading. This strategy is part of the immune system reflecting our conscious intention of keeping the body alive. Without this strategy, malignant cancer would exceed the current 33% estimated rate.

What about getting cancer, then? Does this have a link with our intentional self? Do people get cancer because they intend to? Certainly not. Life presents us lessons to learn from. We are not always in control over those lessons, although we can invite them by not learning the lessons the first time around. Should we not learn any particular lesson, life confronts us with the lesson again—until we learn it.

In many cases, a cancer growth can be a physical manifestation of a particular decision we made in the past, rejecting nature's course. That is a lesson in itself. Perhaps we decided to enjoy puffing smoke in the form of a cigarette though we knew it was not good for us. Maybe we did not know it would cause cancer, but we knew it was bad for us because we could not run anymore without wheezing. Instead of listening to our body and learning the lesson then that this is not good for the body, we decided we wanted to look cool, and feel the minor rush from nicotine. A few years later, we pay for that decision in the form of lung cancer. The lung cancer is the lesson, teaching us the lessons we need to learn.

Or perhaps we simply do not want to live in the world anymore. Our kids are gone and our spouse is dead, and we live day to day with nothing to live for. Maybe we are alone in the house with no one we can exchange love with. In this case, cancer may be part of the body's cells expressing the lack of a strong desire to continue living. In this case, the immune system slows down. Does it do this by itself? No. Again, the immune system is driven by the inner self through the mind's programming features.

Medical doctors—especially those from cancer treatment centers—have documented that cancer survival tends to be positively related to having strong family support. In other words, strong family bonds create a greater intention to keep the body alive, if even for a few more years. This observation has been made over many decades of medicine. It is one reason why bedside family visits are considered so important in hospitals today—even at the risk of infection. Because the immune system is ultimately driven by the intentions of the inner self, a greater connection with people will increase the inner self's determination to remain in the body. This in turn stimulates the immune system.

This mechanism is the purpose for, and the reason for the wild success of Paul Newman's *Hole in the Wall Gang* camps. Thousands of children with metastasizing, lethal forms of cancer—have out-lived their expected survival rates simply by coming together to share with other children within an environment of care and love. There have been cases where a child had a month or two to live attending one of these camps and going into complete remission shortly afterward. Though not proven, this mission by Mr. Newman probably saved more lives on a percentage basis than chemotherapy has.

The human cell is quite adaptive, but it becomes weakened when it must become too adaptive. Even a minor disturbance can force an adaptation of cellular genetic structure to accommodate the disturbance. This happens every day, as our bodies adapt to the various changes that our environment presents to us. Our bodies learn to adapt to chemotoxins, pollution, lack of food or nutrition, and dehydration. In the case of a toxic chemical, the adaptive stress leads to either detoxification or adaptive response. In the former case, the body must initiate an inflammatory response, often requiring a certain level of sacrifice by the individual while the body detoxifies. This might be a swelling, a cold, an allergy attack or otherwise. Sneezing, fever, coughing or immobilizing inflammation is a sacrifice by the inner self. In the later case—the adaptive process—the cell must begin to operate under duress and its DNA and RNA functions must develop procedures for these altered mechanisms. This in turn forces the DNA sequencing to be altered slightly—mutate—to facilitate these new mechanisms.

In the case of a lack of nutrients or water for extended periods, the DNA, RNA or cell organelle function may be forced to adapt to a condition where the cell operates with less fuel. The first nutrient deficiency to damage the cell is oxygen. Without oxygen, our cells will starve for energy and will not be able to function. This can take place within minutes. The second most dangerous nutrient deficiency is water. Should the cell not have enough water, it will begin to deteriorate. A lack of adequate hydration for any duration will stimulate the release of histamine to help regulate water usage, which will deplete immune system function and drive up inflammatory activity. Histamine will stimulate antidiuretic hormones to control water loss as well as stimulate vasopressin, which controls artery wall pressure and renal water regulation systems. Histamine (H2) will encourage the production of histamine-induced suppressor factor (HSF). HSF in the presence of monocytes appears to result in prostaglandins that suppress lymphocytes, thereby reducing the immune system's effectiveness. Histamine (H1) appears to stimulate arachadonic acid pathways, which encourages greater inflammatory response. The sum total effect of dehydration is thus one of depressing immune function while stimulating hyperinflammatory responsiveness (Batmangheilidj 1990).

Our DNA will undergo direct damage from interfering electromagnetic waveforms from unnatural EMF waveforms themselves. Electromagnetic waveforms originating from alternating currents, including those arising from electronic appliances, cell phones, high transmission power lines and so on will stress the cell's ability to communicate within itself and with other cells and messengers. The cell must then adapt to these new environmental waveforms by making genetic accommodations. The need for chronic adjustment will result in the mutation of DNA. This mutation could turn the cell into a cancerous cell.

Assuming a static DNA molecule with permanent bonds is a model that allows for little flexibility. The accommodation of the cell and genetic information is evidence that the waveform bonding sequencing of DNA can be altered to accommodate external influences. We have seen this evidenced through genetic analysis of various family trees. Should an ancestor have a particular environmental exposure, their adaptation will be passed on to the next generation. This is why we find that the people in cultures that have lived in sunnier regions have higher levels of melanin in their skin cells—giving them darker skin. For those who moved north and lived primarily indoors with long winters, melanin content greatly decreased, leading to whiter skin color. In both cases, today's skin colors are reflected by the genetic accommodation of their ancestors' bodies.

This accommodation is also subject to the inner self's guidance as well. Without the permission from the self and the mind's programming to allow the adaptation, the entire body would drastically respond to the environmental change, resulting in physiological chaos and most likely some form of illness. If we were to move to a location and find it unacceptable for some reason, the self's dislike of the new situation would subtly result in a negative response to the environment. On the other hand, should the self's desire to live in the location outweigh some of the challenges of the new environment, the body's adaptive systems would quickly fall in line and help accommodate the change, even if it had to make some genetic changes.

This is also the reason we find our bodies accommodating so many environmental changes taking place despite obviously being foreign and burdensome to the body's detoxification mechanisms. Why have our bodies adapted to the avalanche of plastics and the plasticizers that come with them over the past three decades? Though the plethora of plastics have certainly increased the burden upon our immune systems, disrupted our hormones and damaged our livers, we have seen little outward allergies, sensitivities or other obvious detoxification due to plastic use. At the same time, we see overwhelming allergic reactions to smog, pollen and other environmental exposures. The difference is that the inner self anticipates the enjoyment of various plastic products and so programs the body for adaptation. Because plastic can be molded to our imagination, creating virtually any shape, tool or play toy, the inner self rebels against the notion that plastic could be harmful to the body. (This does not mean the hormone-disrupting plasticizers will not be having their damaging long-term effects, however.) For many years, smog and cigarette smoking were held in esteem among people. Gradually the science demonstrated that cigarettes were toxic. Now smoking in restaurants is intolerable for many and against the law in some areas. Smokers are frowned upon. People are generally more sensitive to smoking now because the general consciousness regarding smoking has changed. As a result, more of us will sneeze and get watery eyes immediately when in proximity to cigarette smoke.

Our cells are adjusting to new environments all the time. For example if we were to move to a warmer location—with greater solar radiation through contact with infrared radiation—our cells will begin to operate with slower metabolism, allowing the body's core temperature to remain balanced. Though this might stress the cells somewhat, this sort of adapting mechanism is not considered harmful primarily because the sun's rays (except perhaps mid-day UV rays) are considered healthy to the body. However, should our body move into a building where it is bombarded with unnatural amounts of magnetic radiation and toxic chemicals, our cells might react more violently, with allergies and physical stress, as our cells attempt to adapt to this new environment.

As this process continues, an immune function called *tumor necrosis factor* may be stimulated, which will immediately halt the cell's metabolism from within. This may force the stressed cells to die. This part of the body's programming covers the desire of the body to recognize a cell out of control and stamp it out. This essentially keeps the body alive. It is another form of the body's immune system. However, should the mutation damage the signaling capability of TNF, the cell may divide with few if any barriers. It may even form its own proprietary source of circulation to avoid the immune system's attack.

Another possibility is that the genetic damage forces an alteration of DNA waveforms just enough to stimulate the body's immune system. The immune system identifies the slight alteration as inconsistent with the rest of the body's cells. When a T-cell electromagnetically scans a cell to make sure it is healthy, genetic alterations will be identified as "foreign." Once this ID takes place, the immune system specifies cytokine instructions to kill the cell. The body's cell-mediated immunity launches an inflammatory response to rid the body of the altered cells. Should this occur over a wide range of cells in the same territory, this is autoimmune syndrome.

Incidentally and ironically, modern medicine's solution to autoimmune disorders is to try to stop the symptoms by interrupting the pathways of inflammation and immune response. This solution merely weakens the entire immune system. It would be analogous to killing our dog because he barked at a thief who was invading our home.

Botanicals provide the key to a more harmonic method of enhancing the immune system. Plants have metabolism and immune systems that collectively produce particular biochemicals to respond to environmental challenges. For example, many plants produce polyphenol molecules that help protect the plant from being burned by the sun. These same pigments also help the body from the damaging effects of the sun. There are hundreds of known polyphenols, including catechins, flavonols, flavones, anthocyanidins, bioflavonoids and isoflavonoids. Each has a particular immune function within the plant to resist disease or environmental stressors. Each of these biochemicals exerts a similar activity—of assisting the immune system—in humans. Both organisms—the plant and the human—utilize the same biochemistry to conduct intentional survival.

Mushrooms are another example. They produce particular polysaccharides like beta-glucans that help protect them from invading bacteria and viruses. Mushroom scientist Paul Stamets and author of a number of books on the subject, has pointed out that recent mushroom research is showing certain mushrooms have unique antimicrobial effects. Mushroom extracts are showing strong activity against bacteria such as *E. coli, staphylococcus,* and *tuberculosis* strains, and a wide variety of viruses from pox to flu viruses (Stamets 2005). Some of this new evidence is based upon testing by the National Institute of Allergy and Infectious Diseases (NIAID) over the past few years. Over 2,000,000 samples of various agents were submitted to NIAID. The samples Mr. Stamets submitted were one of the few natural agents that illustrated true anti-pox activity, according to Dr. John A. Secrist III who oversaw the program. When humans eat these mushrooms, our immune systems utilize the same genetic information assembled by the mushroom to combat invaders to assist our immune systems in combating similar viruses and bacteria.

The dramatic conclusion regarding the harmonic synchrony between our bodies' immune systems and those of planet earth is that we are best served by consuming those botanicals grown close to our home. Because those botanicals have developed particular immune biochemicals to resist the invaders of our local region, our own immune systems are stimulated more precisely to fending off those same local invaders. This is an example of nature's ultimate conscious orchestration: In a natural scenario, our bodies are tuned to the conscious organisms living around us. Just as the plant and its flower are perfectly tuned to attract the pollinating honeybee, our bodies are (or can be) tuned to those plants, waters, sun, and atmosphere surrounding us. We can dryly consider this a convenient product of evolution, which of course it is. Yet we must not forget that within those living organisms surrounding us are also conscious individuals—who also seek the survival of their temporary bodies.

Utilizing waveform fingerprinting, the immune system uses a translation and matching process analogous to sound communication. If we were to listen to a French-speaking person, we could immediately know they were a foreigner just from hearing their language. Even if they tried to speak English, we could probably tell they were a foreigner by the accent. In the same way, the immune cell can immediately know whether a tissue cell is a foreigner. If the language of the cell is different, the immune cell knows immediately there is a problem. Should a cell begin to emit different waveforms, it will be noticeable to immune cell censors coursing through the bloodstream and lymphatic fluids. Though science sees cellular communication in hard biochemical binding, cells communicate like tiny radio satellites: Though cells might lie pretty close to other cells, they are still separated by interstitial fluids. Cells do not touch. Although ligands can stimulate receptors chemically, this is not always required. Hormones and other biochemical messengers also relay more information through the transmission and reception of subtle waveforms.

This waveform scanning process also occurs with and between bacteria. Some bacteria like probiotics are considered symbiotic with the body. Thus, they do not provoke an immune response like invading bacteria do. Probiotic bacteria emit waveform signals the immune cells recognize. Invading bacteria—like mutated cells—emit signals the immune system considers foreign. This ability of bacteria to communicate has been the subject of increasing study as colonies of bacteria have been observed responding to a particular situation as a group suddenly. This characteristic has been described previously as quorum sensing. Apparently, some form of communication between separate bacteria dwelling within an independent medium causes the bacteria colony to act in concert as a group.

Researchers have observed biochemical environment changes concurrent with quorum sensing events. The assumption of biochemical changes causing the quorum-sensing event presents a challenge. What stimulated the biochemical change in the first place? If we assume a biochemical response with no initiator, we find ourselves in a quandary. With no initiator, we have no practical rationale for the event at all. If we assume, for example, a particular environmental event initiated the quorum sensing, this would not require a quorum at all. Each bacterium would simply turn on like multiple light switches. There would be no biological mechanism occurring. For this reason, biologists agree that quorum sensing takes place through some sort of sensory information exchange.

A sensory exchange of information means that there must not only be a sender and receiver of the information, but there must be a source of the information. Furthermore, this source of the information must have an intentional purpose for transmitting or stimulating the passing of the information. The immune system is defined by such a state. We see clearly that the cells and cytokines of the immune system are transmitting and exchanging information regarding what is foreign and what is not, and what should be eliminated and what should be protected. This type of critical information exchange has an ultimate purpose. It is not a chaotic cycle of events. There is a definite purpose for the storage of information on particular antigens, creating strategies to exploit the weaknesses of invaders, and developing process for eliminating infected cells. The purpose is the survival of the body for a specific period of time. For whose benefit does this purpose serve, we might ask. It is for the ultimate benefit of the living being occupying the body. Therefore, the immune system is a tool or vehicle for the inner self. This is no ordinary tool, however. This is a tool with specific information exchange, memory storage, and acute analysis and investigation mechanisms.

What other part of the conscious anatomy executes these sorts of functions? The mind also retains memories, investigates, examines and analyzes.

The bottom line is that there is little difference between our intentions translating to mental strategies to build faster cars or jets and our intentions of enjoying the physical body translating to immune strategies to deal with toxins, viruses and invading microorganisms. The immune system is simply another branch of our mind—a tool for the intentional self to utilize. We might consider its programming somewhat autonomic like the reflex arc. Still, this programming nevertheless operates within the constructs of the conscious and changeable mind.

We might suppose that the immune system does not have a conscious component. This cannot be further from the truth. If we want to avoid our body getting ill during an exposure, we will consciously undertake many immunity strategies. These may include washing our hands frequently, eating well, drinking plenty of fluids, exercising, taking detoxification botanicals and avoiding others who are sick. As we become aware of particular viruses "going around," our immune systems simply extend this strategy and will begin producing more antibodies to those types of infections. This does not necessarily require a conscious effort. It is no mistake that the immune system's activities are perfectly aligned with the conscious activities of the self to avoid disease and stay healthy. Like the reflex arc, these are pre-programmed metabolic responses. It is the emotional, intentional self who is ultimately behind this programming. Whether the programming is picked up from the passage of antibodies from mama through the placenta or cervix, from vaccination response, or from the response following exposure, the intentional self ultimately authorizes and stimulates the immune system relative to our desire to remain in the body.

Chapter Six

Planet Probiotic

There are ten times more probiotic bacteria in our bodies than cells. This means our bodies are more bacterial than cellular. Friendly bacteria make up about 70% of our immune system. Researchers are now suggesting that the DNA of our probiotic bacteria—the *micronome*—may be more important than our cellular DNA genome in predicting future disease models.

Like a planet, the human body houses huge populations of conscious unicellular life forms. About one hundred trillion bacteria live in the body's digestive system. The body can contain thousands of different strains. About twenty or thirty species make up about 75% of the population. These are our resident strains, which stay with our bodies for the duration. The majority of these live in colon, although billions live in the mouth and the small intestine. Other populations of bacteria and yeast can also live within joints, under the armpits, under the toenails, in the vagina, between the toes, and among the body's various other nooks and body cavities.

Microorganisms living within our bodies may be either *pro*biotic or *patho*biotic. A probiotic is a microorganism living within the body while contributing positively to the body's health. These friendly bacteria also are also called *intestinal flora* or *eubiotics*—meaning "healthful." The pathobiotic is a microorganism that harms or impedes the body in one way or another. A healthy body contains a substantially greater number of probiotics than pathobiotics, while a diseased body likely contains more pathobiotic than probiotic populations.

Our first major encounter with large populations of bacteria comes when our baby body descends the cervix and emerges from the vagina. During this birthing journey—assuming a healthy mother—we are exposed to numerous strains of future resident probiotics. This first *inoculation* provides an advanced immune shield to keep populations of pathobiotics at bay. The inoculation process does not end here, however.

Our body establishes its resident strains during the first year to eighteen months. These are accomplished from a combination of breast-feeding (early mother's colostrum may contain up to 40% probiotics) and putting everything in our mouth, from our parent's fingers to anything we find as we are crawling around the ground. These activities provide a host of different bacteria—both pathobiotic and probiotic.

Early breast milk is abundant in *bifidobacteria* (family *Bifidobacteriaceae*), assuming the mother is not taking antibiotics. Healthy strains of *bifidobacteria* typically colonize our body first and set up an environment for other groups of bacteria such as *lactobacilli* to more easily be established.

Picking up a good variety of probiotic species is a crucial part of the establishment of our body's immune system. Many of the probiotic strains we ingest as infants become permanent residents. They line the digestive tract to protect against infection. They are also incubated in parts of the body's lymphatic system. The vermiform appendix, for example, was observed in 2007 by researchers at Duke University as housing resident probiotic strains, and releasing them into the cecum during increased infection. It seems that finally the purpose for the mysterious appendix has been discovered after decades of surgical removal. We propose that further research will eventually unveil that other lymph ducts like the tonsils also incubate probiotic strains.

Gaining our early probiotic strains from the environment may appear difficult to understand, as we have been taught that dirt is infectious. Rather, natural soils contain huge populations of various bacteria. Many of these are spore-forming *soil-based organisms.* Some soil-based organisms or SBOs can become probiotic populations after early ingestion. Others, which may be less healthy to the body, will train the immune system and probiotic colonies to counteract those strains in the future. This training mechanism is critical to the body's future immunity. This means those important infantile occupations—crawling on all fours, eating dirt, making mud pies, having food fights, playing tag and so on—all come together to deliver a stronger immune system.

This has been confirmed by recent research illustrating that infants raised in sterile environments are more likely to suffer from allergies, infections and food sensitivities. Parents should consider living in a natural setting or at least outings to natural environments like pesticide free parks to provide the exposure to pathogens and future probiotic colonies.

The most common probiotics include *bacteroides, bifidobacteria, eubacterium, fusobacteria, lactobacilli, Peptococaceae, Rheumanococcus and Streptococcus.* Some of these bacteria live peacefully together. Most struggle with other colonies, and mark clearly defined territories. Probiotics within the same colony usually specialize in particular functions. Some work together to help break down foods, and some guard and protect their territory. As they protect against pathobiotics, many will produce a number of *natural antibiotics* designed to reduce the populations of competitors. At the same time, some of their antibiotic secretions aid the body's immune system by stimulating T-cell and B-cell activity.

Many will release antibiotic secretions called *bacteriocins* that selectively reduce the growth of other pathogens, including yeasts and pathobiotics. In other words, their antibiotic secretions—unlike many pharmaceutical antibiotics—can selectively damage certain strains of pathobiotics and not others. Many probiotics also produce lactic acid, acetic acid, hydrogen peroxide, lactoperoxidase, lipopolysaccharides, and a number of other antibacterial substances. Lactic acid, for example, helps acidify the intestines and prevent harmful bacteria overgrowth.

Most bacteria also manufacture waste products. Some of these are toxic and some of them are beneficial. Pathobiotics manufacture substances that increase the risk of disease by raising the body's toxicity level in addition to infecting cells. Various immunological diseases directly or indirectly stem from the waste streams of pathobiotics. Harmful bacteria can overload the liver and lymph systems with toxins. The toxins produced by bacteria are referred to as *endotoxins*—a technical name for poop. Bacteria defecate just as does any living organism. Probiotic waste is either healthy or inconsequential to the body in comparison.

In 2003, researchers (Gionchetti *et al.*) at the University of Bologna in Italy reported a study of probiotic administration among patients suffering from Crohn's disease, ulcerative colitis or pouchitis. The study focused on patients after having undergone an ileostomy closure. Three grams or 900 billion probiotic bacteria per day (a blend of eight *lactobacilli* and *bifidobacteria*) or a placebo were given to 40 patients. Of the 20 patients given probiotics, only 10% experienced an acute pouchitis episode (a result of colitis), versus 40% of the 20 patients given a placebo. This statistically significant difference indicates the important role that probiotic bacteria play, and their ability to reduce intestinal inflammatory diseases.

Most bacteria in the digestive tract are anaerobic. This means they live without the need for oxygen. They can thus live in the darkest, bleakest regions of our bodies—including areas with little circulation. Not all biotics are anaerobic however—some are aerobic and thus require oxygen. These species will live in regions where they can more easily obtain oxygen—including the mouth, the stomach and the vagina. We might compare this to some species on the earth walking on the land and breathing oxygen, while others—like plants—utilize carbon dioxide.

Probiotics are called "friendly" also because they help us digest food and they secrete beneficial nutritional products. Unbelievably, probiotics are a good source of a number of essential nutrients. They can manufacture biotin, thiamin (B1), riboflavin (B2), niacin (B3), pantothenic acid (B5), pyridoxine (B6), cobalamine (B12), folic acid, vitamin A and vitamin K. Their lactic acid secretions also increase the assimilation of minerals that require acid for absorption, such as copper, calcium, iron, magnesium and manganese among many others.

Probiotics are also critical to nutrient absorption. They break down amino acid content from fatty acids. They break apart bile acids. They can convert polyphenols from plant materials into assimilable molecules. They also aid in soluble fiber fermentation, yielding digestible fatty acids and sugars. Among many other digestive tasks, they also work to increase the bioavailability of calcium.

They assist in peristalsis—the rhythmic motion of the digestive tract—by helping move intestinal contents through the system. They also produce antifungal substances such as acidophillin, bifidin and hydrogen peroxide, which counteract the growth of not-so-friendly yeasts. Probiotic hydrogen peroxide secretions are also oxygenating, providing free radical scavenging. In addition, they can manufacture some essential fatty acids, and are the source of 5-10% of all short-chained fatty acids essential for healthy immune system function.

Probiotics directly and indirectly break down toxins utilizing biochemical secretions and colonizing activities. Some probiotics have been found to have antitumor and anticancer effects within the body. Many will prevent assimilation of toxins like mercury, chemicals and irradiated elements by helping to bind these toxins. They are also instrumental in preventing cellular degeneration and associated diseases, which can burden our bodies as they age. Through their various mechanisms, probiotics help normalize serum levels of cholesterol and triglycerides. Some probiotics even break down and rebuild hormones. They can increase resistance to food poisoning. They can increase the productivity of the spleen and thymus—the key organs of the immune system.

Probiotics are necessary components to healthy intestinal mucosa. Their populations dwell along and within the intestinal mucosa lining, providing a protective barrier to assist in the process of filtering and digesting toxins and other matter prior to their encountering the intestinal barrier cells. This mechanism helps protect the *brush* barrier cells and keep the mucosal lining of our intestines from damage that might be caused by foreign molecules coming from our foods and metabolites. Damage to the brush cells of the intestinal lining is the prime cause for a number of irritable bowel disorders.

To illustrate this, forty patients with ulcerative colitis and pouchitis were followed in a placebo-controlled, randomized study (Madsen 2001). Patients receiving six grams a day of a formula consisting of three strains of *Bifidobacterium*, four *Lactobacillus* and one *Streptococcus* strain experienced a relapse rate of 20 percent, compared to 100 percent among the control group.

Probiotics will also compete with pathogenic organisms for nutrients. Assuming good numbers, this strategy can check pathobiotic growth substantially. Probiotics will also stimulate the production of various immune system cells. For this reason, research indicates some 80% of our immune system is located within and around the digestive tract, and probiotics are a big part of that 80%.

The Invasion

Dysbiosis is a state where the body is lacking probiotics, or is overgrown with pathobiotic populations. This is usually a concurrent situation. Many disorders can be traced back to dysbiosis. Some are direct and obvious, and some are not so obvious, and often appear as other disorders. In general, most digestive disorders are either caused by or accompanied by a lack of balanced intestinal probiotic populations. We can usually detect *putrefaction dysbiosis* from the incidence of slow bowel movement, B vitamin deficiency, depression, diarrhea, fatigue, memory loss, numbing of hands and feet, sleep disturbances and muscle weakness. Many of these disorders and others are often due directly to the overgrowth of pathobiotics. These bacteria can burden the blood stream with waste products and neurotoxins; infecting cells, joints, nerves, brain tissues and other regions of the body.

Another overgrowth issue is *fermentation dysbiosis*. This is often evidenced by bloating, constipation, diarrhea, fatigue, and gas; and faulty digestion of carbohydrates, grains, and fiber. This is also a result of overgrowth, but in this type, yeasts are also among the overgrowth populations. As we know from bread baking, yeast will ferment in warm, humid environments.

In 2004, Allen *et al.* published a review of twenty-three studies that trialed probiotics on patients with acute diarrhea. These twenty-three studies were randomized and controlled, carefully chosen to meet stringent criteria. Together the review gathered data on 1917 patients in countries with low infant mortality rates. The overall conclusion of this review was that probiotics reduced the risk and duration of diarrhea by an average of 30.48 hours, with 95% confidence.

In a study done by Rosenfeldt, *et al.* (2002), sixty-nine children hospitalized with rotavirus enteritis were given probiotics *L. rhamnosus* or *L. reuteri* twice per day for five days or a placebo. The probiotic treatment group had a reduced period of rotavirus excretion and reduced hospital stays and duration. Another group of forty-three children with mild gastroenteritis recruited from day care centers had a faster reduction (76 hours versus 116 hours) of diarrhea among the probiotic treatment group.

A body with low probiotic populations will create havoc for the immune system. *Deficiency dysbiosis* is related to an absence of probiotics, leading to damaged intestinal mucosa. This can lead to irritable bowel syndrome, food sensitivities, and intestinal permeability. The lack of probiotics allows the intestinal wall to come into contact with foreign molecules. This can open up the junctions between the intestinal brush barrier cells. This can in turn lead to the entry of these toxins along with larger more complex food particles into the bloodstream—such as larger peptides and protein molecules. Because these molecules are not normally found in the blood stream, the immune system identifies them as antigens. The body then launches an inflammatory immune response, leading to *sensitization dysbiosis.* Linked to probiotic deficiency, sensitization causes food intolerances, food allergies, chemical and food sensitivities, acne, connective tissue disease and psoriasis. Intestinal permeability has also been suspected in a variety of lung and joint infections.

In 2002, a Swiss study (Glück and Gebbers 2003) recruited 209 health adults. Upon examination, 119 were found to have nasal-cavity inhabitation of either *Staphylococcus aureus, Streptococcus pneumoniae* or *b-hemolytic Streptococci,* all potential pathogens. Sixty-eight of these adults consumed a probiotic beverage containing *L. rhamnosus GG, L. acidophilus 145, S. thermophilus* and *Bifidobacterium sp. B420* each day for three weeks. A control group consumed standard yogurt containing only *S. thermophilus* and *L. bulgaricus* at lower dosages per day. After three weeks, exams of all subjects showed that infection rates among the probiotic group dropped 19% while little or no change occurred in the control group.

The obvious signs of dysbiosis include hormonal imbalances and mood swings, high cholesterol, vitamin B deficiencies, frequent gas and bloating, indigestion, irritable bowels, bruising of the skin, constipation, diarrhea, vaginal infections, lowered sex hormones, prostate enlargement, food sensitivities, chemical sensitivities, bladder infections, allergies, rhinovirus and rotavirus infections, influenza, and various histamine-related inflammatory syndromes such as rashes and skin irritation.

Illustrating the connection between probiotics and skin irritations, Denmark children ages 1-13 were diagnosed with atopic dermatitis and tested in a double blind, placebo-controlled crossover study (Rosenfeldt *et al.* 2003). Freeze-dried *L. rhaminosus* 19070-2 and *L. reuteri* DSM 122460 probiotics were administered for six weeks. The children were then examined for symptoms, and 56% reported improved eczema compared to 15% among the control group.

Colonies and Territories

The two most important groups of friendly bacteria are *lactobacilli* and *bifidobacteria*. *Lactobacilli* are primarily found in the small intestine. *Lactobacilli* will typically lower the pH of the intestine by converting long-chain saccharides to lactic acid. This effectively inhibits pathogen growth. Meanwhile, *bifidobacteria* are primarily found in the colon. They also colonize in great numbers, inhabiting large sections of the colon and staying close to the intestinal wall. Here they work with the body to help process our waste matter and help break down remaining micronutrients. Infants typically begin with *Bifidobacterium infantis* colonies. With age, these colonies are joined by other species of *bifidobacteria,* including *Bifidobacterium longum* and *Bifidobacterium brevis* among others.

Some of the specific benefits of *bifidobacteria* include the manufacture of all-important B-vitamins; the inhibition of yeasts and nitrate-producing bacteria; the production of acids to balance pH; the lessening of antibiotic side effects; the prevention of toxin absorption; and the regulation of peristalsis.

The benefits of *Lactobacillus acidophilus* include their ability to inhibit *Candida albicans* overgrowth, which can invade various tissues of the body if unchecked. They also inhibit *Escherichia coli,* which can be fatal in large enough populations. They can also inhibit the growth of *Helicobacter pylori*—implicated in ulcers; *Salmonella*—a genus of deadly infectious bacteria; and *Shigella* and *Staphylococcus*—both potentially lethal infectious bacteria. It should be noted that *L. acidophilus'* ability to block these infectious agents will depend upon the size of each colony. In the case of infection (as with any disorder mentioned in this book) a health professional should be consulted.

Lactobacillus acidophilus will also lessen antibiotic side-effects; aid lactose absorption; help the absorption of various other nutrients; help maintain the intestinal wall; help balance the pH of the upper intestinal tract; create a hostile environment for invading yeasts; and inhibit urinary tract and vaginal infections. Reports have shown the *L. acidophilus* species will specifically inhibit antibiotic-induced yeast infections. One report showed lactobacilli produce four different antibiotic substances: *acidolin, acidolphilin, lactocidin* and *bacteriocin.*

The digestive effect of *L. acidophilus* is to aid absorption of nutrients. In a study sponsored by India's National Institute of Nutrition (Saran *et al.* 2002), 100 malnourished two- to five-year old children were fed either 50ml fermented curd containing *L. acidophilus* or a placebo for six months. Significantly more weight gains (1.3 vs. .81 kg) and height gains (3.2 versus 1.7 cm) were noted from the group ingesting the probiotic compared to the control group, which ingested a similar curd without *L. acidophilus.* In addition, fewer cases of diarrhea (21 versus 35) and fever (30 versus 44) resulted. The authors of the study suggested that probiotics aided in the repair of damaged intestinal epithelium due to gastrointestinal infection and lack of proper nutrition. They also suggested *L. acidophilus* assisted in promoting intestinal cellular repair.

Lactobacillus casei bacteria have been reported to reduce skin inflammation while increasing immunity. This seems to be accomplished by regulating the immune system's CHS, CD8 and T cell responsiveness.

Lactobacillus bulgaricus bacteria assist in *bifidobacteria* colony growth. They have also have shown antitumor and anticancer effects, and they produce antibiotic and antiviral substances. *L. bulgaricus* bacteria have been reported to have anti-herpes effects as well.

Another important probiotic microorganism is *Saccharomyces boulardii. S. boulardii* is yeast, rendering a variety of preventative and therapeutic benefits to the body planet. Yet should this or another yeast colony grow too large, it can quickly become a burden to the body due to the yeasts' dietary needs (primarily sugar) and waste products. *S. boulardii* is known to enhance IgA—the antibody immunoglobulin focused on skin and mucosal membrane immunity. This is likely why this biotic helps clear skin disorders. *S. boulardii* also helps control diarrhea, and has been shown to be helpful in Crohn's Disease and irritable bowel issues. *S. boulardii* has been shown to be useful in combating cholera bacteria as well.

Bacillus subtilis microorganisms were used for centuries by Arabs for dysentery. They were discovered in camel dung. They are also prevalent in many soils. *B. subtilis* was isolated and used first by the Germans in 1941 for dysentery among troops. The strain is known as one of the most immune-stimulating bacteria available. It activates IgM—blood and lymph immunoglobulins associated with the body's first response for a number of infections; IgG—body fluid antibodies which respond to bacteria and viruses; and IgA antibody activity. *B. subtilis* bacteria are used commonly throughout Germany, France and Israel to repel infection.

Streptococcus thermophilus is a temporary microorganism in the body. Its colonies will typically inhabit the system for a few weeks, setting up a healthy environment to support the more permanent colonies. *S. thermophilus* also produces a number of different antibiotic substances.

Soil-based organisms have also become controversial in the discussion regarding probiotics. There has been a strong contingent promoting soil-based organisms as probiotic supplements. It should be known, however, that these soil-based organisms are typically spore-formers. These are the same kind of organisms that cause pathogenic bacteria growth. They also can grow at incredible speeds and threaten our resident probiotic colonies.

This is not the case during infancy. By exposure to soil-based organisms, babies gain the body's exposure to a number of bacteria species. The young, fresh immune system memorizes these, and learns to mount an immune response that someday will prevent a fatal infection. Adults, on the other hand, may not have the strong immune systems that babies have. As a result, if a human ingests too many of these organisms, there may be a significant overgrowth of aggressive and pathogenic bacteria.

At the same time, soil-based organisms provide a variety of benefits to plants. They are important benefactors for healthy gardens. In the soil, these tiny microbes support plant growth by assisting in the production of a number of nutrients. They also help plants produce phospholipids, which assist and stimulate further plant growth. SBO colonies grow exponentially around roots. Carefully washing fresh plants and roots will dramatically reduce our exposure to these SBOs. At the same time, however, a small amount of exposure to minimal populations during adulthood may be a positive thing, as our immune systems continue to mark and memorize the various organisms that threaten our systems.

A minimal amount of SBO populations, under control, may also help eliminate accumulated putrefaction in intestinal mucosa. They have been observed breaking down hydrocarbons and other molecules, allowing better absorption of difficult-to-digest foods. SBOs can aggressively attack, engulf and ingest other pathogens such as *Candida albicans, Candida parapsilosis, Penicillium frequens, Penicillium notatum, Mucor racemosus, Aspergillus niger* and others. Some SBO strains may work symbiotically with other probiotics. SBOs can also stimulate alpha interferon production. They stimulate "non-addressed" B-lymphocytes, increasing immune response reserves. SBOs also manufacture *lactoferrin*—iron-binding protein. People who lack lactoferrin may absorb too much iron, which can accumulate around the body, becoming a toxic burden. Certain SBO strains, such as *Bacillus coagulans,* are considered probiotics, but all SBOs should be considered more aggressive than probiotic *lactobaccilli* and *bifidobacteria* species. Without a few of these more aggressive 'wild' SBO probiotics, however, our immune systems will not be as strong.

Feeding the Masses

One might wonder why and how there are so many little creatures living within our bodies. Yes, it sounds a bit creepy, but the fact is, our health depends upon different populations of probiotics that depend upon our body's internal environment and the nutritional content of our diet. Just as we thrive off the cycles of the sun and the nutrition of the earth, our probiotics depend upon regular eating habits and wholesome food. Just as we stand comfortably on an earth that oscillates with rotational spin, magnetic fields and alternating weather currents, our probiotics thrive within the human body's oscillating nervous energy, thermal conditions, intestinal peristalsis, heart beat, oxygen flow and so many other rhythmic cycles. All of these mechanisms are as important to the lives of probiotic populations as the movements of the earth and solar system are to the human colonies on planet earth.

Ulcers and intestinal polyps might be compared to the earth's volcanic activity, for example. The bleeding eruption of an ulcer or polyp is as dangerous to the many probiotic colonies as a volcanic eruption would be to those living in a volcano region. Certainly, this means that these bacteria have become connected to our dietary habits and our stress factors. When we eat healthy foods and maintain low levels of stress, this is conducive to a relaxed and healthy probiotic environment. As indicated in research by Dr. Backster and others on bacteria, bacteria can recognize events and even intentions that affect their welfare, even from remote distances. This tendency to recognize actions and decisions that affect their welfare only means that our probiotic bacteria are consciously "in tune" with our daily habits and activities.

Clinically, there are many reports from patients that opportunistic yeast and bacterial infections (*Candida* and lyme disease, for example) immediately multiply following stressful episodes, for example. Many lyme and candida patients report of a growing recognition of the seemingly conscious responses of these creatures. This leads to the possibility that these intentional organisms may indirectly drive the patient to crave sugars and other foods that allow their colonies to grow. This appears consistent with the volumes of bacteria research, revealing that bacteria endeavor for survival and can easily recognize threats and survival aids. This is also consistent with the well-accepted quorum sensing abilities that bacteria colonies have, leading to communal responses to environmental cues.

Noting the undoubtedly conscious nature of these microorganisms, we can change the paradigm of physical health. It is not only important to have established populations of probiotic colonies. We must also harmonize our conscious activities with the needs of the populations of probiotic bacteria that dwell within. By offering a balanced environment for these creatures, they will thrive, and help our bodies thrive as well.

Various strategies can accomplish this. One is lowering our external stressor levels. This means we slow down and relax. We try not to over-react to things. We try to reduce the amount of electromagnetic radiation levels around us by not putting our laptop on our laps and not standing too close to a running microwave or television. This also means trying to establish and stay with regular eating and sleeping patterns. Going to bed around the same time, and eating around the same time every day will create a regular and comfortable internal environment.

One of the important factors to establish this balance is making sure probiotic colonies have the right mix of nutrients. Healthy nutrition for probiotics is often called *prebiotics.* Certainly, some (antibiotic) herbs and roots are not so helpful to probiotic colonies. Nevertheless, most other natural, fibrous unrefined plant-based foods provide healthy nutrition for probiotics. Some foods are particularly beneficial for *bifidobacteria* and *lactobacilli* populations. These are the fructooligosachharides, also referred to as FOS. Some FOS-containing foods are Jerusalem artichoke, onions, chicory, garlic, leeks, bananas, fruit, soybeans, burdock root, asparagus, maple sugar, whole rye and whole wheat among others. 2.75 grams of FOS alone will dramatically increase *bifidobacteria* populations assuming resident colonies. FOS is also antagonistic to toxic microorganism genera such as *Salmonella, Listeria, Campylobacter, Shigella* and *Vibrio*—which tend to thrive from refined sugars. FOS is a mostly indigestible sugar that can cause digestive disturbance in some people. Such a digestive disturbance is likely caused by an absence of healthy probiotic colonies.

Inulin is considered a powerful prebiotic. Functioning very much like FOS, inulin is a natural substance derived primarily from the roots of plants. Plants use inulin to store energy. Inulin is a soluble fiber, and it has special sugar groups called oligosaccharides. Although not necessarily the rule, we can generalize that most root crops are good providers of inulin.

Plant foods also provide another element for nourishing our probiotics: These are the polyphenols. Polyphenols are groups of biochemicals produced in plants that include lignans, tannins, reservatrol, and flavonoids. There is some uncertainty as to which of these are most helpful to probiotic populations. However, a preponderance of scientific literature indicates that probiotics are best preserved by a diet of plant-based natural foods with plenty of phytonutrients, while meat diets promote pathogenic bacteria.

Breeding Grounds

As discussed, nature provides many avenues of entry for probiotics. These include breastfeeding, the birthing canal, and all the stuff a baby puts into its mouth. To this we can add that raw fruits and vegetables train the immune system against and supply a few SBOs. We certainly encourage the washing of store-bought fresh fruits and vegetables. We might suggest, however, that a personal garden of organic fruits and vegetables can be a wonderful ongoing source for both prebiotics and SBOs.

Because yogurt is usually produced using *L. burglarious, L. thermophilus* and sometimes *L. acidophilus,* it is certainly a good source of probiotics. However, we should clarify that pasteurization kills many probiotics. This means that commercial yogurts that pasteurize the yogurt after it has curded will have lost most or all of those probiotics used to convert the milk to yogurt. Some producers pasteurize the milk first and then make the yogurt. Still others add probiotics following pasteurization. The last two are recommended. Of course, the best way to get healthy cultures is to make fresh yogurt at home.

It is quite simple to make yogurt: After heating a pot of milk to 180 degrees F (82 C) momentarily, we can add a half-cup of starter (active yogurt from a previous batch or an active commercial yogurt) into the milk after it cools to about 105 degrees F (40 C). After stirring thoroughly, we can put the container in a warm, clean, dry place, with a towel or loose seal over the container. The mixture will sour and gel in about six hours. Then we can jar and refrigerate.

Other good sources of probiotics include foods fermented with healthy bacteria. These include cheddar cheese, cottage cheese, sauerkraut, kefir, lassi (Indian fruit smoothie usually made with mango and yogurt), amasake (Japanese sweet rice drink), miso (contains 161 strains of aerobic bacteria), tempeh, tamari and soy sauce. Tamari and soy sauce should be brewed without solvents in order to retain the biotic cultures, however—unlikely in many commercial versions.

Extinction

How do we decimate a healthy probiotic population? Very easily. In fact, much of our modern culture's lifestyle provides deterrents to the survival of these precious populations. An abundance of stress can lop off big numbers and stunt colony growth. Under stress, our vagus nerve will translate stress to digestive functions. During anxious consciousness, our peristalsis wave rhythms will not be coherent. They will pulse at different times, creating an unpredictable, uneasy environment. We might compare this situation to post-earthquake tremors that keep the population unnerved for days following a big quake. Under stress, the digestive tract will also not be given enough blood to carry nutrients and cycle toxins. Our digestive tract will slow in its content of mucoid membrane and bile salts. This 'environmental crisis' will force our probiotic colonies to tolerate an increasingly inhospitable internal atmosphere.

In addition, without a balanced natural diet with plenty of plant-based foods, we will effectively starve or under-nourish many probiotic populations. Foods lacking in fiber, high in trans-fats, high in refined sugar and low in nutrient content discourage probiotic growth. A diet high in animal-proteins has been shown to increase pathobiotics and decrease healthy flora such as *bifidobacteria* as well. This is due to putrification. The slow movement of meat through the digestive tract and the subsequent acidification of intestinal pH allow the overgrowth of pathogenic, gram-negative bacteria. Furthermore, the meat itself may also introduce pathobiotics into the system.

A variety of manufactured chemicals added to many foods, including preservatives and food color agents, also hamper the growth of probiotic populations. Preservatives, remember, are added to foods to specifically deter bacterial growth and eliminate food spoilage. The problem with this strategy is that foods containing preservatives will also retard our own probiotic (bacteria) populations.

Medications such as oral contraceptives, NSAIDS, corticosteroids, and so many other chemical pharmaceuticals can kill off or shrink probiotic populations. Antacids and acid-blockers are destructive to probiotics because low HCL production opens the stomach to various invading pathobiotics. These destructive bacterial colonies can quickly reduce probiotic colonies. This possibly is increased in a body also suffering from weakened immunity. As invading bacteria begin to win these battles, probiotic populations will be effectively overrun by pathobiotic colonies. The HCL content in the stomach is a critical gatekeeper for the intestinal tract giving protection to probiotics.

We might ask how probiotics get through this stomach acid gate themselves. The body puts up shields against invading organisms with various antibody immune responses and HCL. Probiotic entry is still difficult because of gastrin, but our immune system will not launch an inflammatory response against probiotic colonies, because they are helpful to the body. This is the other half of a mutually beneficial relationship. The conscious body also remembers the good guys. As for the stomach's HCL, both probiotics and pathobiotics can be slipped through with meals, when HCL levels are diluted. The probiotics do not have the same kind of barriers of entry as pathobiotics. It is for this reason that many traditional diets have included probiotic foods taken near the end or during a larger meal—such as the lassi of India, the sauerkraut of Germany and the kefir of Bulgaria. These traditional cultures may not have had the microscopes to perceive the organisms, but they saw the positive results obtained through nature's fermentation processes.

By far the worst enemy to healthy probiotic populations is antibiotic medications. A week's course of pharmaceutical grade antibiotics will practically kill a gut's entire probiotic population. Imagine, not only killing off invading bacteria, but also killing off trillions of symbiotic probiotic colonies that have attached and colonized over decades. We wonder why we have such an overwhelming surge of autoimmune disease among western societies. As we are killing our probiotics, we are killing off our body's ability to digest food properly. The symbiotic relationship probiotics have with our body's immune system evaporates with such a mass probiotic die-off, leaving our immune system and intestines in disarray as they try to adapt to the 'scorched earth' consequence of antibiotics.

Unbelievably, this situation has been known to the cattle industry for many years. As cattlemen began dosing cattle with profuse amounts of antibiotics to keep the cattle alive, cattle began dying of malnutrition—even though they were eating enough. Because cattle could be slaughtered and examined immediately, it was not hard to find out that the lack of microorganisms caused by the antibiotic dosing killed off their probiotic populations, preventing the animals from digesting food properly. This has led to a decrease in antibiotic dosing and even probiotic supplementation. Despite this, rigorous antibiotic dosing continues in this occupation, primarily because cattle are often imprisoned in unhygienic feedlots where pathogenic bacteria congregate. Without antibiotic dosing, entire herds of cattle can die of bacterial infection.

Furthermore, without good probiotic populations, the cells among many mucosal linings like the nose, the esophagus, urinary tract and the intestinal tract—begin to alter. This is because the environment surrounding these cells changes due to the removal of the probiotic populations in that region. The scanning immune system begins to recognize that many cells have adapted abnormal processes to adjust to the lack of probiotics. This precipitates a change in the genetic expression of these cells. When a cell must adapt to a changing environment, its epigenetic DNA expression mirrors its adjustment. This mutation subtly changes the identity of the cell, which stimulates the immune system's inflammatory response to rid the body of these mutated cells. This pattern is apparent in autoimmune diseases including Crohn's disease, irritable bowel syndrome, allergies, arthritis, interstitial cystitis and many other new disorders. The loss of the body's probiotic colonies is not necessarily implicated in every autoimmune disorder. Still, it should, at the very least, be considered a participating factor.

Probiotic populations can play a dramatic role in the incidence of food sensitivities and food allergies. Without probiotic colonies positioned along the intestinal wall, large food particles can become absorbed into the bloodstream. Once absorbed, these larger-than-normal molecules are subject to attack by the body's immune response. During this inflammatory response, histamines are generated, which cause the sinus cavities to explode with sneezing and watering of the eyes.

Another autoimmune and infectious issue related to a loss of probiotics is the bacterial invasion of joints and organs around the body. Should the protective layer of probiotic colonies along the intestinal wall become diminished, pathobiotics can escape into the bloodstream. Once into the bloodstream, the bacteria can infect various parts of the body, including the heart, the liver, the kidneys and even the joints. Only recently has medical research demonstrated that many arthritic conditions can be at least sometimes attributed to infectious bacteria. The bacteria is thought to have traveled through the bloodstream and interstitial fluids, gradually making their way to the synovial membranes in an attempt to hide from the immune cells and proteins wandering the blood and lymphatic system. Once pathobiotics accumulate in the joints they will multiply. They may also become identified by the body's defense systems. Once identified, the body launches an inflammatory attack, resulting in the swelling and pain associated with this debilitating, degenerative disease.

A number of reputable health experts have concluded that a variety of internal diseases may result from or be related to unbalanced microflora. Research is beginning to support this conclusion, as studies have shown that *bifidobacteria* have the ability to protect against tumor development and prevent or remove enzyme processes linked to tumor growth. Research from Canada has recently shown that *Lactobacillus rhaminosus* has been linked to the increase of natural killer cells from the spleen. As discussed previously, NK cells prevent tumor formation by self-destructing cancerous cells. *Streptococcus thermophilus* was also shown to reduce or delay tumor development in animal research.

Supplemental Colonization

One of the misnomers in the probiotic discussion is that probiotic supplementation will result in replacement of resident strains. The research, however, has not shown this. The research has so far shown that almost any strain added either from the diet or through supplementation after the childhood years will pass through the body after about ten days.

This does not mean that supplementation has no benefits. Supplemented probiotics rearrange the landscape by killing pathogenic bacteria and creating a lactic acid *fermbiotic* environment for our resident strains to grow.

It is important to note that large genetic differences exist within different strains of the same bacteria species. Various *L. acidophilus* strains can differ up to 20% genetically, for example. In fact, some strains may not grow well in some people, while they might colonize prolifically in others. This can also relate to lifestyle choices, food choices and our local environment. For this reason, it is important not to rely upon one brand of probiotic supplements. In other words, we should rotate brands of probiotics to some degree. As we complete one bottle, we can move to another brand. There are a few very good probiotic supplements out there now, and most have a unique assortment of species and strains. As discussed, all supplemental species are transitory. It is important to give multiple species the opportunity to attack different types of pathobiotics. It is also helpful if the strain has been tested and confirmed to grow safely in humans. Human-friendly strains are standardized, identified and cataloged within the *American Type Culture Collection* (ATTC) or *Collection Nationale de Cultures de Microorganismes* at the Institut Pasteur in France. The majority of probiotic supplements sold in the U.S. are listed in the ATTC.

There are also a few other considerations to insure good probiotic supplementation. Each supplementation should supply both *Lactobacillus* and *Bifidobacterium* species because these two each reside in different intestinal regions, where they balance their exclusive populations.

Practically any encapsulated probiotic will require refrigeration for CFU viability, even if the label says otherwise. There only a couple of probiotic packages that do not require refrigeration. These are the enclosed shells and the tablets containing a patented intestinal delivery system. This should be evident from the label.

Some probiotic supplements also contain FOS, providing immediate food for the bacteria. This may slightly improve survival and colonization. However, a whole plant-based diet will better supply all the FOS needed, as we have discussed. While supplemented FOS is okay, most supplements do not supply the quantities necessary to provide much lasting benefit. Supplemented FOS can also cause bloating in some people.

Supplements with too many different species of bacteria can cause competition between strains, which can limit growth. It is probably best to limit the supplement to about three to five species, and take that supplement exclusively (after a meal) until it is finished before starting on a different one. Note also that *L. bulgaricus* and *L. thermophilus* are the only truly cooperative bacteria. Freeze-dried versions of *L. acidophilus* and

Bifidobacterium are probably a good idea. This will keep them from competing within the supplement jar or capsule. Freeze-drying puts microflora into suspended animation, making them dormant until coming into contact with water. For this reason, gelatin capsules are not recommended, as they have high moisture content. Veg-caps are drier and better, but not as dry as the shells or intestinal delivery system tablets. Note also that these latter two versions also allow for better survival though the stomach acids.

A good dosage for preventive measures can be one to five billion CFUs ("colony forming units") of each species per day. Total intake during a therapeutic phase can be between fifteen and thirty billion CFUs. Maintenance doses can be five to fifteen billion CFUs per day. This assumes freeze-dried supplements and the typical strains. There are a few strains, such as *Bacillus coagulans,* that are more resistant to stomach acid. The spore-former *B. coagulans* will resist stomach acid more than most protein-membrane probiotics. *B. coagulans* thus requires smaller doses—say 200-300 million CFUs. Like most supplemented probiotics, *B. coagulans* will typically survive no more than about 10 days in the intestines. During that time, however, they will enable larger colonization by resident probiotic strains, while controlling pathobiotics with profuse secretions of lactic acid, antibiotics and immunostimulatory biochemicals. This should also bear caution, as these colonies may then muscle out resident strains.

Travelers can take probiotics before and while traveling to avoid reactions to strange microbes in foreign food and water. People who must take antibiotics for life-threatening reasons can alternate doses of probiotics in between the antibiotic dose. The probiotic dose can be at least two hours before or after the antibiotic dose. *B. infantis* can be a good supplement of choice for babies.

Probiotic Consciousness

Clive Backster's work illustrated a unique cognition and communication between life forms and living intentions. Dr. Backster called this *primary perception.* Biologists have also found that bacteria communicate perception with quorum sensing. This research and others have confirmed that bacteria—whether pathogenic or probiotic—are conscious organisms, each maintaining individuality and a desire to survive. This indicates that each is also host to a unique inner self. Each inner self within each tiny unicellular body has the same drives we do for happiness, survival and love. Certainly, bacteria may not be as aware and conscious of the larger physical world as we might. Still, we know they are aware because we see that they react to danger or threats. We also know they have sensory perception and the ability to communicate to each other.

We also know that colonies of specific probiotics are selective in their production of antibiotics. Some will directly see a need for reducing specific pathogens, such as *E. coli, Salmonella, Candida* and other infectious overgrowths. This ability of probiotics to produce selective antibiotics might seem unbelievable. Yet it has been confirmed in numerous experiments. What makes this fact seem more unbelievable is modern science's continued sterile, impersonal view of existence. In reality, our entire physical body, down to every cell and molecule, is driven by individuality and consciousness. Our immune system has the ability to selectively identify, focus and respond to particular bacteria, viruses, cells and toxins with a specificity, intelligence, memory, and appropriateness. The immune system's cells and proteins can somehow single out—among an environment of trillions of microorganisms—which ones are foreign and potentially damaging to the body, and which ones are useful to the body.

In the same way, every cell is selectively programmed to absorb certain nutrients, partake in particular activities and even divide and die at the opportune time—perfectly synchronized with the needs of the greater body. This type of intelligent behavior is driven by the intentional desires of the inner self who drives not only the operations of the body, but oversees the environment of trillions of microorganisms, which are also operating within the same overall mission of the body. These microorganisms essentially become the surrogates of the conscious inner self. This of course assumes a minimal of conflicts between the inner self, the body and its microorganisms. With conflict, we find stress, and with stress we see diminished populations.

We now understand that we can connect every cell of our body via common DNA expression through epigenetics. These are the crystallizing radio-transceivers of the cell. How do we connect the independent bacterium with the needs of the body? The bacteria's DNA is certainly different from our DNA. A bacterium is also a separate living organism.

The answer to this question lies within the complexities of consciousness and quorum sensing. Just as we learn to adapt and (hopefully) care for our planet by seeing the environmental signs of stress (such as global warming), our bacteria can sense our body's environment, and respond appropriately. Through quorum sensing, they can construct and communicate common strategies to repel invaders and assist in the process of digestion. This is again the result of consciousness. We do the same thing with radio and television communications as we broadcast strategies to save our planet.

The inner self within each of our probiotic partners are independent entities, and they take transient journeys through our hosting physical body. Maintaining the health of the host body is only possible if we have a mutual respect for these probiotics and their environment. This kind of focus will lead to a healthy, conscious, and symbiotic relationship.

Chapter Seven

Waves of Brain and Mind

The sciences of psychology and mental health have a rather obtuse history. Psychological disorders such as depression and anxiety were considered and treated in Ayurvedic medicine, ancient Chinese medicine, the Egyptian healing arts, and the medicines of the Greeks and Romans. In the middle ages, however, a religious fanaticism took hold of Europe, which led to the widespread belief that mental disease was the result of demonic possession.

There is a significant amount of knowledge and research on the mind over the thousands of years of traditional medicine amongst those cultures. Psychology and psychiatry as a science is considered today to have arose only during the late nineteenth century: A limited view to say the least. Wilhelm Wundt is thus considered the father of modern psychological research. He founded an 1879 laboratory at the University of Leipzig—where he was a professor. Two years later, he founded the first European psychology journal, and wrote a number of books on the subject. Professor Wundt's *structuralism* model of the mind proposed a dividing of the mind into various parts, with each part performing different tasks. This theory later gave way to the modern theories of *functionalism* and *behaviorism.*

The role of the unconscious part of the mind has been studied for thousands of years. The Greeks were known to use hypnosis, and they studied the undercurrent of the mind, together with the dreamscape. The art of hypnosis was somewhat lost, however, until it was revived by Franz Mesmer in the eighteenth century. Mesmer's proposal was that hypnosis was created by a force of nature called *animal magnetism,* which overwhelmed his subjects as they encountered magnets—adjusting the body's tidal influences. Interestingly, Mesmer also proposed that life moves through the body via thousands of tiny channels. The flow of life through these channels, he thought, was subject to various environmental influences, including spiritual forces and the movement of planets. One might wonder whether Mesmer studied the ancient Ayurvedic and/or Chinese systems. Nonetheless, hypnotism became controversial to say the least.

It was not until the respected Scottish surgeon James Braid announced hypnotism as genuine in the 1840s that the hypnotic trance was accepted as anything other than a form of hysteria in Europe and America. Hypnosis was largely overlooked during the years following. Its use as a form of treatment only became more prominent in the late nineteenth century and the early twentieth century. Today it is widely used.

The concept that prevailed in the nineteenth century was one describing the mind as consisting of different levels of sections. A number of theories were proposed on the nature and functions of these portions. Probably the most famous were those of Dr. Pierre Marie Félix Janet and Dr. Sigmund Freud, both prominent psychologists during the late nineteenth and early twentieth century. Janet is attributed to have arrived at the theory of the mind being divided into *conscious, unconscious* and *preconscious* parts. In the 1920s, Freud proposed the mind contained three different components: the *ego*, the *super-ego* and the *id.* Freud's theory took center stage as a possible explanation of various behavioral problems confronting physicians and psychologists since that time. Both Freud and Janet gathered a great deal of information through hypnotism. By hypnotizing people, Freud and Janet *regressed* them to re-experience the behavior or thinking that occurred prior to a current disorder. Though many insights and disease pathologies came out of this research, it was generally regarded as having fallen short of proving the existence of the three parts of the mind.

The proposal regarding mental disease stemming from the three sections of the mind was rooted in the assumption that the mind is constantly in conflict. Freud proposed that a conflict between these three parts of the mind creates mental disturbance, while a balance between them creates mental health. He proposed that the id is the unconscious source encouraging the gratification of desires, rooted in the most basic desires of survival. Meanwhile the super-ego supposedly stands in opposition with these desires, acting as the conscience. The ego supposedly mediates between the id and super-ego, presenting the conscious portion of the mind to the world. The science of psychology has accepted the assumption of a conscious and subconscious apportionment of the mind. However, various ancillary theories have been presented over the years since Janet and Freud.

Unsatisfied with the ability to change a person's behavior using hypnotism, Janet and Freud embarked on their now-famous methods of *psychoanalysis.* These methods are still used today by psychologists and psychiatrists, and are actually quite basic: The patient is simply encouraged to discuss problems and issues the patient feels is related to the dilemma at hand.

The process of hypnosis for psychological treatment is based upon the use of *autosuggestion.* The process usually begins with the hypnotist positioning before the patient and suggesting the patient is becoming sleepy and relaxed. Sometimes distractive rhythmic devices are used, the most famous of which is a small pendulum. As the trust in the hypnotist develops within the patient, the patient dozes off into a state of *suggestibility*—being open to suggestion. During this time, the patient may be clearly aware of the events transpiring—or not, depending upon the suggestions of the hypnotist. Depending upon the type of hypnosis given, the patient may also be drawn into a deeper state where the patient may not be able to recall the hypnosis episode consciously. This has often been described as an altered state of consciousness.

One discipline, which has its roots in Freud and hypnotism, is *autogenics*, introduced by Dr. Malcolm Caruthers in the 1970s. The word autogenic refers to something generated from within. The *autogenic training system* consisted of becoming aware of the body's autonomic nervous system, and being able to control both sympathetic and parasympathetic physical responses to stress. This was accomplished primarily through visualization techniques.

Another important psychological system, also deeply steeped in these concepts of the conscious and unconscious mind was behaviorism. Research into behavior modification was made famous by the work of Ivan Pavlov, who in the early twentieth century worked with both animals and humans to understand how the mind can connect pleasure and pain with particular *triggers,* which bring about a trained response. The dog-salivation experiments of Pavlov's dog experiments are quite famous, and they have given birth to a number of behavioral psychological theories and practices. One of the more notable behavioral theorists is B. F. Skinner. Professor Skinner's research into conditioning and behavior modification has become a foundation for many of the psychological theories assumed today.

A distant relative of behaviorism is functionalism. This concept was advanced by Dr. Alan Turing. In 1950 Dr. Turing laid out the fundamentals of the theory with his article *Computing Machinery and Intelligence.* Dr. Turing proposed that the mind is a learning machine of sorts, accumulating experience throughout ones lifetime.

Of course, behavior modification and conditioning—or *operant conditioning*—has been commonly used by parents, teachers and authoritarians over the duration of human existence. This system is also embedded into the natural world. It is not hard to observe that as we experience events and the consequences of our actions, we begin to learn that certain activities have better results than do others. This realization theoretically changes our behavior, leading to a gradual process of evolution. Those who do not adjust their behavior or learn the lessons, on the other hand, are destined to face a recurrence of those lessons until they are learned.

After many years of hypnotherapy, the fundamental mechanisms—along with the supposed conscious and unconscious mind themselves—are still considered mysterious by western science. Some propose suggestibility is simply a state of mind and hypnosis is simply the succumbing to suggestion. However, there is enough documented evidence of hypnotized patients retrieving historical information not accessible when conscious to consider the alternatives. This lends credence to the position of the mind held by the ancient sciences.

The Mind Map

Over the past couple of decades, the study of the mind has been directed towards the electromagnetic properties of the brain's neurons. This trend towards a physiological interpretation of the mind through the transduction of electrical activity between neurons necessitates the assumption that the mind and brain are one and the same. The primary means for research promoting this assumption has been the use of various radiative imaging systems such as electroencephalography (EEG), magnetoencephalography (MEG), magnetic resonance (MRI), positron emission tomography (PET), and computed tomography using x-rays. These imaging systems each focus on different waveform attributes of brain neurons, as they are altered by these different forms of radiation.

This mapping of the brain was pioneered during the 1920s by Dr. Wilder Penfield, who touched various parts of subjects' brains with electrode sensors while they lay conscious on the operating table prior to or following brain surgery. Dr. Penfield began noticing commonalities between patient responses as he touched certain parts of the brain. Dr. Penfield accumulated enough data over time to develop a map of the various cortex regions and sensory regions. Dr. Penfield co-authored the landmark *Epilepsy and the Functional Anatomy of the Human Brain* (1951) with Dr. Herbert Jasper, a reference still used today.

Dr. Penfield's research focused on epileptics initially. He observed that certain parts of the brain were more active than others during certain types of thoughts, memories, and/or behaviors. Dr. Penfield found that if he stimulated a part of the brain with the electrode, he could provoke a particular type of memory. This led to Dr. Penfield and the rest of the medical community surmising that memory is retained within particular specialized brain cells within certain regions. Furthermore, he concluded that particular parts of the brain specialized in certain types of thoughts or activities. The subsequent mapping not only identified functional parts of the brain. It also identified which types of memories were theoretically stored within that particular region. These mapped locations were called *engrams.*

In the 1940s, a psychologist named Dr. Karl Lashley conducted research that contradicted this notion that memories were located in specific brain neurons. Dr. Lashley trained mice to particular tasks and then removed different parts of their brains. He then reintroduced the mice to the same circumstances, and found that despite brain cell areas associated with those memories being removed, they were still able to remember the tasks learned prior to the surgery. Furthermore, even when most of the rats' brains were removed, the rats were unexpectedly still able to remember what was taught to them prior to the surgery.

A prominent neuroscientist Dr. Karl Pribran followed this research with many years of study on memory and engrams. Dr. Pribran's initial research focused on the frontal cortex of monkeys and cats, and his research identified specific areas of the brain associated with particular cognitive functions. However, he was intrigued by repeated results—like Dr. Lashley—indicating that when specific neurons or regions were removed or severed, cognition predominantly continued. For example, he found when the optic nerve was severed, an animal could still perceive an image in detail. This led to Dr. Pribran's conclusion that perception and cognition went deeper than simply particular brain neurons and brain regions.

Years earlier, Dr. Lashley had entertained the notion of a wave interference pattern for memories. Dr. Pribran, worked closely with renowned physicists Dr. David Bohm and Dr. Dennis Gabor—the 1971 Nobel laureate in physics. Together they arrived at the notion that cognition and memory were related to the mechanics of wave transmission. Using *Fourier analysis*—in which sine wave function is calculated within the context of the action, the *holonomic brain model of cognitive function* was born. This theory was proposed along the lines of the *Gabor function,* which was put forth by Dr. Gabor to propose the natural existence of the hologram within light (Pribran 1991).

When we examine some of the expansive research done in the field of brainwaves, we see how both brain function and the mind are closely related to rhythmic wave mechanics. The electroencephalogram measures the voltage potential differences among different regions of the brain. These voltage differences result in a wave formation, which can range in wavelength, frequency and amplitude among a collection of neurons. These brainwaves are not single units in themselves. They are surges of collective interference patterns created by the billions of reflecting waves of billions of neurons, cells and the various other waveforms large and small moving through the body.

Delta waves cycle from one to three hertz, and tend to predominate during NREM (non-rapid eye movement) sleep, and some meditation. During this type of sleep, dreaming is minimal and the body is often in motion. Delta waves tend to resonate more actively in the frontal cortex. Delta waves correlate with an increase in the production and circulation of growth hormone. One of growth hormone's more important attributes within the body is its ability to advance the healing and regeneration process.

Theta waves cycle at four to seven hertz and dominate during mid-stage sleeping. Theta waves are more elusive, but are very active during memory retrieval and consolidation during sleep. They also become more active in creative endeavors and behavior modification during waking hours. The hippocampus appears to actively accommodate and transduce these waves. Observations have noted peak hippocampus activity during predominantly theta wave periods. The hippocampus is associated with spatial recognition and short-term memory consolidation.

Alpha waves will cycle at eight to thirteen cycles per second, and are dominant during light sleep and dreaming, as well as some meditation states. Alpha waves are seen dominant during memorization tasks, especially those related to words, persons and visual impressions.

They tend to be most prominent at the back of the skull and towards the side of the body most favored by the organism. The earth's predominating waveforms cycle in the alpha range. This is called the *Schumann resonance,* discovered by Dr. Winfried Otto Schumann in 1952. The earth has several Schumann Resonance nodes, including the alpha level eight hertz (rounded), fourteen hertz, twenty hertz, twenty-six hertz, thirty-two hertz, thirty-nine hertz and forty-five hertz. The harmonic here is approximately six to eight hertz. Audio testing has concluded that listening to an eighth hertz beat will increase alpha brainwave levels. This essentially establishes a harmonic between the body's wave activity and the earth's.

Beta waves will cycle at fourteen to thirty hertz and are dominant during active, waking consciousness. These waves tend to be prominent towards the front of the brain on the side predominating during that activity. Beta waves reflect a state of focused attention and activity. A lack of beta waves during waking hours—or lower frequency beta waves—tends to occur with a lack of focus or concentration. On the other hand, as the brainwave levels increase toward the higher range of beta and into the gamma range at over thirty cycles per second, a higher level of focus and concentration occurs.

Gamma waves are higher frequency brain waves, and are often referred to as high-frequency beta waves. Gamma waves predominate during intense problem solving and focused learning. Gamma waves cycle at thirty to sixty hertz. Recent research has determined that gamma waves will be synchronized and coded by phase within the visual cortex. This phase shifting creates a coherence mechanism—a sorting process where gamma waves with the same phases are segregated and commingled. The resulting sorting process allows the gamma waves to interfere and provide associations of particular thoughts, images or impressions of sensual information.

High gamma waves cycle from sixty to two hundred hertz, and have only become obvious to researchers using more sensitive equipment. These brainwaves are seen during the most intense cognitive functions. The slower waves of theta, delta and alpha tend to resonate with distinct physical attributes. The high gamma waves tend to relate to higher states, and tend to be more diverse in their connection points and locations around the regions of the central nervous system. In one study of eight subjects, for example, high gamma brainwave activity increased during the practice of *pranayama*—a method of concentrated meditative breath control (Vialatte *et al.* 2008).

Another type of brainwaves were found using sensitive microelectrodes. These have been termed *ripples*. Ripples are high frequency oscillations that appear to be generated in the hippocampus. They have been observed oscillating with the negative portion of slower brainwaves. Ripples appear to transduce through the medial temporal lobe, notably between the hippocampus and the rhinal cortex—a region associated with the processing of explicit memory recall. Explicit memory includes active intentional recall during conscious cognition. In other words, ripples appear to function as informational waveform 'bites' used to access recent, conscious memories and instructions. It is part of our active information biocommunication system.

The discovery of ripples augments our position that EEG research has tended to oversimplify the role of brain waveforms that oscillate through the various neurons. The brain's mapping has focused on larger regions of the brain. There are still intra-neuronal networks that function on a more subtle basis. For example, a central pivoting exchange factor of the brain's networking system includes the *pyramidal neuron networks*. Pyramidal neurons lie within the cortex regions of the brain. Regions more dense with pyramidal neurons are often collectively referred to as the *neocortex*. Here their densities can be as high as 75%. Researchers have estimated the total number of pyramidal neurons in the brain to be in the neighborhood of fifteen to twenty billion. These specialized neurons crystallize and transduce waveform signals between the cortices and the rest of the central nervous system. Some of these signals have different frequency attributes. They appear to transduce through the polar gateway systems of ion channels. These are not unlike the on-off states of computer machine code, except there is typically more than one type of on-off state among each gateway, to allow for feedback loops. Another, more dimensional description of this transduction is called *signal coupling.* This is when multiple waveforms are "coupled" to create a unique pattern. We might refer to this as a *multiple wave interference model.*

Research has clocked the brain's activity has speeds of between 1/1000 and 10/1000 of a second, which would convert to 100-1000 meters/second. As these frequencies relate to the wave nature of the electrical activity of the brain, they also imply that there is a rhythmic function to the mechanics of the mind. The fact that the frequency increases as our mind becomes more active indicates that higher activity exerts a greater wave speed.

Certainly if we consider how instantaneous reactions and thoughts move around the body, we are talking not only about speed. We are dealing with a network broadcasting system allowing for nearly instantaneous communication. Not that this communication system is not linear as well; it is linear yet still global: concurrently spreading into the vast territories of organs, tissues and muscles. Allopathy compares all of this activity moving through the body to electricity. We would rather compare this biocommunication process to the network access of a website to billions of browsers connected on the internet. This certainly requires an information technology quite a bit more complicated than a home electricity circuit. This type of technology utilizes a mechanism of simultaneous information data coherence.

One example of how multiple waveform coherence works is the *potassium channels*—discovered several decades ago. Potassium channels are specialized proteins found in brain neurons, which regulate the voltage moving between neurons around the brain. As we look closer at these channels, we find they oscillate between gateway states, regulating ionic electrical pulses. These channels provide just one of the conduits for transmitting information. As we examine the instructional pathways connecting neurons together with the physical activity of the body, we can conclude these circuits crystallize and broadcast complex waveforms, disseminating conscious intention from one part of the body throughout various regions of the anatomy.

These pathways for waveform broadcasting from one part of the brain to another appear to be necessary for the mind to develop complete images. Multiple researchers have confirmed that neurons of the visual cortex do not readily pick the full spectrum of frequencies necessary to form a complete image of what we perceive. The ramification of this is significant, simply because we typically assume that what we perceive is "out there" in the physical domain. We assume that we are receiving a complete picture.

Russian scientist Dr. Nikolai Bernstein performed film studies on human perception for several decades in the mid-twentieth century, illustrating that human movement could be translated into wave patterns using Fourier calculations. This is illustrated as we watch television or a movie. When we perceive movement on the TV or movie screen, we are not actually seeing any movement. We are merely seeing a series of still pictures flashed in sequence faster than we can consciously notice. Between the flashed images is a significant dead space or dark image. Our minds fill in the blanks and create the illusion of movement.

The work of neuroscientist Dr. Russell DeValois focused on this element of visual perception over the past several of decades. His research papers documented how the mind integrates batches of visual inputs such as color and motion. His years of groundbreaking research culminated in a 1990 compendium *Spatial Vision*, co-authored with his wife Kathleen—also a professor in the subject. His memorial quoted him describing his lifetime's work in visual perception as, *"the physiological and anatomical organization underlying visual perception. In particular, how wavelength information is analyzed and encoded, the contribution of wavelength and luminance information to spatial vision, and how spatial information is analyzed and encoded in the visual nervous system."*

In one study performed by Dr. DeValois at the University of California at Berkeley, the responses of cats and monkeys were analyzed while responding to visual checkerboard patterns. Rather than responding to the patterns themselves, the animals responded to the interference patterns created by the complementary aspects of the design, consistent with Fourier-calculated interference waves.

The work of Dr. Fergus Campbell at Cambridge University has confirmed that the human cerebral cortex picks up particular frequencies and not others. The cerebral component neurons are 'tuned' to specific wavelengths and frequencies. Dr. Pribran also confirmed this in his research on cats and monkeys. During these tests, it became apparent that combinations of waves of particular frequencies were being received, processed and converted into perceived images as they were combined with internally created waveforms. These internal waveforms are drawn from memory through a hierarchical cortical mapping sorting process.

In the 1970s, Dr. Benjamin Libet began researching decision-making and brain electrical response at the University of California at San Francisco. His goal was to explore a concept first introduced by Luder Deeke and Hans Kurnhuber called *bereitschafts-potential*—which translates to *readiness potential.* In Dr. Libet's studies, human volunteers hooked up to an electroencephalograph were told to perform activities such as button pressing or finger flicking. Dr. Libet's research compared three points in time: When the subject consciously made the decision to press the button; when the button was pressed; and when brainwaves indicated an instruction from the motor cortex was made using the EEG. As expected, the conscious decision preceded the button pushing by an average of about 200 milliseconds (or 150 milliseconds considering a 50 msec margin of error). Surprisingly, however, the brainwaves associated with the instruction to press the bottom actually preceded the subject's conscious decision to take the action. Stunned by these results, Dr. Libet and others spent several years confirming the results. Several scientific articles documented the findings (Libet *et al.* 1983; Libet 1985). These results indicated that the action somehow was not originating from the conscious mind, but must be coming from a deeper source. Still, as Dr. Libet wrote in 2003, the gap between the conscious mind and the physical act gives the conscious mind an ability to *"block or veto the process, resulting in no motor act."* This, Dr. Libet said, is confirmed by the common experience of consciously blocking urges incompatible with social acceptability.

In 2004—more than two decades after his groundbreaking discovery—Dr. Libet proposed a theory based on his and others' research in this area. He called this the *conscious mental field* theory. This theory proposed the mind is a sphere of activity bridging the various rhythmic pulsing of physical nerve cells with the subjective conscious experience. He described this subjective experience as an outgrowth of the various pulses, a sort of gathering or convergence of various inputs.

A neuron is made up of a cell body with a nucleus, and two types of nerve fibers that extend outward from the cell body. The fibers include *dendrites,* which conduct informational waveforms into the neural cell body. *Axons,* on the other hand, project waveforms outward, away from the cell body. Most neurons have multiple dendrites that spider outward making several connections. Sensory nerves typically have only one dendrite, however. Sensory nerves are also typically longer—sometimes measuring up to a meter in length. Dendrites act as receptors. They are tuned into the pulsed waveform messages that pass from neuron to neuron. They carry this rhythmic information into the neuron cell body where it may be translated or even transmuted before being conducted or broadcasted. In some cases, the neuron may simply conduct and amplify the waveform.

In addition to specialized sensory neurons referred to as *afferent nerves,* there are also motor neurons, which are usually referred to as *efferent neurons.* The efferent or motor neurons are designed to carry instructional waveforms outward through the central nervous system to specific skeletal or organ cells. In these locations, these cells respond as instructed by the information provided by these waveform interference patterns. We note this because a single waveform does not necessarily contain enough information to drive a complex motor process. It takes a waveform combination to affect these specialized cells. Some are stimulated into metabolism responses, secretions, or contractions. Because they are stimulated by the efferent neurons, these cells are called *effectors.*

The intentional self ultimately stimulates the effector neurons through the facilities offered by the neural network. The neural network generally has three basic types of processes: The first is to receive and translate afferent sensory waveforms from the senses and environment. The second is to project instructional waveform combinations outward through the appropriate neural tracts. The third process of the neural net is to prioritize, sort and catalog memories and various autonomic programs.

The brain grows and develops in the body from a tubular canal called the *neural tube.* The entire brain is made up of billions of neurons. These are networked into bundles of groupings, which include *nerve tracts, gyri, fissures, sulci* and *cerebrum lobes.* These groupings of specialized neurons work conjunctively to accomplish specialized tasks, while transmitting information back and forth through neural superhighways. The locations of these nerve groupings will be common. Most nerve functions thus have location *plasticity.* Plasticity is the ability of the organism to move or reorganize the location or processes involved in accomplishing particular tasks. In other words, should one location not be able to function, the organism will relocate the function to another region of the brain.

The self primarily utilizes the brain's functions through the frontal cortex. Here the various waveforms provided by the senses and the body's feedback are observed by the self. The self utilizes a command center called the prefrontal cortex to respond to these images. This is located towards the front of the brain, behind and on top of the forehead, almost the precise position described by *Ayurveda* as the region between the sixth and seventh *chakra* regions—the *soma chakra.* Indeed this region provides a gateway for the self to not only observe the condition of the body and the environment, but also submit executive orders in response. For these reasons, researchers have determined that the frontal lobes are stimulated during the processing of decisions related to right and wrong, the prioritization of consequences, and logical thinking. Through the prefrontal region, the self expresses personality and submits executive orders.

The *motor cortex* lies just behind the frontal cortex as we comb back over the head. It normally resides within a band of neural grey matter (neuron cells) that wrap around the top of the head onto the two sides. Here physical instructions from the frontal cortex begin their transduction towards execution. Within the motor cortex reside specialized networks of neurons, each network coordinated with specific types of motor activity. The *premotor* region contains billions of specialized *mirroring* neurons, which mirror and sort the executive decisions transmitted from the frontal cortex. Behind the premotor cortex is the *primary motor cortex*. This region contains specialized neurons that are able to broadcast specific neural waveforms out through the neural network for specific parts of the body. One section will govern the toes, while another will govern the feet, and so on. This organized vertical arrangement of specialized motor neurons is also referred to as the *homunculus motor* region, because each location is connected to specific body locations.

Behind the region of the motor cortex neurons is another set of regions grouped into what is called the *sensory cortex*. This region has several individual cortices, and spreads from the top of the head (*parietal lobe*) through the back of the head (*occipital lobe*) and along the sides (*temporal lobe*). Among these lobes lie the *visual cortex*, the *auditory cortex,* the *olfactory cortex,* the *postcentral gyrus,* and the *gustatory cortex*. In these respective regions, the various incoming sensory waveforms are translated and processed. The first three cortices—the visual, auditory and olfactory—are self-explanatory, being the centers that process waveforms of seeing, hearing and smelling, respectively. The postcentral gyrus processes the sensory waveforms of touch and balance, while the gustatory cortex processes taste waveforms from the tongue. Into each sensory cortex, specialized neural tracts conduct in and blend waveforms from the sense organs. The interference patterns of these waveforms blend together to provide an image screen of sorts for the self to observe.

The critical limbic system is positioned inside these cortex regions, towards the center of the brain. The limbic system is made up of the thalamus, the hypothalamus, the hippocampus, the cingulates, the fomix and the amygdala. Each of these has a slightly different function, but together they translate waveform data from the body in to be processed for memory and observance by the self. The limbic system's role is to prioritize and sort information according to crystallized neural programming. The hypothalamus and thalamus are the central translation system for waveforms traveling between the brain and the rest of the body. They also stimulate endocrine release of hormones and neurotransmitters, and translate incoming communications from around the body. The cingulates are programmed to govern the autonomic systems such as the heartbeat, breathing, hunger, and so on. The amygdala on the other hand, provides a gateway to the lower *chakra* centers, channeling the self's focus upon survival into fear and anger into the information processing. The hippocampus sorts and prioritizes all this information for memory storage. The fomix channels the waveform information from the hippocampus through a circuitry of memory processing (called the *Papex circuit)*, which we will examine in detail. Together the limbic system provides a translation and staging service for waveform information. We might compare the limbic system to a computer's operating system. The software might be stored in a particular location within the computer. Nevertheless, its programming instructions govern information translation, assembly, prioritization, storage, and transmission out to processing among peripheral devices and specialized programs.

The brain receives several types of input. The first is called *exteroception*, which means information gathered by the five basic senses of hearing, taste, smell, vision and touch. *Interoception* is the reception of signals received by the internal neurons, such as pain and other internal responses. The third reception type is *proprioception,* which is the internal feedback mechanism gauging coordinated movements, balance and motor efficiency—often referred to as *kinesthesia.* Meanwhile *equilibrioception* is the feedback of motor balance information, which is coordinated with waveforms passing through the vestibular system. *Nociception* is the reception of pain signals that accompany a threat of damage to tissues or cells. Finally, *thermoception* is the sensing of heat or coldness within the body. Other interoceptions include the sense of time, the esophageal senses and others. A few other sensations have been proposed, though most could also be considered a subset of interoception.

Each of these types of signals is associated with a particular region of the brain—though most interact in one respect or another within the limbic system and its components. For example, proprioception appears to resonate at the cerebellum. Thermoception resonates with thermoceptor cells in the hypothalamus. Nociception is thought to biocommunicate through the *anterior cingulated gyrus* (part of the cingulates).

As waveforms are stepped up through neural tracts toward the brain, the waveforms are boosted or converted by neural gateways into waveform configurations that can be managed by the limbic system. It is through the limbic system that various cortex regions are fed interoception from around the body. Programming sequences drive autonomic responses from the cortices primarily via the limbic system as well. As waveforms travel through the limbic system, the amygdale—channeling survival concerns of the self—is able to interact and alter these waveforms on their route to the particular cortex. This emotional interference system also works in reverse. Even if a particular decision is being channeled from the motor cortex to initiate a particular response in the body, the amygdale can alter or influence that instructional waveform as it moves back through the limbic system on its way out to stimulate particular motor nerve centers and endocrine responses (initiated primarily through the hypothalamus-pituitary pathway). In this way, motor responses may be exaggerated or muted through fear responses or other emotional responses.

Research has demonstrated an ionic channel based electrochemical *beta-adrenergic modulation* (Strange and Dolan 2006) facility within the amygdale. This modulation process requires a sophisticated level of waveform collaboration between the sensual inputs coming from the cortices and those arising from the mind web. As mentioned, the amygdale sorts images or impressions with an emotional or fearful perspective, which provides a sorting and priority criteria to the information. Research has concluded that by pegging information with emotional criteria, greater memory recall is established as compared to images without emotional tags (Dolcos *et al.* 2006).

This blending and transduction system could be compared to the internet or worldwide web. The internet or 'web' accomplishes a peer-accepted platform for the convergence of a variety of information gateways—or website portals. The convergence of all these website portals through the internet platform allows a particular user with a computer to choose to view any of the information portals. On the internet, the computer operator can choose to view a sorted compilation of websites through a search engine. The search terms are of course decided by the computer operator. In the case of the mind's web, the viewer is the self, and the gateways are the various types of pathways for waveform information being received and retained by the billions of brain cells. The limbic system offers to the self a platform where these information waves can be sorted and compiled. The self uses the sorting facility of the mind to program the search terms and the priorities for search compilation. In acquisition mode, once a search string is established, the limbic system coordinates a search through the standing waves of the various neuron gateways to locate information with similar waveform specifications.

The hippocampus is a central locator and search center to the mind's web. We might compare it to the placement of information throughout a hard disk, or even the assembly of information by search engine spiders. Located on each side of the brain in the temporal lobe, information from the senses and the body are converted by the hippocampus through a complex staging process. As was first published in a 1957 report by Scoville and Milner and later confirmed by Squire *et al.* (1991) along with other researchers, when the hippocampus becomes damaged, the first symptom is typically disorientation, memory acquisition loss, and recall deficiency. This is also evidenced in cases of encephalitis, where the hippocampus does not receive enough oxygen. When the hippocampus is damaged, new memories cannot be retained or recalled.

Within the hippocampus is an intricate pathway called the *Papex circuit* for electromagnetic rhythms, which can be likened to the cochlear passageway that stages and converts air pressure waves into electromagnetic nerve pulses. In the hippocampal pathway, waveforms from the cortical field (*entohinal cortex, perihinal cortex, cerebral cortex,* and so on), the subcortical field (*amygdale, broca, claustrum, substantia innominata,* and so on) mix with pulses from the thalamus and hypothalamus. These pulses are channeled through the *perforant path* consisting of three regions of the *dentate gyrus.* The signals pass through the CA3 and CA1 regions and on to the *subiculum* and *parahippocampal gyrus.* Here, between the subiculum and the parahippocampal gyrus, information in the form of interference waveform patterns is processed and translated to higher frequency waveforms—and broadcast into the neural net for storage or processing. In all, this circuit vets, tags and prioritizes information, preparing it to be cataloged. The various regions of the brain are also identified during this circuitry, which also identifies potential storage locations for information. In this way, the various neural networks of the different regions of the brain are mapped for waveform information storage and further processing.

In the pathway for visual impressions, for example, waveform combinations of different frequencies strike the retina and pass through the LGM to the visual cortex. Here in the cortex, waveforms drawn from memory through the amygdale are combined with internal stimuli waveforms and the LGM waveform data to create impression waveform interference patterns. These interference patterns create the specific information images for the self to see. We might compare this with creating an image by blending light rays of different colors and shapes onto a dark screen. Alone each light ray does not create much of an image, but together the different rays and colors can create a more complete image on the screen.

The images the self observes within the cortex are thus altered by context and history. The waveforms from the amygdale and memory alter the interference patterns. This accounts for the expression that we 'see what we want to see.' The interference patterns from these different sources eventually deliver convincing impressions to the hippocampus. Because the cortex combines all these waveforms together, the waveform information is forever altered. This creates the reality that each of us actually perceives a slightly different world around us.

In order to attempt to 'standardize' our perception, the self will seek confirmation from others. Information is thus gathered from others and the different forms of media. This creates a feedback loop between the amygdale, the hippocampus, and the cortices to constantly adjust our perception of reality towards the apparent perception of others. This is an intentional process because the self is constantly seeking affirmation from others in our never-ending quest for love and fulfillment.

Mapped brain regions also sort and translate incoming waveforms from the hippocampus. These are ultimately governed and coordinated by the prefrontal cortex. The intentions of the self stimulate a form of waveform programming mechanism that modulates neuron channels for particular waveform biocommunications. This creates a sorting system among those programmed neurons. The ion channel gateway states, neurotransmitter fluid content, and even genetic structures within the neuron may be manipulated by the executive initiatives programmed by the mind—under the intentions of the self. Many pre-programmed responses are crystallized within our static DNA. Still, neurons accommodate the executive authority of the inner self, expressed and translated through the prefrontal cortex and communicated via messenger pathways.

Chakras have been described in esoteric terms in much of the literature. However, we should realize that the *chakras* are inseparable from the waveform translating gateways existing within key networking regions of the brain and central nervous system. This is why the first five elemental *chakras* are described as regions aligned along the spine, and the last two within the brain. While not all neural tracts are *chakras*, all *chakras* utilize neural tracts to translate and transmit waveform conversions. These neural gateways of the *chakras* each accommodate a different medium and type of waveform, as we have described. Each also utilizes other pathways outside the neural system.

The limbic system is a part of the sixth *chakra* energy center, for example. Here waveforms from all over the body are converged and translated together with remodeled waves from the sensory cortices and the various feedback centers throughout the body. After translation, the limbic system coordinates instructions out to the body, together with a reflective broadcasting of waveform signals to the frontal cortex for executive review. Should the self respond to these inputs, executive waves are fed back to the body through the limbic system and the motor cortex. Here again the limbic system is acting as a transfer station, stimulating the release of various hormones through the hypothalamus and pituitary gland, which cascade through the various glands of the endocrine system. This provides the feedback pathway of executive instruction that Dr. Libet's research illustrated, allowing conscious decisions to take place after (programmed) responsive nerve impulses are detected.

Ultimately, it is the inner self—utilizing the various equipment of the brain—who initiates executive action. Once converted through the prefrontal and frontal cortices, this is accomplished directly through executive stimulation of the motor cortex and limbic system. This is like a car driver who sets up the proper cruise control speed, then removes his foot from the gas pedal. The cruise control will maintain the speed of the car by accelerating up hills and decelerating down hills automatically. However, should the driver decide to change speeds, avert running into the car ahead, or even stop the car, the driver can immediately take over the gas pedal and control the car's speed directly. In the same way, the self is driving the vehicle of the body, through both autonomic programming and executive control. Most autonomic functions can be manipulated directly should the self consciously intend to change them. In some cases, this takes practice, as biofeedback research illustrates. This conscious insertion of executive command can be initiated even during an autonomic response, just as the car driver can hit the gas pedal at any time to change the car's speed while it is running on cruise control.

As waveform messages from sensory nerves combine with physiology feedback and enter the brain's mapping network through the limbic system, they can be observed by the self on the interference 'screens' of a particular cortex or a combination of cortices. (The self can also manipulate, prioritize and distort these incoming physiological waveforms through the amygdale, however.) As they blend in the cortex, the self is able to review the waveforms and if need be, respond with intention. By this time, however, the programming already in place to process the particular situation is also ready to respond. Should a conscious 'executive' decision be made by the self, instructional waveforms are initiated through the prefrontal cortex. These are channeled through the motor cortex, which formats the waveforms for the hypothalamus. The hypothalamus in turn transduces these waveforms into physical response through the endocrine system and central nervous system. These instructional messengers may also contain a stop order to override whatever other instructions may already be in place.

Autonomic responses are established through initialized intentions and a subsequent programming of key web hubs by the mind. Most of these intentions are related to the survival of the body, translated from the self's fear of dying. This fear becomes translated into various scenarios that stimulate the programming features of mind. The programming waveforms stimulated by the mind are stored in neurons just as memories are, in the form of standing waves, crystallized by ionic molecular polarity and bonding sequences. Some autonomic programs are more permanently 'wired' into the standing waveforms that make up DNA bonds. These 'hard-wired' programs ultimately are passed on to the body's successors through the DNA.

These 'coded' standing waveforms with neurons are activated by certain types of waveforms incoming through sensory nerves and from interoception translated through the hypothalamus and thalamus. As information moves through this network, the neural programming indirectly relays the self's ultimate intentions of keeping the body alive with specific autonomic responses. The information will also be stepped up to the mind's web for viewing through the cortices. When we burn our finger, our autonomic programming will immediately respond by pulling the hand away. The self will also be able to view the incoming information separately, and initiate a separate, conscious response, such as tending to the injury or turning off the flame.

The self's recognition of information within the frontal cortex (or *mind screen*) is called *cognition.* In humans and primates, the central interface or bridge between the incoming impulse pathways of the nervous system and executive control is located in the *dorsolateral prefrontal cortex* (Otani 2002). It is here waveforms are examined, responded to and their responses relayed onto the motor cortex. Simultaneously, goal-directed intentions from the self stimulate the broadcast of waveform messages back into the neural net through the frontal cortex. Instructive waveforms are simultaneously pulsed through the hypothalamus, the specific regions of the motor cortex, and then the lower *chakras*. These instructive waveforms together stimulate the various elemental channels to respond. In other words, the body is not shocked or jerked into motion solely from pulses moving out from the brain. There are several pathways of activity initiated during a full-body response. The body's endocrine systems are stimulated. The body's heat-producing centers are stimulated. The body's insulin and energy releasing centers are stimulated. The body's pacemaker, vasomotor, perfusive and respirative functions all are simultaneously stimulated into immediate response. How else could the body react so instantaneously and thoroughly from head to toe following an intentional decision? We certainly have to characterize the chemical binding process as too cumbersome to exclusively provide these broadcasting mechanisms.

The connection between the cognitive functions of higher decision-making and the mind screen web are illustrated by the size of the frontal lobe cortex areas of the brain in more evolved organisms. Behavioral studies with animals and humans have also confirmed that complex executive functions with goal-directed behavior, language and higher cognition in general is associated with a larger, more developed prefrontal cortex (Fuster 2002). The developed frontal lobe cortex enables the self to command a greater volume of switchboard control and the ability to specify intention through a complex mental capacity. We also note that all highly evolved organisms also have advanced backbones and high-energy entry-points to carry out full-body *chakra* responses. As for less evolved organisms, we still find key neural points that transduce that self's intentions, albeit less complexly.

Neurotransmitter Conduction

As we examine the incoming waveforms received by the neural cell body through the neuron dendrites, we note the dendrites do not actually touch. They are not connected in the physical sense. Rather, between them exists a space called the *synapse*. The synapse contains a special chemistry called the *neurotransmitter fluid*. The neurotransmitter chemistry provides the medium for the waveform pulses traveling between neurons. Through this chemistry, waves of various frequencies are transmitted, moving information from one neuron to another, and as described above, enabling a broadcasting of the information through various other channels around the body.

This tiny sea of neurotransmitter fluid contains various biochemical components, most of which are ionic in nature. These ions combine with the protein neurotransmitters to create a system that drives an electromagnetic *synaptic potential*. Each CNS neuron can range in synapse count. Some might have several thousand while others have significantly less. Through these synapses, each neuron may be firing up to 100,000 electromagnetic pulse inputs into this fluid at one time. Depending upon its particular makeup at the time, the fluid will provide a combination of *excitatory potential* and *inhibitory potential.* This balance serves to escort or conduct waveform information from one nerve to another, while at the same time dampening or filtering these waveforms to prevent overload and over-stimulation. This process might well be compared to the process of transistors and resisters we see in integrated circuits. Neurotransmitters are tremendous semiconductors. Their delicate ionic balance precisely buffer and conduct waveform biocommunications within neurotransmitter fluids.

Two examples of neurotransmitters are acetylcholine and adrenaline (or epinephrine). These two messenger substances conduct and/or magnify specific wave rhythms, which reflect either programmed (autonomic) intention or conscious intention. Acetylcholine will modulate an instruction to muscle fibers to contract, while adrenaline will modulate instructions that perpetuate the 'fight or flight' response: Causing a quickening of heart rate and blood flow, immediate motor muscle response, visual acuity, and so on. Each of these biochemicals conducts particular types of waveforms. They will affect the neurotransmitter fluid, but they also interact with waveforms outside the confines of the fluid. For example, acetylcholine also stimulates skeletal muscle cells directly. This means the intentional response and programming to protect the body in specific ways is being conducted through these messenger molecules—and they are effectively translating that information into physical response.

Neurotransmitters and their cousins the hormones are secreted by various glands of the body. Epinephrine, for example, is secreted by the adrenal gland. Sex hormones are secreted by the gonads and ovaries. Metabolic hormones are secreted by the thyroid. Most secretions of the body follow a chain of command, however. Their secretions are stimulated by other secreted messengers produced by the pituitary gland. The pituitary gland is the master gland stimulating most of the various neurochemical messengers. This master gland not only responds to the stimulation of the hypothalamus and cortices, but also resonates with the higher frequencies of the *chakra* programming.

The pituitary gland is about the size of a cherry. It is located behind the eyes in a depression of the sphenoid bone, just behind where the optic nerves cross. It is also lying within the region of the sixth *chakra.* The pituitary produces hormone messengers that directly stimulate the body, such as growth hormone (GH), vasopressin, oxytocin and others. The pituitary gland connects to the hypothalamus by the *infudibulum,* a stalk of portal veins and nerves tracts. It is through this stalk the pituitary gland's activities are regulated by the hypothalamus. The hypothalamus sends *releasing hormones* to the pituitary. This regulatory process might be considered a balancing or filtering mechanism, compiling various waveforms into a balanced set of instructions.

Neurotransmitter chemistry acts as a conductor for these informational waveforms. There are many types of neurotransmitters. Some neurotransmitters such as epinephrine and glutamate increase transmission, while others such as dopamine subdue transmission. Other neurotransmitters—such as acetylcholine—facilitate muscle stimulation response, while others—such as serotonin—facilitate biocommunication of emotion and mood responses between nerves. The specific neurotransmitter chemistry provides a medium for particular types of wave transmissions, allowing the endocrine system (where most neurotransmitters are produced) to exert some feedback control into the process of conducting information around the body.

The biochemistry is intricate in this biocommunication process. We must be careful not to confuse chemicals with waves, however. Waves are informational, and conduct through chemicals. Their interference patterns can be stored within biochemicals in the form of standing waves between atoms. This is why biomolecules have unique properties. Biochemicals serve primarily as echo chambers, reflecting the informational waveforms being transmitted around the body. We might compare this to hearing a radio playing a song broadcast from a distant station. The radio does not contain the song, nor is it the source of the radiowaves that are being broadcast to millions of radios from the same radio station. The radio does not contain the singer either. Rather, the radio is simply a conducting vehicle, which temporary crystallizes and transforms the radiowaves into the speaker sounds that we can hear. In the same way, biochemicals reacting throughout the body during metabolism are merely vehicles of wave conduction. Waves and their informational interference patterns are being broadcast in multiple bandwidths through biomolecular processes.

Neurotransmitter conduction also might be compared to opening our eyes under water. Were we to dive into a river during a rain storm and attempt to open our eyes and look through its murky, muddy waters, we would not see much. We would be lucky to see our hand in front of our face underneath the muddy brown waters. That same river during a warm summer day might be so clear that we could see the bottom ten feet down. The difference between seeing within the two rivers is due to the muddy river mud being stirred up by the rain and stormy weather. It is not that our vision has gotten worse.

In the same way, an imbalanced chemistry in the neurotransmitter fluid will alter the waveforms passing from neuron to neuron. Some chemicals will interfere in the transmission of waves through the fluid. Certain chemicals affect neurotransmitter fluids in such a way that can subdue or distort the biocommunications as they are conducted across the neurotransmitter chemistry.

Case in point: When we drink alcohol, the alcohol will affect the chemistry of the synaptic junction—the neurotransmitter fluid—in such a way that distorts the electrical signals that travel from one neuron to another. This creates a situation where the brain cells controlling motor functions receive slow or even inaccurate signals. As these are stepped up into the neural net, the distorted signals create an unrealistic impression of the circumstances. This distorts perception, leading to coordination impairment, irrational behavior and mood swings: A potentially disastrous combination.

The key role of the neurotransmitter is to create an electrical potential for the waveform. This creates a bridge of sorts for the wave to transverse. The type of neurotransmitter also dictates which type of channel gateway will be opened on the post-synaptic nerve—the receiving nerve. The type of ion channel will typically dictate what kind of information will be transduced through the linkage of neurons.

One of the more interesting players in neurotransmitter biochemistry is GABA, which stands for *gamma-aminobutyric acid.* GABA is considered an inhibitory neurotransmitter in that it slightly slows down the wave conduction. This actually has a positive effect upon the synaptic transmissions, allowing nerve signals to pass through without as much distortion. GABA appears to be manufactured in the brain. GABA is known for its calming, regulating, and clear-thinking effects upon the brain and nervous system. Research has indicated that various mood disorders like depression, anxiety and even insomnia are related to the body having lower GABA levels within the neurotransmitter fluid. Epileptics typically have insufficient amounts of this neurotransmitter as well. Many of the popular anti-depressant pharmaceuticals increase the levels of GABA. It should be noted, however, that these drugs also produce various side effects as well.

Healthy amounts of GABA in the neurotransmitter fluid have been shown to accompany a state of physical relaxation with greater alertness. This state naturally also facilitates the conductance of alpha brainwaves. GABA research has confirmed that this molecule will induce increases in alpha brainwaves. In one study, L-theanine (a GABA precursor) was given to thirteen subjects. Electroencephalography examinations were conducted, and each recipient was observed having heightened alpha waves and reduced beta waves (beta waves are associated with nervousness and anxiety while alpha waves accompany increased concentration) (Abdou 2006).

Abdou's research also demonstrated the effect chemical neurotransmitters have upon the biocommunication of fear around the body. Two groups of eight volunteers were divided into a non-GABA (placebo) group and a GABA group. Both groups were monitored for IgA immunoglobulin levels following the crossing of a suspension bridge. Because IgA levels tend to shut down during anxious or fearful moments as the adrenal gland prepares for 'fight or flight,' this test illustrated GABA's effects upon fear-based immune response. The GABA group had normal IgA levels while the non-GABA group experienced significantly lower IgA levels. It was thus concluded that GABA levels are associated with reducing inappropriate fear responses as well as facilitating alpha waves.

As we assess this last trial, we can conclude that GABA created a calming or clearing effect upon the neurotransmitter fluid, which allowed the subjects to realistically assess the dangers involved. Using the senses to realistically assess the strength of the bridge and the likelihood of the bridge actually collapsing would be considered a clear-headed response. On the other hand, a heightened fear of falling simply by looking down (acrophobia) would not be considered a realistic assessment of the situation simply because the bridge could be easily crossed and was obviously strong enough to handle all of the walkers.

GABA provides a neurotransmitter environment at the synapse allowing a clearer and less distorted broadcasting of waveform information through the neural pathways. This allows the information to flow more clearly between the mind, the neural network and the sense organs. We might wonder how a seemingly simple biochemical molecule has such a drastic affect upon perception.

Microtubular Waves

During the 1970s, Dr. Stewart Hamerhoff from the University of Arizona, and Dr. Kunio Yasue and Dr. Mari Jibu from the Okayama University began researching the pathway of conscious activity between neural cells. One of the mysteries they probed in independent research was how anesthesia agents such as chloroform and nitrous oxide could disable the consciousness of a patient. Through their respective research, they independently discovered that conscious activity within the body had to do with a curious matrix of twisted spiral filaments they called *tubulins.* These tubulins are arranged into networked pathways that wind through the neural cells in three-dimensional protein spirals called *microtubules.* These microtubules appear to be conducting tracts for waveform activity. The research illustrated that the microtubules make up a previously unseen network for subtle waveform biocommunication through the neural net (Hameroff 1974; Hameroff 1982; Hameroff *et al.* 1984; Hameroff 1987; Hameroff and Penrose 1996).

As the larger waveforms of the physical realm are processed and transmitted through dendrites, they conduct through the neurotransmitters between the synapses. As they are conducted through this medium, the waveforms meet with other waveforms traveling within the neural network. This convergence creates coherent interference patterns. The resonating results of these interference patterns are then transmitted through the subtle network of the microtubules. In this state, these subtle waveforms are 'stepped up' to a higher frequency format. These subtle high frequency waveforms in turn create holographic wave patterns, which are ultimately reflected (or mirrored) onto the 'screens' of the cortices. Once on the screens, these holograms interact with others to create a 'picture' of the body and the world around us. The self interacts with these cortices through the primary screening device of the frontal cortex to view this holographic 'picture.'

Within these microtubules also travel the various subtle waveforms that conduct the intentions of the self through the body. The discovery of these microtubule pathways confirms much of the ancient wisdom of the *nadis* and *meridians.* These channels were also described as being pathways for living energy flow. We might consider nerve tracts as pathways of lower-frequency reflexive waveforms, while the microtubules broadcast higher-frequency, complex information waves.

We might compare the microtubular process of projecting wave interference patterns onto the mind to the recording of a musical composition in a modern studio. The studio producer will record the guitar onto one track, the piano onto another track, the drums onto another and the voice onto another track. The producer may even overlay background singers' voices onto other tracks. Then using these various individual sounds, the producer will assemble all the tracks together at particular sound levels to form the entire piece of music. This is often referred to as a *composition.* Each track makes up a piece of the total song. To listen to each track alone without the other tracks will sound wierd. In much the same way, the mind captures the various waveform frequencies coming through the microtubular network, neural net and biochemical messengers—combining them to form unified holographic images of the outside world.

One of the basic principles of holography is that each part mirrors the entire image. This is accomplished through a splitting of waves as they interfere, creating a multitude of waves, each containing all the information via the composition of waveforms. Using waveform interference, the mind orchestrates holographic assembly in both directions. The mind reflects its images semiconducted through particular neurons. The mind also stimulates effector neurons to act reflectively in response to the intentions of the self. The mind projects the whole image using the various cortex images, each assembling waveforms from different locations. This collection of images is broadcast through crystallized neuron pathways. Each neuron is constructed with the appropriate crystal DNA structure, ion channel system and microtubules, giving it the ability to join with others to relay multiple waveform interference patterns simultaneously.

The Memory Net

Modern neuroscience divides memory into short-term and long-term processes. Long-term memory is further divided into three types: *Episodic*—when memories are unique to the time and place; *semantic*—when memories involve concepts or learning; and *procedural*—when memories revolve around skills. Episodic memories relate to events that happened in the past, or people we knew from the past. Semantic memories relate more to concept understanding. Procedural memories relate to remembering how to ride a bike, write or use a telephone.

Interestingly, memory loss of one type will not typically accompany the loss of another type. Thus in many amnesia cases, long-term memory may appear erased while short-term memory is retained. The person may forget older events yet continue to remember what just happened.

Furthermore, all too frequently one type of long-term memory may be lost while another type may be retained. For example, a person may suffer the loss of their episodic memory—forgetting their name, family, school history, phone number, birth date and other personal details or events of the past. At the same time they may remember how to write, drive, talk on the phone and even retain concepts such as how economic markets work.

Often a particular trauma or event may cause the forgetfulness of either what happened just before the event, or what happened just after the event. The former case is referred to as *retrograde amnesia*—a loss of memory just prior to a trauma. The latter is referred to as *anterograde amnesia*—a loss of memory just after a trauma. Both may also occur. The causes of these types of forgetfulness are considered quite mysterious. This is because memory has been miscalculated.

There are other types of memory loss. Many are unconnected to any particular event, while others follow injury to particular brain regions or involve trauma. Trauma-associated amnesia may or may not involve physical injury. It may follow a head injury or automobile accident. Traumatic amnesia may also follow a witnessing of a traumatic event, or may involve abuse. Rape is an example of traumatic amnesia involving abuse. *Psychogenic* or *dissociative fugue* is another type of memory loss, which also may occur following a trauma, and may result in a person re-identifying him- or herself as someone else, and even taking an unexpected trip to a place previously unknown. Other events that can cause memory loss include alcohol and drug related blackouts, and *Wernicke-Korsakoff's,* which is thought to be caused by thiamin deficiency.

A more common type of amnesia involves the loss of memory of a particular event. This may be the forgetting of certain childhood events, for example. Forgetting certain events may also be referred to as traumatic memory loss. Many of us forget events in the distant past that were not necessarily traumatic as well. It is not unusual for us to forget our younger childhood events. We also may recall something without remembering how we knew it—called *source amnesia.*

One illness overwhelming modern medicine and capturing research attention is *Alzheimer's disease.* The first documented case of AD was discovered by a Bavarian psychiatrist named Dr. Alois Alzheimer. Dr. Alzheimer treated a 51-year old patient who suffered from memory loss and hallucinations. The patient, "Auguste D" was frequently delirious and had extreme short-term memory deficit. She complained of having "lost myself." She was committed to the Frankfurt asylum in 1901 and died five years later. Autopsy revealed a sticky plaque among brain cells and nerve tissue entanglement. The disease was named after the diagnosis given by Dr. Alzheimer, and this variant of dementia became associated with physical damage to the brain apparently relating to a build-up of beta amyloid plaque among certain regions of the brain. The definite cause of AD has not been determined, although there appear to be a number of potential contributing factors, including stress, heavy metal toxicity, and certain diets. Recent research seems to point at a lack of phosphatidylserine among brain cell membranes as well.

This sort of research contributes to our notion that memory is chemical-based. The frontal and medial temporal lobe is the prevailing theory for long-term memory storage location—based on EGG and magnetic resonance scans. Still, researchers have observed numerous instances where memories are retained when specific regions of the brain thought to control a particular type of memory are removed or incapacitated. This occurred in hemicortication surgeries—a frequent treatment of childhood epilepsy for many years. Episodic memories were retained even through the brain regions thought to be involved were removed. We must therefore question the assumption that memories are specific to particular neurons. Yet we still need to address the fact that many memory losses occur following brain damage to particular locations. What is going on here?

The first clue is that most of these cases are specific to short-term memory loss. Long-term memories remain a mystery. In one study (Piolino *et al.* 2006), thirteen patients with early stage dementia, ten patients with semantic dementia and fifteen patients with frontotemporal dementia were compared to assess the connection between memory loss and damage to the medial temporal lobe. One of the central areas of focus in this study was the *autobiographical amnesia of episodic memories,* or the lack of ability to acquire or remember events of ones past. The results of this study concluded no consistency between memory loss and frontal lobe impairment. In some cases, short-term memories were difficult to acquire as a whole, and in other cases, the memory acquisition depended upon the details and importance of the event. In many cases, long-term "remote" memories were retained and preserved while short-term details and events were not. This led the study authors to support a newer theory called the *multiple trace theory,* which says that memory acquisition occurs through more than one physical mechanism, and can be stored in multiple locations.

In a similar study (Matuszewski *et al.* 2006) on autobiographical episodic memory loss among frontotemporal dementia patients, near learning abilities with semantic memories revealed a shifting executive function with multiple processes. As for other possible models of memory acquisition, several studies have indicated that the hippocampus complex was significantly involved in the storage and recall of recent memories, but not for older memories. Other research has offered evidence that the hippocampal complex is responsible for autobiographical episodic memory and special memory, but the storage of other types of memory was shifted to other locations (Nadel and Moscovitch 1997).

In a 2002 report (Nester *et al.*) published in *Neuropsychologia* on autobiographical memories among semantic dementia patients, the preservation of recent memories and the loss of remote memories supported the trace theory of memory retention and acquisition. This report confirms, as so many animal studies have, that memories are not chemically retained within specific neurons. We can logically compare memories to data stored on a computer's hard drive. However, modern science has yet to locate the program, the language nor the methods used to categorize, place and retain memories.

This is because modern science does not understand the most basic understandings of living biology. Again, we first must know who the driver of the vehicle of the body is. From there we must understand the means for the operation of the vehicle. Just as a car's driver uses the wheel, the clutch and the gas pedal to move the car, the driver of the body also utilizes particular equipment to drive the body. The reality is, the mind is the software of the brain, and the brain assembles information as programmed by the mind. The self dictates the functioning of the mind through conscious intention: desire.

This was clearly exposed in a study of memory-challenged patients with different brain disorders (Thomas-Anterion 2000). Twelve Alzheimer's disease patients and twelve frontotemporal dementia patients with functionally similar semantic memory, logical memory and retrograde memory test scores were studied for antegrade verbal memory and frontal lobe activity. Despite similar memory acquisition scores and types of memory loss, physiological brain function occurred in different locations among the subjects. This illustrated flexibility in brain region utilization, quite similar to practical daily living: Should we be unable to pick up something with one hand, we will quickly adjust and pick up the item with the other hand. In the same way, the self, using the utility of the mind, can often accomplish the same purpose using different neurons, cortices and/or limbic components.

Should the intent to remember exist, memory can be retained using a variety of external physical mechanisms as well. Humans have indeed resorted to various tools to replace or augment memory function for thousands of years. For example, a person may retain memories within a diary to assist in the recall of particular thoughts, emotions and events. Projects or objectives may be recorded onto daily planners, or onto digital voice recorders for later recall. Most students and businesspeople carry notebooks to every class and meeting to assist with the retention and recall of lectures and discussions. These external memory devices replace or augment limited memorization abilities. They also illustrate an intention to remember.

The memory experiments by Dr. Wilder Penfield at the Montreal Neurological Institute in the 1970s clearly illustrated that memories typically accompanied emotions and intentions. When Dr. Penfield's weak electrical currents excited locations within the brain, the subject would recall historical facts associated with past experiences. Their recollections included songs connected to feelings from the past, aromas connected to experiences, people connected to personal relationships, and events connected to other emotional events. Dry information such as what score a person received twenty years ago on a test or sporting event might seem like raw data, but even this data are connected to personal intentions to win or receive a good score. Without an emotional, intentional attachment, the ability to recall that event subsides as the self's intention to remember it weakens.

What this tells us is that memory is impossible without emotion or consciousness. Memory studies have shown that when a person is emotionally involved in a particular incident or detail, the recall rate of that incident or detail is significantly higher. Furthermore, as the event converts to longer-term memory, if it has no emotional attachment, it is typically sorted out during our consolidation process—which typically takes place as we sleep. In order to remember trivial details, those subjects who connect the detail to a colorful, emotional or funny association will dramatically increase the likelihood of recalling it later.

Certainly, without consciousness there would be no need for memory or recall. We might think that a robot must have a memory in order to store its programming information. However, we also know that no robot would be built without an original conscious intention. Without consciousness, there would be no purpose for a robot. The robot, then, is simply a surrogate of a conscious person's purpose and intention. This is precisely what the physical body is.

From these points, we can logically conclude that the inner self utilizes the physical elements of the brain for memory retention and recall, but only by utilizing the programming of the mind. This also means that damage to the hardware may also destroy the organism's ability to recall and apply those memories. Memorization and recall may be shifted to a variety of brain regions and even external tools. The hardware is still necessary, however. This is because memories are waveform interference patterns linked to emotion. Yes, the waveforms are crystallized within groups of resonating neurons. However, the memories will not be retrievable without conscious intention. Should those brain cells become damaged, those memories may become difficult to retrieve. The retrieval difficulty is due to a drop in the link between the inner self and those interference patterns. The standing waveforms may still be there, but the emotional tie to those waveform patterns will be severed.

This is not to say the self has no memory without the body. This is clearly evidenced by near death experiences and past life regression research. The self has the ability to recall events without the tools of the brain's neurons. The real question is whether once the self has moved on from a particular body; does the self retain any real intent to remember events related to the petty details of that former body's history? Without the body's existence, what good would remembering these details be to us? Memories may provide interesting conversation or perhaps pathological interest (as Drs. Freud and Janet might have), but have little application to the self's emotional situation once the body has decomposed. We can just imagine how confusing life would be if we each could harken back at will to the different physical bodies we have lived within. We would be simply remembering the traumatic events leading to the death of that body, along with various details that would serve us only with regrets and the missing of loved ones who are probably still around us in different bodies anyway (as loved ones and family members often transmigrate together). Currently it is difficult to remember all the names, dates, appointments and other details of *this* life, let alone past ones. Imagine the overload if we could mix memories of different lifetimes together at will.

Consistent with many of the ancient sciences, the self has another identity transcendental to this physical dimension. This identity has the ability to retain and remember everything in the past and present, assuming the self is not locked up within the confines of the false identification within a physical body. Just as a dark movie theatre blocks our ability to see what is going on around us as we focus upon a movie, our absorption into our mind and present physical body buries our ability to recall events of previous lifetimes. Because memories are part of the self's learning process, we still intuitively draw upon the learning experiences of previous lifetimes without the mind being involved in the memory of that lifetime. We will elaborate on this innate ability to retain and learn from the past as we discuss the "subconsciousness" later.

The self might have the ultimate ability to learn and grow from the events that take place here. The waveform patterns crystallized by brain neurons linked to emotions are what we might call *virtual memories,* or more accurately, *holographic memories.* In other words, the memorized details we associate with emotional intentions are related to the accommodation of our desires. We remember the type of information that we feel will contribute to our enjoyment of our body the most. This takes place on several levels, but it is certainly tied to our intention to accomplish happiness within the physical world.

The sensual information we absorb with our senses is transmitted via waveform mechanics. Our senses convert waveforms from one medium into waveforms that can travel within the medium of the neural biology. As these waveform pulses are stepped into higher frequency waveforms, they are transmitted through the various neural pathways, including the microtubules, as we have discussed. These waveforms come together within our cortices to create coherent interference patterns, which tie together with the brainwaves arising from our limbic system. Together these interference patterns create networks of standing waveform patterns that bond molecule and ion sequences within our neurons. They accumulate to create a web of networked waveforms.

This might be compared to looking at a pond after many stones have been tossed into it. The confluence of intersecting and interfering ripples contain the data that reveal the original event to an intelligent observer. The interference patterns reveal whether a single stone or multiple stones were thrown in. They may reveal how large the stones were, how long ago they were thrown in and how far apart the stones were thrown in. Even one of the stones' waves, ripped up by interference patterns, can be followed back to the original stone throws, because they have each become interconnected through the medium of the pond. In this way, the ripples and waves of the stone throws are all interconnected into a web of waveforms.

In the case of the mental web, we are speaking of a convergence of millions of sensory, neural and brain waveforms all interacting within the system. This wave interaction keeps each memory associated with various other events and memories. This interactive pattern might also be compared to that of a spider's web—weaved and linked with silk strands interlaced into a sturdy net. One strand alone will not hold much. Networked together, they are strong. In the same way, our holographic memory retention is based upon a linking of emotions with sensory images, all wrapped together by the intention to succeed and enjoy the physical body. As some strands become older or less important, they gradually become pushed further away from the priority strands that are tied to the current events now central to our current goals. These older memories might still available in the grand web of interlocking waveforms. However, they become increasingly difficult for us to recall, as they fade from our intentional priorities.

For this reason, we find it fairly easy to replace actual memories with forged memories. The forged memories are inserted through emotional intention. This intention holds the forged memories in place, and after awhile the mind sees no difference between the forged and the real memories.

The reason tumors in the hippocampus have been known to cause amnesia is because the hippocampus is a conversion tool used by the mind to transmute event waveform combinations from one type to another. The ability of the limbic system to translate impulses into the memory web map and also access that map—translating the webbed memories back into physical recall—has been damaged. In the same way, if we got cancer of the vocal cords, we would not be able to convert our thoughts into words. Losing the conversion tool does not bode well for that activity. The bridge between the physical waveforms of the neural net and the subtle mapping of those rhythms has been broken. As research has indicated, should another part of the limbic system be available for web building and should the intent remain, the self may still be able to shift that function elsewhere, though it will be difficult. It is easier to shift cortex functions because there are several cortex regions situated around the brain, each having similarly structured neurons.

We can compare the mapping technology of the memory web or net to the tracking location system of a computer hard drive memory disk. The computer hardware is compared to the limbic system, which coordinates the mapping and retrieval of particular memory waveforms. The hippocampus, hypothalamus and amygdale work together with the rest of the limbic system to coordinate the storage and retrieval of particular informational waveforms. These are of course fed in from the senses along with feedback from the body, converted, and then escorted through the particular neurotransmitter messenger relays.

Together this sorted information is both sent to memory and projected in the frontal cortex for the self to view. Together these waveforms create a harmonic coherence, because the events are strung together by our emotional intent. Our intentions are thus inserted into the sorting process of the limbic system. The waveform synchronization is finally projected upon the mind screen web for the self's direct interaction. The self's feedback from this viewing becomes tied together historically using the formatting and storage mechanisms of the hippocampus and prefrontal cortex. This reformatting sorts specific types of waveform patterns to resonate with other historical information, tying them together within the particular region of the brain that resonates with that wave format.

Each memory waveform or set of interference waveforms is held in resonance and crystallized within a region of neural cell molecules. Protein crystal semiconductors provide the platform for these waveform combinations to be retained in standing waves. Though this statement might deceive us into thinking the memories are contained in the neuron chemistry, this is immediately refutable. Research has illustrated that when we sleep, the mind quietly shuffles and reprioritizes the memory banks, aligning them with the self's current objectives. Less important memories are shuffled out, while memories considered more critical to the self are retained. The rejected memories are discarded, yet those neurons remain, albeit with newly crystallized waveform interference patterns.

Mental Programming

The inner self is separate from the mind. The inner self is the instigator of the mind's programming, and the viewer of its networked mapping system. By understanding how the mind is interfaced and utilized by the self, and how its intentions program the brain's functions, we can better understand how the mind is utilized by the self. We can understand how physical events affect the mind, and how life's various traumas and addictions can become embedded into the mind. As we will discuss later, this information can assist us in the healing of these issues.

The goals and intentions of the inner self are converted to practical strategies by the mind. The mind is a subtle programming tool that compares to the operating system program of a computer. The design of the mind is set up to embrace the instructions of the inner self, and design a process to most effectively execute those instructions. Because the mind operates within the construct of waveform mechanics, it is designed to manipulate and coordinate waveforms. Utilizing this ability gives the mind the opportunity to sort the waveforms that accomplish its programming goals. It prioritizes the various wave patterns moving through the body, and assembles various concoctions based on the data it receives.

The mind is a quick learner. From birth, the mind utilizes the incoming wave patterns from the senses to sort through the nature of the outside environment. It also utilizes the various feedback impulses from within the body to coordinate particular physiological activities. The similarity between the mind's mechanism and artificial intelligence software is uncanny. The mind works almost precisely the same way. Artificial intelligence may seem to be running on automatic, but its programs were designed by conscious programmers. The mind is also programmed by a conscious programmer. Just as in artificial intelligence, the mind's programming can also respond to its inputs and outputs. We might better compare this to a robot that follows the commands of a particular operator. Once given the commands, the programming set up in the robot by its builder will work to achieve those commands. The mind's programming accomplishes the same kind of results.

Initially the self might have broad commands for the mind. The primary directives of the self are typically to enjoy physical life and obtain love. This is because the self is constantly seeking these two primary goals: pleasure and love. Based on these two primary commands, the mind develops various strategies to manipulate the body and the environment to accomplish these realities. If one strategy is unsuccessful in fulfilling the self's ultimate goals, the mind will then develop yet another strategy. These are called *concoctions.* They are the mind's recipes for accomplishing the goals of the self.

Because these strategies or concoctions of the mind are frequently reviewed by the inner self, the self becomes deeply involved and even committed to the concoctions of the mind. As the self becomes committed to the mind's strategies, determination develops. As the self becomes determined, the self will rest its hopes of accomplishing its primary directives by achieving the mind's current strategic concoctions.

A good example illustrating this is how our primary directive for obtaining true love evolves within the mind's various strategies. In the beginning of life within a particular body, the self attempts to receive true love from the body's parents. After a few years of trying to please the body's parents without achieving the satisfaction of true love, the inner self feeds back to the mind that parental love is not achieving the primary directive. As a result, the mind concocts—after observing others playing and laughing with their friends—that achieving certain relationships with others should complete the directive. During youth, friendships with playmates may subsequently become the goal. Once these relationships still do not satisfy the primary directive of the inner self, achieving a relationship with the opposite sex may become the current concoction of the mind. The mind develops various strategies to accomplish this, such as becoming successful in sports, school, popularity, and so on—all in an attempt to attract the opposite sex. Once a girlfriend/boyfriend relationship is achieved, after some time again the self will not be satisfied. The primary directive of pure love is not reached. The mind may then contrive that maybe marriage will accomplish the goal. *Maybe if we possessed the other person…* We soon discover that these relationships do not accomplish the primary directive either. The mind may then be directed to look elsewhere for the attention and admiration of others in its attempt to gain the love the self needs. To accomplish this, the mind develops strategies such as becoming successful in a particular career or skill. This strategy is based upon the observation that others who have become successful have achieved the admiration of others. The mind concludes that if we can be seen as a success by others, we will achieve their love—

again a failed assumption, as the many suicides by famous people have shown us.

As the self feeds back to the mind that we still have not accomplished the fulfillment we need, the mind will immediately develop yet another strategy. On this goes. The mind keeps concocting new strategies. Once one strategy fails, another is concocted to replace it.

This same process works for the other primary directive: pleasure. The self is constantly looking for pleasure, and this is fed into the mind to try to achieve pleasure in the physical world. The mind concocts various strategies to achieve pleasure. During the early years, this may consist of getting certain toys and games. Later on, the concoctions will become more complex, including obtaining wealth, a new house or perhaps living in a location that is appears to the mind to be more beautiful or warmer than the body's current location. These larger concoctions are filled in with more immediate concoctions such as eating a tasty meal, having sex, watching a movie or television, or listening to a particular song or concert. These strategies large and small are developed by the mind, and because the self wants to achieve the directive, the body follows suit to accomplish those strategies. With each successive failure, the mind immediately comes up with yet another new strategy.

Each strategy of the mind assumes success. Hence, the self anticipates that once a particular concoction of the mind is accomplished, the goal will be met. As we can observe in our own lives and in the lives of others, the mind's concoctions never seem to satisfy either of the two central intentions of the self for achieving love and pleasure. The problem lies with the non-physical self looking for fulfillment within a physical realm.

As the mind programs the body to accomplish each successive concoction, it also facilitates innumerable sub-programs—or sub-concoctions. These are also ultimately intended to facilitate accomplishing the central intentions of the inner self. These sub-programs can range from working out or training the body to accomplish specific strengths and functionality to the body's autonomic nervous responses. These also include sub-features such as pulling the hand away from a fire to avoid losing the hand. If the hand is lost, many of the primary concoctions of the mind will be hindered. These sub-routines are developed with the self's ultimate goals in mind, but they accomplish the tasks of basic survival. These tasks have thus been categorized as instinct.

Biologists like to consider survival activities as instinctive, since many species seem to inherently seek survival with similar techniques. These are simply sub-routines of the mental concoctions to keep the body alive, however. This can be seen in cases where children were raised by animals—called *feral children.* As the syndrome—*Mowgli syndrome*—goes, the child turns out emulating the chief caregiver—be that an animal or handicapped parent. The mind of the child develops concoctions and sub-concoctions based on the perceptions and choices made available through living with the animal pack. This is also applicable to a child trained in a terrorist camp-school. They will come out with dramatically different strategies to achieve pleasure and love.

As the body is programmed by the mind, its metabolic activities are orchestrated together with the routing of sensual inputs, memory and the instigation of feedback. The body can be said to be a reflection of the mind's programming. The mind does not create the body, as is proposed by some. The body's functions are shaped and steered by the mind, however. The mind certainly has the ability to direct the body to attempt to achieve its particular concocted strategies. We can also say that without that direction the body-person would probably not have achieved that result. However, the mind still does not control the outcome. The mind does not create or control the outcome, and those who profess this view are simply deceiving others in an attempt to achieve their own objectives.

This conclusion can be arrived at quite logically. Despite the desire, the mind cannot control the weather. The mind cannot control what others say. The mind cannot control the outcome of events. Attractive semantics used by some self-help "gurus" will claim that the only reason the mind may not control the outcome is due to some defect of thinking. Where is the defect of thinking when the weather is boiling hot or freezing cold and there is no ability to get out of this circumstance? Despite our mental attempts to change the weather, we simply cannot. Yes, we can pack our bags and travel to a better location. This decision will come at a cost, however. There will be consequences our mind cannot control. The next location is likely to also have its weather problems as well. The mind simply cannot change certain physical realities.

The mind also cannot avoid trauma. Does the mind create the trauma of rape or other physical abuses? Is there some defect in that mind that has somehow attracted that event to the person—as the law of attraction might imply? This is not only an absurd notion, but it is cruel. Its implication is that all the suffering in the world is caused by our mental derangement.

Rather, traumatic events are learning experiences. The outcome is dependent upon whether the inner self learns what the trauma is supposed to teach. The body may be experiencing a particular traumatic event. However, the inner self only experiences the trauma to the extent the self is connected with the body and has committed to those related concoctions. If the self can release from these concoctions and detach from those strategies, the trauma will heal because the inner self will have redirected the mind and body with new intentions.

Let us explain further using a practical experience. Let us say that after one thanksgiving a family decides to purchase a live turkey and raise it through the year, and eat it for thanksgiving the following year. The family puts the turkey into the backyard and duly feeds the bird and makes sure it is warm and cozy at night. The young girl in the family oversees the care of the turkey and begins to pet and coo the bird. The little girl and the turkey become close over the year. The day before thanksgiving, her father yanks the beautiful bird by the neck and cuts its head off while the girl is watching. She is traumatized by this event.

There are two possible outcomes to this trauma. In one, the trauma continues to haunt the little girl until she becomes an adult, and every thanksgiving when she sits down to her turkey dinner, she is still haunted by the event. In the other outcome, the little girl, feeling sick at how animals are unnecessarily killed for food, decides to become vegetarian. For the rest of her life the girl is not haunted by the bird, rather she has learned something significant from the event, and has evolved and made changes that empower her learning experience. She learns from this event, and the changes she makes remove the trauma from the situation.

This example illustrates how we can either grow or shrink from trauma. This is our choice—the inner self has the power to make changes in direction, or not. Therefore, continuing traumas are symptomatic of a lack of change despite life teaching us to change. Why is this? Simply because life was designed—actually programmed—by the Almighty to teach us to grow and progress through this lifetime, towards our higher purpose.

Why are some of us experiencing more trauma than others, then? In reality, every body experiences traumatic events. It is our lack of preparation for the event that makes it traumatic. For this reason, even unexpected loud sounds can become traumatic for a person who is not expecting the sound. This is often referred to as *acoustic shock*.

The particular traumas we face depend upon our prior decisions and activities. Actions that inflicted cruelty or pain upon others will return reciprocal reactions either later in this life or into the next. This is the ultimate design of the universe. In family psychology, there is a form of discipline called *learning by consequence*. This is described as a child being given specific consequences related to specific actions rather than unrelated punishment such as spanking. In the design of the universe, our decisions and actions result in precise consequences—our current situation thus perfectly mirrors a combination of our current consciousness and what we have done in the past.

This reality has been confirmed in many past life regression studies. In many studies, subjects' current fears or dilemmas can be related precisely to an activity they took part in within a past embodiment. The experience of the trauma allows the self to work through the issue, and resolve it by making the appropriate changes. If the self committed suffering upon others in a previous life, it will have to work through a similar trauma in this life. Once the trauma is experienced, the self can potentially grow and develop from the experience. Having experienced that traumatic event, the prudent self makes a determination not to ever commit that experience upon another—knowing what it feels like. This determination is often made regardless of whether the person consciously realizes that the trauma happened because of an action they took in the past. The inner self will understand this in a deeper way, however. Through the decision to not partake in that activity, we have essentially learned the lesson, which will automatically resolve the trauma.

If we do not adequately grow from a trauma, it will likely bear upon us as a conflict to resolve later. As such, following a traumatic event, some of us will negatively retain the memory of the trauma. Most will seek to escape or release from this disturbing web of traumatic events. Often these attempts only serve to exacerbate the issues, as the intent to escape the memory causes a resurfacing of the disturbing memory. However, nature's system is designed to force the self into a resolution with the trauma. This can render a change in direction, resulting in growth and evolution. If that change does not take place, there will likely be a continuing disturbance, or at least a buried trauma, which will emerge later to be reckoned with.

An example illustrating this burying mechanism is the use of *propranolol*—a pharmaceutical drug developed in the 1950s for depression. Propranolol works by blocking the reception of epinephrine on beta-adrenergic nerve receptors. When the epinephrine messenger receptors are blocked, the mind can better disengage from stress because the feedback-response channels through which the limbic system and prefrontal cortex operate are inhibited, temporarily disengaging parts of the neural memory net.

Recent research on propranolol has revealed an additional unintentional effect, however: Clinical results have indicated that a person can also more easily release from past physical or emotional traumas by taking propranolol. Researchers observing these effects have documented women able to release from rape trauma and soldiers able to release from the battlefield traumas, for example.

This use of propranolol has become controversial. Many ethics scientists have protested that using a synthetic drug to remove or disconnect from past trauma interferes with the natural learning process inherent in nature's mechanisms of remembering and resolving historical traumas. They correctly propose that without this natural mechanism, our ability to grow and evolve is stunted.

Both sides of this issue certainly have respectable positions. It is critical we learn and grow from our experiences. No one likes to see someone else suffer from their particular traumas. The question here is whether propranolol—like alcohol and many other mind-altering drugs—simply delays the trauma from being worked through—the lack of which may cause a later unforeseen fall-out. In the case of alcohol, which is used by many to escape from reality through similar biochemical mechanisms, more damage is eventually done by the attempted escape. While the alcoholic may wish the world will get better and problems will dissolve, the problems simply worsen. Family and friends of the alcoholic simply become increasingly hurt and disaffected, and during drunken rages, the alcoholic may damage these relationships and create more problems. This in turn only makes the situation worse. This situation is illustrated by the large populations of homeless alcoholics. These people choose to try to escape from life's traumas. Ironically, the escape only aggravated those problems into full-blown disasters. Instead of improving the situation by our escaping from it, the problematic situation will be worsened and the traumas will still need to be reconciled along with the need for physical withdrawal. The recovering alcoholic will have to deal with the problems caused by the alcohol in addition to resolving the trauma.

We might compare this again to the computer. In the case of propranolol, the blocking of epinephrine's waveform reception would be equivalent to shutting down a problem part of a computer's hard drive in order for the operator to be temporarily blocked from accessing its data. The problem data is still there. It will not resolve itself.

Release: This is what we try to do with drinking, taking drugs, watching TV or otherwise getting lost in some other diversion. We want to release from the anxieties and stresses of this world. We want to disengage ourselves from the traumas of life: From our job, from a difficult relationship, or from tough family situations. Periodically, most of us need escape. Some of us might partake in some of the destructive forms of escape as mentioned above. Others will simply exercise or go for a walk in the woods for release. Still others might garden, go shopping or go to a movie.

These types of release all certainly might work temporarily. Chemical releases such as alcohol or drug use are based upon the blocking or modulating of synaptic neurotransmitters, which change the waveform pathways through the nerves. When the synaptic receptors are blocked by the introduction of alcohol into the system, the channels are blocked. This means the mind cannot gain access to the critical mapping information needed to recalibrate with physical reality. The mind becomes slightly disconnected with the body. This provides a temporary release. However, the self also loses considerable control over the body, including many autonomic functions necessary to maintain health and detoxification. As a result, there are multiple physiological disorders associated with alcoholism, including liver disease.

There are positive forms of conscious release as mentioned: Exercise, gardening, reading, giving and so many others. By doing something to refocus our attention onto something other than the cause of the anxiety, it is possible to disengage naturally. Focusing elsewhere naturally releases our mind's focus onto problematic areas. As documented in a study by Westman and Eden (1997), satisfactory vacations by clerks lead to a reduction of stress and job burnout. A vacation is a redirection of our attention—focusing the mind from one thing to another, which is a process of selective intention. Along with this redirection of focus naturally comes a redirection of the self towards the concoctions of the mind. A vacation can naturally bring awareness of different approaches and a means to possibly accomplish the self's directives differently.

Selective Steering

It is apparent that the self has the ability to be selective. The self has the ability to choose its cortex viewing priorities. Reflecting this, the limbic system's memory storage sorting facilities can also be directed with selectivity. This is why we remember interesting things more than boring things. This is also why we can forget traumatic events during childhood while remembering all too clearly the traumatic events that unfolded during adolescence or adulthood. During times of childhood trauma, the inner self can more easily disconnect from the event. This ease of disconnection helps the memory fade. A trauma occurring later in life will have a lot more emotional attachment than a trauma occurring during youth. For this reason, it is clinically more difficult to resolve traumas that occur after 5-7 years of age.

We might consider how children can run around laughing and playing, and when they fall—especially if they are playing a game they enjoy—they may simply jump up and keep playing. They may hardly notice the scrapes and scratches—or the pain—of the trauma. The child may even avoid Mom's first aid application—intended to avoid infection and speed healing. In the child's eyes, this might just interfere with the remainder of the game. It is likely this child will completely forget this trauma as he or she quickly learns not to repeat the fall. However, an adult falling with the same intensity will likely cause a significantly more amount of trauma. An adult will typically be focused on the pain, concerned about how it might endanger the various plans—or concoctions—of the mind. The adult will thus be overly concerned with the healing process, and trying to prevent infection in its aftermath. An adult would probably stop the game to wash-up and bandage the wound. The focus would immediately shift from the game to the injury and the pain, reinforcing the trauma of the pain. The adult would likely walk off the field for the day to tend to the injury.

This type of focus also contributes to our ability to remember one person's name while forgetting another's. It is not that the person whose name we forgot did not interest us: Their name simply did not capture our attention and focus at the moment. Our mind was engaged in processing other items that took priority over the name. The mind is the programming tool of the inner self, and though it might seem a bit out of control at times, its sub-routines directly or indirectly respond to the interests of the self. Should we exert a determined effort to remember names, however, it would be another story. We would likely employ various *mnemonic* tools such as creating a funny picture to associate with the person's name. These intentional insertions are stimulated by the self, but are executed through the amygdala. Once the mind creates that funny picture it is inserted by the amygdala into the limbic system, which exchanges a holographic image with the frontal cortex. The self thus becomes emotionally involved directly in the process of viewing a holographic representation of the name via this mechanism. This intentional viewing triggers a priority sort of the memory within the hippocampus— enabling better retention and recall of the name.

The processes of the mind work through a combination of programming, design, and the intentional steering by the self. The self may drive or direct the mind, but does not necessarily control the design of the mechanism. There are some benefits from this. Imagine a situation where a person remembered every trauma experienced during their lifetime: The pain of being enclosed in the womb; the trauma of being born; the challenges of growing up; the pain of every accident or physical injury. Each of these events is certainly traumatic. If we were to remember every one vividly, we would be tormented to say the least. Again, the reason why we do not remember these traumas is because while they were happening, we were focused elsewhere. These traumas were not interfering with current concoctions.

The interaction between the self and the amygdala—the emotional center of the limbic system—and the memory-oriented regions of the limbic system such as hippocampus, hypothalamus and the visual cortex have been shown in a number of EEG and magnetic resonance studies. Meanwhile it appears the prefrontal cortex—often referred to as the *seat of cognitive control*—is able modulate these waveform interactions. This modulation provides an ability to interfere in the memory web process, thereby effecting memory suppression or repression.

During research performed in the Department of Psychology at the University of Colorado (Depue *et al.* 2006), subjects were shown faces paired with either pictures or other faces—some neutral and some disturbing. After repetition and memorization, the subjects underwent brain MRIs while being asked to either recall an image paired with a particular face, or suppress the image. This gave researchers the ability to trace the regions of the brain involved with both memory recall and suppression. The study concluded firstly that people are able to successfully suppress disturbing images on request. This is a substantial point. In addition, MRI scans demonstrated the involvement of the prefrontal cortex in memory suppression. The inner self has a considerable amount of control over our memories, using the prefrontal cortex to exercise this control.

This relationship between memory and formulating pictures has been taught for many decades by a number of memory experts. Some have written and lectured on the process of using this method to build *super-memories.* There also have been many demonstrations by those who have utilized these methods and developed super-memories. The basic technique is to connect the detail to be remembered to an interesting image and/or story. This creates an emotional connection with the detail. A number of details can thus be memorized by linking them together into a series of images to create a funny or unique story.

Forgetting is not necessarily a bad thing. An example to consider is Solomon Shereshevskii (1886-1958), a Russian journalist who seemed to remember just about everything. Solomon could remember extensive lists of numbers, facts, details, names and faces. He was truly one of history's greatest memorizers. His method of remembering such detail, it was later discovered, was due to his ability to connect each fact or figure to a three-dimensional visual picture. Doing this would allow him to relate each fact to not only a particular visual picture, but one that had personal character. This inserted emotion into the memory sorting process. Over time, Solomon had various problems with his super-memory however. He would not recognize acquaintances years after meeting them because their faces and expressions had changed as they aged—he had simply remembered their earlier images too clearly, it seemed. He was also tormented with the amount of details he retained, and as a result spent his later years in daydreams and reveries, as his vivid memories clouded over new experiences.

This all implies the use of a subtle conscious sorting process. When we consider computer memory, for example, data is not being recorded onto silicon. Silicon is acting as a *conductor* for the arrangements of 0s and 1s. These assembled messages are magnetically recorded onto a hard drive tape or disk. If we were to remove that hard drive from the computer and look at it, we will not see any data. We might see a tiny round disk inside of the drive case—like a miniature CD. If we pulled out the disk from the case and looked at it, we still would not see any information. This is because the information is magnetically stored onto the surface of the disk. Hard drive disks are coated with a metal alloy like iron oxide or cobalt alloy. The surface is divided into tiny magnetic regions, each separated to enable a polarizing of the molecules on the surface of the disk. A single polar magnetized molecule contains no information in itself. Nor is the information contained on the magnetic reader. The combinations of polarity contain the message, which are meaningless until they are compiled and converted by the software. These on or off *permutations* must first be arranged into a sequence code into machine code by a translation program in the CPU. This code is then translated into operating system instructions that feed information back to the operator via the monitor.

In the same way, although the physical anatomy of brain gyrus, neurons and the various organs of the limbic system appear to contain the information and memory that resonates through them, they are no more containing our memories than the metal computer box contains any data. Informational waveforms resonate *through* the neurons, where they are crystallized, translated and broadcast into the neural net: It is the translation of the waveform interference patterns that creates the information.

Where is the Mind?

Western science has been struggling with the location of the mind for thousands of years. The Greek physician Galen of Pergamon (129-210 BC) struggled with the then-accepted *cardiocentric theory*—which proposed that the seat of the mind is in the heart. Galen produced a number of anatomical experiments with vivisection, illustrating the difference between the central nervous system and the arterial system. Despite some intense debate among the Stoics and others following Galen's experiments, there was increasing acceptance that the central nervous system played an integral role in the mind's processes. Yet from these ancient times to the modern day, researchers are still speculating and debating on the precise location of the mind.

The planarian worm *(Dugesia dorotocephala)* was Dr. James McConnell's favorite lab subject for his learning and conditioning studies begun in 1955. In one test, Dr. McConnell subjected a group of planaria to bright light followed by a mild electric shock. The shock would make the worms curl up in pain. This light-and-shock sequence was repeated hundreds of times for reinforcement. Eventually the worms would immediately curl up once the light was turned on, with or without a shock. This illustrated not only the worms' conscious attempts to avoid pain (a concept avoided by science), but also their ability to remember the circumstances surrounding the pain. Where were these memories stored?

The planaria worm has a tiny brain and central nervous system, just as most humans and animals have. However, these worms have an incredible ability to reproduce immediately upon being cut or sliced. This is commonly referred to as *regeneration.* Not all sliced worms regenerate on both ends. Most will at least regenerate at the tail end. Many amphibians also have this ability—they will typically regenerate a limb following its amputation. The planarian worm however, can be cut in half and each half will develop into a physically complete organism. This is thought to occur through a regeneration of the head on the tail side of the split. Each side then will develop a full body, tail and head.

In order to test for the location of memory, Dr. McConnell sliced the planarians into two pieces, in the middle of the body, between the head and tail. Assuming memory was stored in the head end where the central nervous system is, the head side regeneration should remember the light-shock training and curl up, while the tail-sided regeneration would not remember the shock treatment.

Not so fast. Contrary to this assumption, both regenerated worm halves remembered the training, and in many cases the tail-generated worms remembered the training better than the brain-side worm did. This research theoretically indicated that memory was not necessarily stored in the brain (McConnell *et al.* 1960).

This research underscores some of the studies referenced earlier, showing continuing memory and cognition despite partial brain removal or damage to loci known for particular functions. In Mishkin (1978) and Mumby *et al.* (1992), for example, surgical removal of the amygdala and hippocampus resulted either in minor memory impairment or none at all. Vargha-Khadem and Polkey (1992) reviewed multiple studies of hemidecortication—the removal of at least half of the brain. Full cognitive recovery following hemidecortication resulted in more than 80% of all subjects.

Magnetic imaging of human patients following brain damage have confirmed the movement of mental functions from one part of the brain to the other. This has resulted in the theory of brain plasticity, as discussed earlier. It is not difficult to logically conclude that if mental function moves from one part of the brain to another, the mind must have a composition separate from the brain tissues. Truly, this composition has continued to baffle researchers. Imaging can locate electromagnetic activity indicating cognition, memory and decision-making—the executive activities—within the brain. Electromagnetic activity may also indicate active regions and pathways during particular thought activity. Yet the precise location and composition of the mind and memory has remained mysterious.

We should consider also that the brain is not restricted to the gray matter within the skull. This region of the brain is composed of the right and left hemispheres of the *cerebrum*, the *cerebellum*, and the *brain stem*—composed of the *midbrain*, the *pons* and *medulla*. Also included in the brain is the *spinal column* and *spinal nerves*. It would thus be more accurate to describe the "brain" as the *central nervous system* or the *neural network,* which expands to the *peripheral nervous system* located throughout the body. The spinal column and spinal nerve system serve as a bridge between the lower activity centers (or *chakras*) and the higher and more subtle waveform translation centers of the brain. From the spinal column radiates various waveforms that stimulate organ activity. These direct pathways from the spine drive the autonomic systems and the programmed response centers throughout the central nervous system.

The virtual link between the senses, the brain and the mind lies hidden within the waveform interference patterns guided by the self through the limbic system and imaging cortices. The inner self's executive processes are generated through the prefrontal cortex and translated through the thalamus, hypothalamus and hippocampal complex to their respective loci. These areas are considered the interbrain. Using a network of subtle and gross conduits, they negotiate the information between the senses and the subtle mind. They also bridge the feedback of the mind's instructions and the initiation of brain and motor function. For this reason, many physicians attribute the amygdala as being the seat of emotion, although removal of it does not prevent emotion to be exhibited. Why is this? This is because emotion arises from the unseen inner self. The limbic system provides an insertion point for emotions to guide and steer the processes of prioritization. However, a surgeon still would not find any emotion within a surgically removed limbic organ.

The neural network is a system of interconnected neurons. Connecting different parts of the anatomy are nerve tracts. Nerve tracts are armored passageways that protect neurons and accelerate wave transmissions. These tracts might be compared to a household network of wire conduits protecting the wires and circuitry. When electricity must travel through underground wires, heavy-duty conduit piping will be used as shielding. These pipe tubes protect the wires from the decomposing elements of the soil. It also protects the local environment from electricity running through the wiring. Nerve tracts serve similar purposes within the body. They provide the sheathing allowing pulsed waveforms to channel throughout the body and interact with multiple waveforms moving via nerves, ion channels and other messenger systems. As they interact, informational messages are created in the form of interference patterns.

Some of the nerve cells among the CNS are specific to particular types of waveforms. Sensory nerves function altogether differently from motor nerves, for example. However, many CNS nerve tracts contain both sensory and motor fibers. A motor nerve radiates nerve impulses from the CNS out to the muscle and organ tissue cells. These motor nerves stimulate specific activity—thus they transmit specific instructional waveforms. Sensory nerves typically transmit in the other direction, carrying information waves from the various organs, tissues and sense organs into the CNS for processing.

The intentional reflections of the self are translated through the mind into physiological instructions. Once translated, they will stimulate both the motor cortex and the thalamus and hypothalamus. The thalamus regulates or adjusts thermogenesis, which controls the body's heat levels, providing a foundation for metabolic activity. Meanwhile the hypothalamus negotiates the sympathetic and parasympathetic activities of the body's autonomic system through the stimulation of the pituitary gland. Via the hypothalamus, the mind dictates control to regulate the functions of the body's metabolic activities through the pathways of the endocrine system. Through the vehicle of the motor cortex, the mind stimulates physical activity. We can thus conclude from these basic physiological cascades—confirmed by many years of research—that the physical interface or conduit between the mind and the physical body is located in the limbic system. This might be compared to the magnetic heads that 'read' the polarity states recorded onto a computer's hard disks.

This cascade of messengers is also regulated by the activities of the pineal gland, which coordinate with the rhythmic SCN cells to secrete melatonin. Melatonin triggers a cascading pathway to slow metabolism, leading to sleep and cell repair. Melatonin levels are balanced by other metabolic messengers stimulated through other command cascades. Examples of these are cortisol and the thyroid hormones.

All of these physical components of the brain and messenger systems are within the perimeter of the mind. The brain is a physical transfer and conversion mechanism. The mind is a holographic echoing mechanism utilizing interference patterns and standing waveforms. The mind sorts and governs, resonating with specific neurons to convert memories and data from waveform interference. The mind is a screening device spread throughout the nervous system, yet centralized amongst the *chakras*. The mind translates the feedback from these central points, and outputs the echoed intentions arising from the intentional self. The mind is quite simply the operating system software and programming utility utilized by the self. The brain is the physical utility used by the mind to translate the code into physical activity and memory.

Dr. Jim Tucker, a professor at the University of Virginia, compares the mind's relationship with the brain and body to a television set (2005). Dr. Tucker explains that while the TV signal is translated through the television set, the signal of television programming originates from a remote location. In the same way, Dr. Tucker explains, the mind is not the brain, but rather, he insists, the signals of the mind are transmitted through the brain.

The neurological research headed up by Dr. Robert Knight illustrated that brainwaves allowed different regions of the brain to appear to communicate using combinations of alpha, beta, gamma and theta waves. According to the research, the synchronization or *coupling* effect of these various waves—together with their timing and frequency—transmit specific information. We can certainly compare the television and television programs, —or the computer and computer software—to the brain and the mind. However, the transfer of the information occurs in precisely the same fashion in all of these cases: Through waveform interference pattern transmission.

As they harmonize with the intentional direction of the self, coherent interference patterns are created: These are *thoughts*. As the mapping system converts instructions from the self through the mind, they are connected indirectly to the rest of the body through the various neurochemical messengers and associated waveform biocommunications. In combination, the mix of neurochemical messengers such as hormones and neurotransmitters provide a feedback and response system, keeping the mindscreen in touch with the rest of the body. For example, nerve pathways from our right arm, elbow, and wrist will travel through the CNS to the upper left hemisphere of the cerebellum—in an area usually referred to as the primary motor region. Meanwhile the sensations from the fingers of our right hand will be received by a lower left side of this region. Our right ankle will travel to an area of the brain further up the left side of this motor area, nearest to the *sagittal sutures*—the division between the hemispheres. The pathways for these messages exist through channels of nerve cells bridged by neurotransmitter fluids, microtubules and ion channels, which accelerate complex messages from the body's remote areas. As the various cranial nerves connect these different brain regions to particular parts of the body, the brain wave channels resonate with certain nerve-ending receptors to facilitate the passage of feedback and response messages. This is comparable to a two-way radio antenna receiving and sending broadcast messages.

This coupling of waveform interference may provide a foundation for an adequate explanation for psi. Parapsychologists such as Dr. Stanley Krippner, and Dr. Michael Persinger have established a magnetic field link with extrasensory perception and dreaming after demonstrating that biomagnetic field changes from solar storms and electrical storms interrupt extrasensory perception. Here telepathics were able to better influence the dreaming of nearby and remote sleepers with geographic visualizations during decreased solar storm activity (Persinger and Krippner, 1989). Both Dr. Persinger and Dr. Krippner independently and with others repeatedly demonstrated geomagnetic effects in dream and psi studies. This indicates the waveform nature of thoughts and dreams—and the similarity between the composition of thoughts and geomagnetic fields.

We find a similar channeling and messaging system with sense perception: Each sensory organ or sensory area of the body will be stimulated by waveform inputs from our environment. These sensations are translated into pulsed waveforms, which conduct through nerve pathways, accelerated by particular neurotransmitters and ion channels toward particular areas of the brain. Upon reaching these brain regions, the sensory pulses are translated into brainwaves, which collide and interact with the various other brainwaves bouncing through the CNS. Coherent interaction among these brainwaves provides a projection observable by the self.

As to the geomagnetic influence upon the brain, mind and thoughts, Dr. Persinger (1989) was able to demonstrate that the earth's geomagnetic condition affected temporal lobe activity. Further investigations have demonstrated that geomagnetic activity also affected melatonin release from the pineal gland. This illustrates that there is a resonance—or harmonic effect—between the external waveforms surrounding our bodies and those waveforms generated through self-direction. The interference patterns created by magnetic and sensory inputs coalesce to influence the mind's imaging systems—ultimately influencing the self's decisions.

The complex exchange of instantaneous waveform pulses moving through the body is nothing short of astounding. Some estimate that over six trillion waveform messages per minute are fired through the nervous system alone—not including the higher frequency microtubule pulses, the various hormonal messaging broadcasts, the intercellular biocommunication and the intracellular network. These waveforms pulsing through the physical layers are all sorted for priority and projected through the mind to be imaged by the self.

Research has illustrated that the left side of the brain is associated with the thoughts relating to logic, language, and mathematics. Meanwhile the right side of the brain has been associated with art, fantasy, and music. Further to this point of specialization, certain regions appear to associate with certain mental skills and particular types of memories. Auditory communication, for example, is associated with the temporal lobe, while written motor skills have been linked with the motor cortex of the frontal lobe. Visual interaction usually utilizes the occipital lobe. Recent neurological research has confirmed that each of these brain functions also run concurrent with particular types of brainwaves. We also know a hierarchy of waveforms is slated to each thought-type. The slower waves like delta and theta tend to accompany sleep and introspection, while faster waves like beta and gamma waves tend to accompany sensual cognition and information transfer.

Without consciousness, organic matter will not develop, grow, or reproduce. Organic matter does not exhibit emotion or mental programming without consciousness being involved. Once consciousness leaves an organism, the body will no longer exhibit growth, fear, emotion, or any type of optional responsiveness.

The hard drive of the mind's memory web has both a subjective and selective tendency. We can see this should we gather various opinions from people. While a group of people may receive the same information through the senses, a variety of perceptions and conclusions will be made by each. Even though the mind may meticulously gather and web together its incoming information, the unique self can shape and prioritize this information through intention.

We know from various research and practical experience that the mind tends to select and choose information as it is being organized and prepared for storage. Research illustrates that the visual cortex will shape and direct spatial visual information as it is being gathered through signaling mechanisms. This process has been termed *retino-cortical mapping* (Johnston 1986).

The entire process of the brain and central nervous system would be impossible without an operator and a power supply driving the sorting operations of the mind. At the end of the day, the self is the operator. The mind is the software and the brain is the CPU. The body is the hardware.

The 'Subconscious' Self

The theories and concepts as proposed by Dr. Janet and Dr. Freud not much more than a century ago included the notion of a subconscious mind. The basis for their conclusions was the use of hypnosis. Under hypnosis, their patients demonstrated an awareness of past behavior and information seemingly unavailable to their conscious minds during their normal awakened states. Like Dr. Stevenson's research over the past few decades, their hypnosis research also demonstrated the possibility of past lives, which they considered unexplainable.

Because our conscious minds appear not to be aware of the subtle memories and programming mechanisms utilized by the mind, the concept of a subconscious mind appeared to adequately explain these phenomena. We must question this assumption, however. What is this mysterious subconsciousness? Why can a person who is brought under trance—which is simply a state of suggestion and trust—suddenly be able to recall things that are not otherwise recalled? How does the programming of the mind otherwise operate beneath the awareness of the conscious mind? Furthermore, what is dreaming? How can these be otherwise explained without the theory of the subconscious mind?

The empirical understanding of the existence of the inner self adequately explains this theoretical subconsciousness seamlessly. It is precisely the positioning of the inner self—the operator—within the body that creates the ability of the mind to submit to the suggestion of hypnosis. The self simply makes a determination to submit to suggestion, and the body and mind follow.

It is the partial shielding or cloaking of the inner self by the veil of misidentification that is responsible for the mysterious nature of the inner self. Furthermore, it is the permanence of the inner self throughout the changing physical body that allows one to be able to recall previous lives under hypnosis.

The relationship between visual pictures, imagination and memory can also be explained within the context of the inner self as the intentional viewer. The mind's holographic pictures are constructed by the combination of the retinal cells, the optic nerve, the LGM, and the visual cortex. We might refer to this as an intentional process called *focus.* Through conscious intent, the self can also stimulate the mind to construct internal pictures. We can aptly refer to this as *imagination.* Through a combination of focus and imagination, intentional pictures are constructed within the mind.

When attached to an intentional picture or image, incoming information can be sorted and stored onto to the neural net. When we connect information with images—including any sensual input such as sound or touch—we are effectively multiplying the number of references within that data. We might compare this with how many search engine spiders prioritize web pages. The spiders will travel the net and tabulate the various cross referencing of websites—and to some extent ranking by intra-website referrals This is because the self tells the mind to prioritize by interest: The more intentional screenings, the higher its priority ranking.

As a result, our retrievable memories of the past are usually connected to events we observed visually, through imagination, or through biofeedback information. We would adequately term these sense perceptions as *impressions.* By capturing focused sounds, smells, touch, or visual impressions on a focused basis, we are effectively increasing the number of impressions that data are attached to.

An example of this attachment between focused impression and raw data is how a song will reconnect us back to a precise time and place of our historical past. Because the song became connected to our intention during this time in our lives, the song will stimulate the recall of vivid memories of those times—sometimes even details otherwise long forgotten.

This can work with pictures just as well. We may see a particular picture and be reminded of the time, place and details surrounding the moment when that picture was taken. The images in the picture stimulated the retrieval of the memories just as the song did.

Why does the memory work better when connected to mental impressions? What is it about a picture, song, or funny story that enables us to retrieve vivid memories?

As we examine the research of dementia and memory loss, we see a substantial amount of evidence connecting the loss of memory with the loss of function among particular regions of the brain or nerve cells. As we have discussed, we have also observed these same regions involved in a constant exchange and echoing of waveform signals during memory storage and recall. A lighting-fast interactive mirroring system allows different regions to check and crosscheck information. This crosschecking allows our minds to validate, confirm, and store information. It also increases the number of impressions the connected data has logged. As the information waves interfere, they form a unique webbing of interactivity, much as if we were to throw several stones into a small pond. Assuming each wave contains unique information and a specific history, the crossing and interaction of multiple waves creates a rich multi-layered view of the history of the stone throws. This is analogous to how a television screen converts various colors, forms, and sounds onto the viewing screen and speakers to image the original broadcast. As information is broadcast into the antenna or cable input, it is also flashed upon the screen.

In a beautiful symphony of homuncular holography, humans have invented and assembled televisions, computers and programs to precisely reflect the functionality of our own human mental programming and web. This simply confirms that our mental and physical programming stems from an intention self. Computers and televisions are simply reflections of our own mental-physical systems.

The use of television and computers are strictly intentional. In the same way, the source of the intentional ability to save and retrieve particular memories is a function of a living, conscious being. We could entertain a programming feature allowing every input to be equally prioritized and accessed. A driving force of intention is still required. We cannot train a dead rat to do tricks. Neither can we expect a dead human to remember names by shouting those names into the ears of the dead body. All the brain regions and brain cells may still be intact in a newly deceased dead body. Yet there is no mind web because there is no intention, and there is no priority or organization of the remaining waveforms because the self has left.

Outside the physical issues and the back-and-forth process of checking and crosschecking between the mind and the neural network lies the conscious intent of the self driving the process of the mind's information processing software. The self ultimately drives the *extent* of the memory saved and retrieved. In other words, while we can typically remember many interesting things about our life and retrieve them quite easily without much effort, we have to make a conscious effort to remember details that are less important to us. If we want to remember details taught in a science class for example, we have to make a concerted effort to repeatedly focus on the information in order to retain it and repeat it later. Simply listening to the lecture and hearing the information once typically does not allow the attachment and recall of massive amounts of unimportant details onto the mind's memory web. We might want good grades, but we may not be interested in the information itself. We do not have any emotional attachment to it. We will have to listen to it, read about it, write it down and then maybe read about it again in hopes that we will somehow connect enough emotion to the information to remember it. If we are able to utilize some of the methods mentioned above—relating the details to unique pictures and funny stories—our ability to remember these details will be better. The remembrance is occurring because the self is connecting emotional intention to the information.

For this same reason, we tend to better remember details about the things that interest us the most. For example, we often see men and boys able to remember the batting averages of their favorite baseball players yet unable to remember the latest economic statistics—even though they saw both on the same television news show. Here the details of intended hobbies and personal missions are placed in a higher priority. We have focused greater intention upon them. As our minds check and crosscheck information—as research indicates is occurring during sleep—the focus is on the areas synchronizing with the intentions of the self.

This is illustrated by a study published in 2005 (Lindstrom *et al.*) concluding that a positive relationship existed between acquiring later-in-life Alzheimer's disease and increased television viewing among middle-aged adults. 135 elderly Alzheimer's cases and 331 healthy (control) subjects were interviewed and classified for television viewing duration during their mid-life years. The results found for each hour per day of mid-life television viewing, Alzheimer's occurrence increased 1.3 times. Conversely, intellectually stimulating activities and social activities were associated with lower Alzheimer's rates. The study's authors concluded that social engagement with others somehow better utilized the neurons at risk of dementia-related disorders.

While watching television, the self's focus becomes increasingly tied to the virtual illusions of the tele-scripted drama, as opposed to the variegated living world around us. These adults presumably reach for their escape from the world by watching television because they prefer to *un-focus* their attention on the living world. (This assumes fictional dramas, not news and documentary programs reflecting reality.) Perhaps the living world provides too many problems or difficulties to solve. Conversely, social activities engage the self's attention onto the real lives and problems of the world. This requires further emotional involvement from the self. Life requires us to prioritize the mass of incoming information. This stresses the neural mechanisms—keeping them better exercised. The real world also stimulates the self to utilize the tools of the mind to solve the problems of the physical world. The research has indeed confirmed that mental exercise creates better cognition and a more resilient memory.

In the case of television watchers, the self's lack of focus and work on real world problems leads to a slow degeneration of biocommunication pathways. Like unused muscles, the neurons are under-utilized. They receive less circulation, less detoxification, less interaction and less activity. This all leads to the slow degeneration of those cells, opening them up to accumulating ameloid beta plaque or a myriad of stifling developments. In the overall picture, however, it is the propensity of the inner self to escape from reality that under-utilizes the brain's biocommunication equipment. Does this mean the self wills or intends the Alzheimer's scenario? Not directly, but just as a sedentary lifestyle perpetuates an inability to adequately move and exercise, the propensity to escape certain physical realities perpetuates an inability to utilize regions of the brain that focus on physical realities.

It has long been held by sleep researchers who have measured the brain's electrical activity during sleep that the higher electrical activity from individual brain neurons indicated the neurons were reassembling and sorting the information received during the day. The neurons were theoretically processing this information into long-term memory. This is referred to as *consolidation.* This theory however has recently been challenged by memory researchers who have noticed the limbic system and interference processes appear to be the focal point of the higher electrical activity. As Dr. John Wixted, professor of Psychology at the University of California at San Diego proposed in 2005, the evidence seems to point to interference mechanics created by activities such as sleep. The process of sleep apparently provokes priorities or images that interfere with the consolidation process of memories. We would contend this is caused by those initial memories not being well-enough synchronized by and to the intentions of the self. For this reason, not all the recent memory is eliminated during sleep. The memories considered more critical to the self are retained. Otherwise, how could we remember those things we consider dear (beyond a day) and forget the other details?

Where do the memory waveform interference patterns go as intention distances them—lowering their relative priority? Where do the waveforms not imaged by the mind go? Do they still exist somewhere? Are they hiding within this subconscious mind?

We contend first, that there is no such thing as a subconscious mind. The conscious mind is a mapping and screening mechanism driven by the self. It is conscious because it is driven by consciousness. The self, however, is of another nature: The self is *composed of* consciousness. Waveform interference patterns continue to exist in the larger realm of consciousness. However, the bridle of misidentification confines the self to those interference patterns intentionally collected and translated by the limbic system, and projected by the mind. The brain and mind are simply tools for intention. This might be comparable to a person going to a lecture and choosing to write down notes on the lecture, even though the person could certainly just listen to the lecture and remember the interesting parts of the lecture. The uninteresting data will likely remain outside the memory web because the self is not interested in it.

This also means that the mind mechanism is limited by and focused onto the intentions of the self. Therefore, the mind will sometimes alter or ignore inputs that do not fit with the intentions of the self. As a result, the self will not want to maintain a memory that might conflict with its attempts to enjoy the physical world. Most traumas are erased from the "conscious" awareness of the mind simply because the self does not want to face those painful experiences. However, if the inner self does not learn and grow from the experience, the self cannot release its focus upon the trauma. As a result, the waveform interference patterns of the trauma event continue to be linked to the emotions of the self—which forces the memory to be retained and linked to those emotions. Linked with these emotions, the memory is prioritized near the top of the standing wave hierarchy, forcing the self to continue to face that memory until it is resolved.

It is only when the trauma has been resolved by the self that the emotion can be removed from the memory. When the emotional link is removed from the memory, it becomes a worthless detail to the self, and the mind eventually consolidates it and reprioritizes it downward. Over time, the reprioritization routine of the mind's programming releases the details and the memory is gradually downgraded within the memory net.

The question becomes; how does the self resolve the trauma? This is accomplished through growth and learning. The self must determine why the event happened. The self must forgive the person who we might be holding responsible. The self must come to an understanding regarding the event and the people involved. The self must learn from the event what was supposed to be learned. As soon as this takes place, the self can detach from the event and move on. This is often communicated by the expression: *"What do I need to learn from this experience?"* If we do not know, we will probably continue to hold onto it.

Reprioritization or consolidation does not eliminate the event. It still exists in waveform interference pattern form. However, ones mental memory of an event is inseparable from intent. As long as there is intent to remember it—or an emotion connected to it—the waveform will be accessible. This might be compared again to the internet. While so many websites might be out there—some even communicating hatred or violence—we choose to only surf the websites we are interested in. We will ignore those others, and even though they may still be there and possibly even accessible, the web surfer will probably not even be aware of their existence.

Although the mind and its programming are set up based upon the intentions of the self, the mind is still different from the self. The mind has its own design, and sometimes the mind can get out of control of the self. As the mind develops its programming, it can take us to places that ultimately we do not want to be. It can be carried away with the directives we have given it. The main directive the self gives the mind is to figure out ways to achieve physical pleasure. The mind begins to concoct various scenarios for physical enjoyment. Sometimes these scenarios will cross the line of decency or morality. The self is clearly aware of these lines. However, the mind will also produce—should the self be open to them—various justifications for the activity to appeal to the morality of the self. We will then be faced with a moral decision on whether to do something or not. As this decision is being made, the mind will continue to throw justifications for the activity on the screen for the self to review. Here is where the evolution of the self becomes critical. Should the self's level of growth be such that we do not understand the consequences of an activity, or should the self's growth not be tempered with the intelligence that physical pleasure will not deliver fulfillment, then the prospect of physical enjoyment may outweigh the consequences of the activity.

Many times nature designs consequences that force a choice between our own pleasure and our relationships. This forces us to consider whether our own pleasure is more important to us than our relationships with others. This conflict between the self's desire for pleasure and the desire to unselfishly love is a constant struggle for the self.

Addiction

In 1950, the American Medical Association officially deemed addiction a disease. It certainly has symptoms and degenerative qualities consistent with a disease. The only problem is that there is no known mechanism of pathology, and no known cure. There is a lot of speculation about how genes play a role in addiction, but still there is no cure: At least none coming from western medical science.

Addiction has been part of human civilization for thousands of years. Today there are dozens of substances considered addictive, including tobacco, caffeine, alcohol, drugs, food, gambling, sex, shopping, and even a new seeming addiction stemming from internet use called *impulse-control disorder*. We propose that the list of addictions covers anything perceived through mental concoction as potentially pleasurable.

This covers a huge territory of activities and substances. Shopping, for example, would include purchasing anything. Food would include eating anything—although some might contend that badly tasting food would probably not be addictive. Still, taste if subjective. Anything that stimulates a feedback response through the limbic system—through the hypothalamus, amygdale, nucleus accumbens and/or prefrontal cortex—has the potential of becoming addictive.

This definition may run contrary to the additive substance's assumed definition of an activity *"having negative consequences and difficult to stop despite the negative consequences."* Under this definition, something healthy would not be considered addictive because there are no negative consequences.

This is a very subjective definition, because what might be considered "healthy" for one person might not be considered healthy for another. A person might become so addicted to a "healthy" substance to the degree that the substance becomes unhealthy due to its over-consumption. Why would the diagnosis change once the substance went over the tipping point if the behavior was the same?

We can give two immediate examples of this: wine and coffee. Research has determined that both wine and coffee contain particular antioxidants like reservatrol in wine and polyphenols in coffee. This of course has fueled those addicted to these substances to justify their intake. Does the apparent healthiness of these constituents make these substances non-addictive? The announcements by health researchers have emphasized words like "in moderation" when describing consumption of these two beverages. Does this mean they are not addictive when only consumed "in moderation?" This begs the question of how a person becomes addicted. Do they not become addicted by beginning to consume these substances "in moderation?" Certainly, we can agree that almost anything, even substances considered "healthy" when consumed in moderation, could potentially be addictive.

Treatment history indicates a fundamental problem with the definition and treatment of this disorder altogether. Over the past 70 years the best of addiction treatments—including behavioral reconditioning and various drug treatments—have only led to about 20% success. This is far less than the placebo effect of 33%. There is thus a good case for saying addiction treatment has been completely unsuccessful.

We can hardly make a solid case for addiction being a physical disorder if the symptoms and behavior covers almost anything we might do, and practically no treatments have been found effective. Perhaps we should revisit the concept of addiction in its entirety. Perhaps it is not a physical disease at all.

When we consider the physiology of addiction, medical technology has observed that the sense of pleasure appears to be related to the release and blocking of the reuptake of the neurotransmitter dopamine between neurons. In most pleasure sensations, GABA and other inhibitory neurotransmitters work conjunctively with the release of dopamine to guide and control the process, rendering a neurotransmitter balance. These guidance neurochemicals work in much the same way that guidance waves operate. They ameliorate the process to prevent a chaotic or uncontrollable situation. This guidance allows the self to maintain some control (or at least influence) over the process. However, should GABA and/or other guiding neurochemicals be blocked, the process may become misguided, and the ability of the self to control the process becomes impaired.

Some of the more addictive substances such as cocaine, alcohol and other drugs block GABA and other guidance neurochemicals because their chemistry turns off the reuptake process. They in effect block the reuptake receptors, preventing the excess dopamine from being dampened or reduced. This excessive dopamine heightens the pleasure response further, which is launched upon the mental screen for the self to observe. This echoing of increased physical pleasure biochemicals further addicts the person to that substance, because the self has programmed the mind with the intention to enjoy, and the feedback of biochemical messengers snares the self into believing that fulfillment will be forthcoming.

Does this mean that we are slaves to the biochemistry of substances? Does this mean that once we take enough of an addictive substance we are lost to the snare of addiction? Certainly not. Simple observation tells us that not everyone becomes addicted to addictive substances, even if they experiment with them to the extent (or greater) that an addict of that substance consumes. One person might experiment heavily with drugs and not become addicted. Another might try once or twice and become completely addicted for many years to come. What is going on here? Do they have different physiologies? Different genes perhaps?

Blood tests and brain scans do not reveal any anatomical or biochemical differences between addicted persons and non-addictive persons. Although gene sequences have been found that suggest a genetic link in alcoholism, there are still large numbers with these same genetic sequences who did not succumb to alcoholism. Additionally we find other large populations without any of these sequences who have succumbed to alcoholism.

To these points, some geneticists propose that those with the alcoholic sequence who did not become alcoholic somehow overcame their genetic disposition. To this, we would simply ask: *who overcame what?* If the supposition is that we are our body and its genetic sequences, then there would be *no one around* to overcome the genes. Like machines, we would follow the codes in our genes. The genetic sequence would result in alcoholism without significant variance. If however, geneticists are proposing that there is somehow a choice in overcoming our body's genetic sequencing, then this introduces a conscious person with the ability to overcome the genetic sequences. This obviously implies the existence of an inner self.

Regarding the genetic sequences and the propensity for the genes to match the alcoholism, we also offer the point that drinking and drug use has been shown to be a learned experience. In societies or families where drinking is not prevalent, we find far less alcoholism, even when there is plenty of alcohol availability. On the other hand, in families where drinking is common, and alcoholism is an accepted reality, the incidence of drinking problems is notably increased. We can see this among cultures as well: Cultures with more casual drinking have more alcoholics.

When we expand these points into the grander field of addiction to any number of activities or substances, we propose that *every one of us has addictive tendencies.* Every one of us seeks pleasure. Thus, any of us could become addicted to any seemingly pleasurable activity or substance.

We must only look at our own lives and tell ourselves truthfully whether we cannot find some activity—"healthy" or not—that we have become attached to doing at one time or another. Furthermore, would these activities not have some possible negative consequences should the consumption or activity become excessive? Should we assume that just about everything done in excess at some point could have a negative consequence, we could easily make a case that each of us has an *addictive personality*. This is simply because the inner self is pleasure seeking by nature.

The answer to this puzzle points to the evidence provided in this book: Each of us has an identity—a transcendental self—separate from the physical body. We are in effect the drivers of this body just as we might drive a car:

Say a man gets into his car to drive across town. The man did not eat that day so he is hungry. Instead of getting something to eat, the man presumes that if his car is full of gas he will also feel full, and will no longer feel hungry. The man goes to the gas station and fills his tank with gas. He drives away from the gas station still feeling hungry.

The man's hunger drives the man to fill up with something. However, because the man is misidentifying with the car, the man is seeking the wrong solution. The man is trying to fill up the wrong thing.

In the case of the addiction, the unfulfilled self is perpetually seeking fulfillment. The self's fulfillment however, comes from a deeper level of existence. When we confuse the self with the body, we erroneously seek fulfillment from elements that cannot fulfill us.

Addiction is simply a refusal to believe a particular physical element will not fulfill us. The programming of the mind assumes that because the body feels good, the self will be satisfied. When we consume the item or have the activity, we are surprised to find we still are not satisfied. That unsatisfaction loops back to the mind's programmed concoction, and assumes we simply need more: *We must not have had enough. Or we must not have done it long enough.*

The programmed concoctions of the mind attaches us to those objects of addiction, with the perpetual idea that the *next time we do them, we will become fulfilled.* This *next time* concoction of the mind's program, combined with the self's innate quest for pleasure, snares one into consistent addictive behavior.

The question we may ask is how one can break the cycle of addictive behavior. The answer is simple: through intelligence. A person simply must realize that the addictive behavior has negative consequences. This is the product of *learning.*

It is a rather simple equation, yet within it lies a more complex lesson. This bears the question of identity and fulfillment. If we assume that our identity is simply this temporary, physical body, then we are trapped within the perpetual search for what *physical thing* will satisfy us. As many of us have experienced, we will try one *thing* after another. With each trial, we will find it unfulfilling, and move to the next *thing.* Maybe food will do it. Maybe a new car will do it. Maybe a new dress or suit will do it. None of these will do it. How about sex? Maybe sex will do it. Or maybe some drugs will do it. How about winning a bet? How about becoming famous? No?

Scientifically, we know none of these *things* bring us fulfillment. How do we know this? Simply by observing that those who have had an abundance of these things have remained unfulfilled.

What do we come away from this learning experience? What do we conclude? (We can also watch and learn from others. We do not have to personally try everything ourselves to learn this.) For some, the conclusion might be that life is simply random and by some quirk, even though we are physical, we cannot for some reason become fulfilled, and life is still meaningless. For others, however, there may be another lesson. Certainly when intelligence combines the lessons with the science, as we have laid out here, a more logical conclusion is rendered: We are spiritual beings in essence—not physical—and fulfillment comes from the activities of that dimension.

Surely most of us can reflect that some of the most fulfilling times of our lives have come during the exchange of love with others. When we deeply care about others, we feel something deeper. We feel a surge of emotion when we feel love for others. For this reason we are drawn to the loving relationships with our families and even the service of others outside our family. Giving of our selves selflessly—loving service—brings to us a deeper type of fulfillment that physical things do not deliver. This reveals the mystery regarding the nature of the inner self: We may be searching for pleasure, but pleasure is ultimately found when we selflessly and lovingly give of ourselves.

Chapter Eight

The Body of Pain

Most of us live our lives trying to avoid pain. Many even grade happiness on how little pain our bodies have. Here we have provided the evidence showing that the body is merely a temporary vehicle for an inner self. As a result, we can know that pain is also temporary. We also know by experience that we each feel pain virtually throughout our physical lives in different degrees. What is pain and how can we live with it?

On a strictly physical basis, pain is transmitted through the nervous system from nerve endings called *nociceptors*. Nociceptors are located around the body, amongst just about every tissue system and organ system. The nociceptor is a waveform receptor. It has a particular threshold of waveform reception, beyond which it stimulates a waveform response—an alarm of sorts—which travels through the nerve channels to the brain. The mind assembles a holographic map of the body using the various waveform inputs from the cortices and *chakras*. This holographic mapping indicates the location of the nociceptor alarm. The specifications of this alarm are reflected onto the mindscreen to be viewed by the inner self. Sometimes the reflection of the pain signal will not exactly locate the pain signal's precise origin—stimulating an approximation of the location. This is called *referred pain*.

Pain has many classifications. It can be acute, chronic, referred, inflammatory, or even phantom. Phantom pain occurs when the pain appears to be coming from a part of the body that was amputated or otherwise lost. This alone indicates a subtle, energetic messaging system going on here. Pain is not as simple as we would like it to be.

The Anatomy of Pain

There are several messages inherent within the design of pain. First and most obvious, pain is nature's way of telling us we need to solve a physical problem. We need to address something that has gone wrong in the body. The solution is most easily related to removing the cause. Sometimes, however, it is too late in the process. The damage has been done. Removing the cause may not remove the pain. This type of pain is caused by inflammation. The damage has stimulated a healing response, and the body is attempting to repair the damage by sending in blood, lymph, macrophages, neutrophils, plasmin and fibrin—likely a combination thereof. If the cause is removed, inflammatory pain will usually subside once the repair process has made substantial progress. Incidentally, nature can assist in this process of repair with inflammation-reducing herbs such as goldenseal, garlic, cayenne, ginseng, turmeric, guggul and others.

If the original cause is not removed, the inflammation may become chronic. Chronic inflammation is the cause of most degenerative and autoimmune disorders. The body is constantly trying to repair damage created by recurring agents. This might be toxic chemicals, poor dietary habits, or many other environmental inputs. As long as this input continues, the body's tissues will continue to be damaged. The inflammation and the pain associated with it will thus continue. It is really quite simple.

In some cases, chronic inflammation may be caused by an infectious agent. Here the infection is the cause. Since the immune system is unable to remove it, the damage it creates causes ongoing inflammation.

Then there is the natural degeneration of the body that comes with age. Degeneration from age can also cause inflammation, although it can be accelerated by poor inputs. As even a healthy body ages, inflammation may gradually outpace the body's ability to repair the damage. This kind of chronic pain is often the result of a lifetime of wear and tear. It is thus unavoidable to some degree. With good inputs of nutrition, water and a less toxic environment, we should be able to decrease the burden on our immune system, thus speeding up the repair process. This in turn aids the body's immune system, decreasing the frequency and intensity of inflammatory pain.

This said, we should get used to the fact that while we might be able to reduce the frequency and intensity of inflammation with exercise and good inputs, despite all our attempts, pain will be unavoidable. Just as a car is built with gauges that feed back oil, gas and heat levels, the body is designed to feed back pain sensations. Like the gauges, pain provides a clear indication on the condition of the body. It also indicates the existence of the viewer of the pain: the inner self.

Dentists and anesthesiologists understand that there is a huge range of pain tolerance between people. Some people are very tolerant and can withstand lots of it. Boxers or rugby players, for example, can tolerate a lot more pain than the average person might. At the dentist's office, some people do not even need Novocain. Others want to be knocked out with nitrous oxide. Some people cannot tolerate even the faintest pain sensations. They exert great effort to avoid it. Others will approach life head on—colliding with painful experiences on their way towards accomplishing their goals. This variance in pain tolerance is because we all have relative degrees of *pain sensitivity* with our bodies.

Indeed, many cultures have varying acceptable notions of pain. Some cultures undertake such traditions as fire walking and body piercing. Other cultures pamper their bodies with air conditioning and hot baths;

whimpering with the slightest of temperature deviation. Soldiers have been known to endure extreme pain, while their rulers have been sensitive to the slightest of discomforts.

Around the world, we also can also see huge variances between tolerances for suffering among different societies. Some countries consider a small percentage of the population being homeless and cold as great suffering. Other societies deal with massive starvation, dehydration, and even mass genocide. Although none of these situations is acceptable in a world where some live in excess, it is easy to see a range of tolerance when it comes to human suffering around the world.

Why such a vast difference in tolerance to pain and suffering? If we were simply chemical machines, and pain was strictly a biological issue, the same amount of pain would affect each of us precisely the same. Yet this is not reality. Such a variance in pain sensitivity can only indicate that some of us—through training, conditioning or otherwise—feel more *connected* or *attached* to our body than do others.

This can be illustrated by measuring *physical consciousness* and pain tolerance together. It is widely accepted amongst anesthesiologists that the less conscious a person is, the less sensitive they will be to pain. This is why invasive surgical anesthesia will usually consist of knocking a person unconscious. Physical consciousness is the level of focus we might have upon our physical body at the time. We must be conscious of something in order to be connected or attached to it after all. This attachment to our body is thus the key element associated with pain sensitivity and tolerance.

If we accept that each of us is the inner self and not our physical body, then we must accept that the pain and suffering our body experiences is not actually happening to *me.* If the pain is not happening to the self, the only way we will dread it is through our misidentification and attachment to the body. In the same way, if we bought a new car we identified with; we would be more sensitive to any scratch or dent it might receive. By being more sensitive about the car, we are focusing more closely upon its value to us. This focus increases our attachment to the car. Now if we had an old banged up car and did not give it much attention, we would hardly be bothered if it got scratched or dented.

We can conclude that a greater focus upon our body (and our misidentification with it) leads to greater pain sensitivity.

The intentions we hold for the physical body are also key considerations for pain sensitivity. Our various plans and expectations to utilize our body to achieve future pleasure will naturally result in a greater concern about anything that might endanger those plans. For example, losing our eyesight would not be so conducive to our future expectations of enjoying visual sensations. In the same way, if we had plans to drive our car across the country, we would be very concerned about how it was running prior to the trip. Any potential engine problem will be met with increased focus and concern.

Physical pain by itself is merely a signal that our body may be in danger. We can respond to each pain as a signal and act upon it; or we can dwell on each an every painful throb, dreading the thought of the pain continuing into the future and endangering our plans for future physical enjoyment.

An example of the relativity of physical pain sensitivity is an athlete who will endure tremendous pain for the sake of winning a race. A competitive long distance runner, for example, will run hundreds of miles per week for many years for the sake of winning that one big race. During their training, the runner may bear upon the body an almost unbearable amount of pain: The kind of pain we could easily compare to being held within a torture chamber. Yet the runner, because he or she is attached to the goal rather than the body's comfort, will endure that pain as a mere byproduct of preparing for the contest. Their attachment to the body's comfort is thus minimized by the purpose of the training. They intend to win, or at least perform well in the race.

On the other hand, a competitive runner determined to avoid pain would not do so well in this race. As soon as any pain or discomfort arose, the runner will slow down or stop to avoid the pain. The winning runner accepts pain as part of the race and thus does not focus on it. The slower runner meanwhile is focused upon avoiding pain. This is due to the slower runner being more attached to the physical body and less attached to winning. The winner's body might feed back more pain signals, but these will not be the winner's focus. The winner's greater focus is upon winning the race—concocting that winning will bring fulfillment. The slower runner concocts that avoiding pain will bring more fulfillment.

Another example of the relative effect of pain is self-mutilation. Today there are millions of kids self-inflicting their bodies. They do this with razors, knives, pins and other painful tools. Surveys on self-mutilation reveal that kids do this in response to their feelings of frustration with the world around them. They feel empty and hopeless. Many describe having a feeling of numbness. Through self-mutilation, they say they hope to achieve a connection to reality. In reviewing many of these cases, researchers have discovered that kids do not feel much pain when they self-inflict. They are more focused on filling their emptiness than on their bodily pain at that moment. Proving this point, many of these same kids have stated that they *do* feel pain when involved in an accidental injury. When not focused on seeking fulfillment from self-mutilation, their typical pain-sensitivity returns.

Self-mutilation is surely an absurdity to most. For most of us, it is difficult to understand why someone would willingly inflict pain upon himself or herself. Some feel the same about athletes like long-distance runners, cyclists, rugby players, and boxers. Some would feel that these people are also a bit insane to allow such pain to be inflicted upon their bodies for the purpose of winning a couple of contests. Athletes and self-mutilators are not much different. They are both simply focused upon achieving particular objectives, which at the moment outweighs the importance of comfort. Their attachment to the intended result overrides the pain.

This detachment also explains how prisoners-of-war can tolerate extreme conditions of torture and survive. During their torture, they are forced to detach from the pain as they focus upon other objectives. As a result, prisoners often pray and become generally focused on their spirituality as they attempt to detach from their current physical circumstances.

We can see the relativity of pain sensitivity elsewhere in our lives. For example, the more attached we are to a particular event or person, the more something affecting that event or person might cause us pain, trauma or frustration. We can see this when people become wrapped up in sporting events—becoming attached to particular teams. In team attachment, a home team loss can significantly disappoint and upset those attached to the team's results. Now if we were not so attached to that team or sport, the loss would not affect us emotionally—even if we lived in the same team's hometown.

Becoming attached to another person can also become a source of pain as well. The more attached we become to that person, the more their death or breakup will cause us pain. The bottom line is that the level of pain we experience is relative to the amount of attachment we have for that person or event.

In the same way, pain is relative to our attachment to our body and the specific intentions we have for the body. Note that physical pain does not actually touch the inner self. Just as a car driver involved in a fender-bender can get out and walk away without a scratch, the inner self can disconnect from the physical body and its various pains and sufferings. This disconnection can be at least partially achieved through our attachment to goals that run contrary to the comfort of our bodies. It can also take place at death, when we are forcibly detached from our body. It can also be accomplished more completely through spiritual activities that bring us inner peace and understanding of a nature beyond the realm of the physical body. In other words, our connection with the pains of our physical body is relative to our attachment and intentions for our physical body. The greater our intentions are focused upon the higher purposes of life—such as spiritual growth—the less sensitive we will be to the various aches and pains of the physical body. We will still feel these pains, however. We cannot simply wish them away.

If we see each pain as lessons to be learned and as opportunities to evolve spiritually, we too will gradually become detached to the body and learn to rise above pain.

Pain Strategies

This does not mean we ignore pain. Again, pain is a purposeful signal that indicates a problem to fix (or a lesson to be learned). Certainly, our response to pain is best related to the type, location, and intensity of our pain. Some types of pain are more critical than others are, and should be responded to in kind. For example, pain and numbness in the left arm or around the heart should be considered more critical than a sore thumb. A few general types of pain and tips to deal with a painful experience:

As for transitory pain, if the pain comes and goes we should note the time, the duration of the painful experience, the location of the pain and the intensity of the pain. If it recurs, then we should make a list of (or think through) the things we have done differently over the past few days, hours or even years. Was there anything we might have done recently to cause this pain? Often the cause will not jump out at us immediately. If it continues, we should write down the time, location and intensity of the pain felt. This is called a *pain diary.* Each time we feel a pain, we can write it down into the diary. With each notation, we can explore the other events that took place around the pain. At some point, this process should help us isolate events or activities that lead to the pain. These events or activities may or may not reveal the direct cause, but they can help us or our health professional better understand possible causes for our pain. Regarding the diary pain intensity, typically intensity is rated from one to ten, with ten being the worst pain imaginable and one being hardly noticeable. Should we use this rating system in our notes, we will gradually be able to understand what activities help the pain and what activities aggravate the pain. By modifying our subsequent behavior, we can eliminate much if not all of this pain.

This process has been shown to be clinically effective for pain patients. Doctors can often make inaccurate assumptions about the causes of our pain. We know pain is often related to inflammation, and chronic inflammation is related to the burdening or weakening of our immune function, or a cause the immune system cannot seem to heal fast enough. Often these are caused by things we can change by changing our habits or lifestyle. Once we discover the cause of the pain, we can design effective strategies to remove the causes or otherwise reduce the pain.

Immediately upon sensing pain, our natural instinct is to rub the spot or move the injury. This is an appropriate response, and we can follow it as long as there is not an open wound or a broken bone involved. Rubbing a wound will increase circulation to the spot and close the feedback loop, which often immediately lessens the pain. This is referred to as *closing the pain gate.* The rubbing will transmit a mild waveform current through the tissues. It can also stimulate the production of endorphins and enkephalins—hormone-neurotransmitters noted for their ability to reduce pain sensitivity. If a smaller wound is open and bleeding, pressure can be applied to stop the bleeding. This will also stimulate a faster clotting reaction, stimulated by increased plasmin activation. The application of pressure can also close the pain gate.

Should our rubbing or pressure application not decrease the pain, then at least we will discover more about the injury. If it is hot, this indicates possibly inflammation due to an injury or infection. In these cases, natural thermal heat or circulation may not help, especially if the injury is swelling excessively. Here we can apply ice, a cold pack or a frozen bag of peas, beans or corn to slow down the inflammatory response. This will constrict the blood vessels and level out the process a bit. Often too much swelling can interrupt the healing process as the tissues become filled with stagnated, under-nourished blood. (Note: Medical attention should be sought for any wound that appears deep and bleeds profusely.)

We would call another type of pain *imbalance pain.* This results from a body that has too much exertion from one set of muscles and joints and too little exertion from other muscles and joints. As we tend to have specific lifestyles, we tend to focus too much on a particular type of movement. This creates strong muscles, ligaments and joints in one direction and weak ones in the other. This results in tightness, spasm, imbalance and joint and ligament injury. The best strategy of course for these types of imbalances is to be constantly working different muscle groups, and trying not to do one particular activity without doing another that is complementary in its muscle group use.

We would call a subset of imbalance pain *sedentary pain.* This results from not moving enough. The modern world is now full of reasons not to move. We have television, computers, movies, automobiles and office desks. Quite simply, when we do not use our muscles they become weaker. The joints also become weaker and prone to inflammatory ailments like arthritis. One of the contributing factors besides a lack of movement is a lack of circulation. Backaches are another rampant result of the sedentary lifestyle. Sitting for long periods keeps the back in one position for an unnaturally long period. The strategy for backaches and sedentary pain in general is balance and movement. We need to walk, stretch, twist, lift, push, climb, dance and jump. For backaches, we need to particularly strengthen the abdominal muscles. A disciplined, everyday strategy of movement, stretching and exercise is necessary to keep the body free from sedentary pain.

Many painful disorders are caused by a lack of natural elements or the toxicity created by the polluting of our local environment, water, food or home atmosphere. It can also be the result of a lack of motion. Many joint and muscle aches are the result of a lack of stretching, walking and movement in general. Researching and removing these environmental toxins is likely to reduce our pain and inflammation even if they are not the direct cause of the disorder. By removing toxins, we decrease the burden on our immune system, increasing our body's ability to fight the new pain and inflammation.

Once we locate the pain source and embark upon a healing process, we can support the process by making various improvements in our posture, activities, or diet. Using different therapeutic methods, we can decrease pain and/or increase our tolerance to it. The first process would be to breathe fully, with either core breathing or abdominal breathing techniques. Complete abdominal breathing will not only better oxygenate the blood stream and increase the healing process, but also stimulate deeper and increasingly introspective thinking, which advances our consciousness and eventual pain control. This can be combined with progressive relaxation techniques to reduce stress. We can also perform guided imagery techniques for relaxation, and meditation. We can also practice transitioning into movements of *Tai Chi* or *Hatha Yoga.* These can be not only relaxing, but can help pull our focus away. We can also use sound therapy and color therapy as was also detailed in *Total Harmonic.* Music and spiritual sounds such as prayer and spiritual chants can help us transcend the pain and put our focus on the bigger issues of life.

During pain episodes, we can set up alternate patterns of relaxing, breathing, and gentle stretching. We might also consider going for a walk in nature during painful episodes. Often simply relaxing our muscles and stress-points will curtail the pain. This can be increased using massage. Professional and friend/partner massages can be extremely beneficial, but self-massage is advised for pain because there is immediate feedback and learning. Another person may increase our pain inadvertently as well.

For chronic pain, our action in response can be directly related to the type and intensity of the pain. We become increasingly concerned with an experience of a constant, intense, and enduring pain. This usually means that there is something incredibly wrong in the body. Something is repeatedly producing inflammation. Again, it is important to note the times of the peaks and valleys of the pain intensity in our pain diary, and be prepared to talk to a health professional and show them these notes. We should carefully consider the advice, and seek second opinions if we are not comfortable with their diagnosis and treatment suggestions. Should we decide to move forward with their treatment, we should be clear on the side effects, and have an emergency plan should those side effects become extensive.

The emphasis in pain response should be to locate the cause and remove that cause. Should we be faced with chronic pain or inflammation and cannot locate a cause or initiate a healing response, or we located the cause but do not know how to heal it, the visit with a local natural health practitioner or other health professional can be used to explore the causes. A visit to the health professional may be more productive if we can bring in our daily log and notes and we can clearly describe the situation and history. With this information, the likelihood of locating the causal relationships and correct healing therapies is dramatically increased. Our consultation with the professional should focus upon the potential causes of the pain and solutions, rather than strictly pain medication. If they do not discuss their opinion of the cause, we should ask what they think could be the cause. Often health professionals will not volunteer their opinions regarding what might have caused an affliction. When pressed, however, they may volunteer some suggestions for possible causes. Sometimes we have to just ask.

Pain medication may be necessary, but the goal of pain medication should be as a stopgap for a short period while the cause of the pain is removed and the body begins to heal. Pain medication will likely not remove the cause of the pain. It can even increase the duration of the pain, as we can lose the incentive to remove the cause. If we can just take a pill and the pain goes away, we will neither learn from the pain nor learn how to remove the cause. Or if we know the cause, we may not develop the discipline needed to change our habits if it is easier just to take the pill. Pain medication may of course also cause dependency.

One of the best health professionals to approach for chronic pain is an acupuncturist. Clinical research on acupuncture has repeatedly shown it to be a successful treatment for pain of all types. Acupuncture has been used successfully for anesthesia for many centuries in China. Acupuncture has little risk and a long history of safety with little or no negative side effects. Acupuncture is a medical science and a medical art. The skill level of each practitioner and his or her connection with that type of pain might vary substantially. Therefore, we might consider going to another acupuncturist if one does not help before we give up altogether on acupuncture. Treatment cost is very low compared to other modalities, and success rates are high in many chronic pain disorders.

Whether we choose an M.D., N.D., acupuncturist (L.Ac., M.Ac. or D.O.M.) or another health professional, we should always be prepared to consider other opinions and ask many questions. We should also feel good about the treatment plan before we embark upon it. If we do not feel comfortable with it, there is usually a good reason.

It is best to not ignore our intuition when it comes to healing. If we are not feeling comfortable, we should first probably discuss this with the health professional treating us at that time. They may be able to remove our hesitations or provide an immediate alternative. If we have some particular information gained from the internet or books, we should ask for the health professional's fax machine or email. We should fax or email the article or web pages and have the professional evaluate and respond to them. If they are not willing to do this, another professional should be approached to discuss these alternatives.

When seeing any professional for pain, we should bring in whatever supplements or medications we are taking, so the doctor can look at the labels and consider what is already being taken before they prescribe others. This is a double concern for western medical doctors: prescribing multiple medications with conflicting mechanisms is happening with greater frequency over the past few decades.

The bottom line is that we can empower ourselves during visits with health professionals. Empowerment strategies include keeping our own medical files, with a copy of every lab, x-ray and treatment plan in it. We can put into this file the medication information sheets we are given, our pain and symptom diaries if we keep them, and any information or research data we gather relating to our pain or medical issue. We can bring this file into every health professional appointment to help substantiate our questions and concerns. This file may also prevent medical errors, which have been increasing. When we bring our file to our visit, we can quickly access our information to show the health professional. This can greatly accelerate the flow and the quality of the information we receive from our health professional. At the end of the day, resolving our pain is our responsibility. Health professionals can offer advice and prescribe treatment, but we must be the ones who provide the effort and make the necessary changes.

Today just about every community has an herbalist or naturopath who can suggest herbal strategies for reducing inflammation and curtailing pain. Many herbalists and naturopaths are well trained and are an excellent resource for general health tips as well. There are also acupuncturists, chiropractors and osteopaths who are well trained in areas of natural healing techniques. Depending upon the urgency of the issue, these professionals can be considered first, as their treatments are typically safer with fewer side effects. Medical doctors can also be sensitive to the needs of the patient and many have become self-taught in a few natural healing strategies. This is different from clinical training with botanicals and homeopathic therapies, however. Due to the restrictive nature of medical school training and licensing requirements, many medical doctors are hesitant to prescribe anything outside of prevailing pharmaceuticals.

Today's medical institutions receive financing from the pharmaceutical industry in a number of ways. Medical licensing and training is heavily influenced by the pharmaceutical industry as a result. Medical school coursework connects pathologies to particular commercial drugs patented by the pharmaceutical industry. Medical schools and hospitals are provided with research grants and other financial incentives to maintain this pharmaceutical-dominated perspective in medical care. Those doctors trained by and affiliated with these organizations are compelled to follow the procedures and prescriptions promoted by those organizations. A medical doctor who decides to treat patients using traditional herbal and other natural therapies will almost certainly face criticism and pressure from their local medical board. They may also be rejected by HMOs and insurance providers, cutting off their supply of patients. Even so, there is an increasing number of courageous medical doctors who support or incorporate natural remedies into their practice. These physicians are not crazy or stupid. They are simply seeing the science and documentation showing the safety and usefulness of nature's remedies.

Natural health professionals generally approach patients substantially different from conventional medical doctors. They will typically allow for more time in their appointment scheduling to listen to the patient's history and understand the potential causes and solutions. Most medical doctors who operate within insurance parameters must turn around patients within 15-20 minutes to keep their practices profitable. This allows little time to understand the patient or understand the causes of their pain. This sort of doctor visit usually results in an immediate assumption of a diagnosis, a quick explanation, followed by a hasty script and a hurried exit for the next waiting patient.

A number of botanicals have been used to relieve pain over thousands of years of traditional medical treatment. These include white willow bark, cayenne, Jamaican dogwood, kava, hops, sage, ginger, turmeric and many others. These have been well documented by herbalists like Dr. James Duke, Dr. Michael Murray, Christopher Hobbs, L.ac. and others. Many of these herbs not only reduce pain, but also speed up the healing process and reduce inflammation. Botanicals typically have many constituents that work synergistically. Ginger is known to have 477 active constituents (Newmark and Schulick 2000). Botanicals provide a balance of constituents by nature's design. One constituent will naturally balance or buffer the effects of another. This allows these *full-spectrum* agents to work synergistically to rebalance the body while reducing pain.

The only caveat about using herbs for pain issues is that they might not be as successful in numbing the pain as completely as medications. This choice goes to the heart of illness and pain, however: With every illness and every pain, there is a lesson—a learning experience. By completely wiping out pain, we remove the learning experience associated with the illness and its future prevention. We remove the disincentive to unhealthy lifestyle choices. This is precisely why a recent study illustrated that most Americans—even if they are suffering from preventable metabolic disorders like type-II diabetes or cardiovascular disease—are still not changing the lifestyles that caused their disorders.

By far the most advantageous way of obtaining herbs according to traditional *Ayurveda* and Chinese medicine is to grow them around our home. As we care for these herbs, they begin to tune in to our body's needs. The specific biomolecular structures they present in their leaves, stems and roots will align more closely with our body's particular biochemistry. This also occurs because we will be sharing a mutual environment. This is illustrated by the constituents that cayenne pepper plants produce in particular areas. Plants produced in regions with specific water contaminants will align their biochemistry with levels of capsaicin and other constituents equipped to better purge the particular local water contaminants. This takes place as the plants' immune system develops particular polysaccharides and polyphenols in response to the particular water. We find this occurs dramatically with mushrooms, as mushrooms tend to develop a resistance to the particular bacteria living in their moist environments. The constituents these organisms produce in turn assist the human immune system to develop strategies specific to combating those infections.

We might ask what this environmental response has to do with responding to a particular person's biochemistry. As we learned from Dr. Backster's research, plants we care for tune into our biology from a biocommunication level. This indicates the propensity to accommodate particular cellular issues as well as environmental issues, making the particular constituents better assimilated and more bioactive. This view might appear speculative, but it is also backed up by empirical research and many centuries of traditional medicine. It also makes sense from a practical basis. Biological research has confirmed that plants in different environments produce different constituents. Producing constituents is an intentional response by the self that dwells within that plant body. Research has also supported that plants can be conscious of humans and even empathetic to them. Despite increasing regulation upon the herbal industry, we still have the freedom to plant whatever healing plant we want around our yards and indoor environments.

Dire Pain

At some point in our lives, we will inevitably find our body in a situation of chronic disease and pain. Should we have the luxury of a clinical response we will likely be presented with a treatment plan that includes aggressive painkillers. What do we do?

The decision to numb the body with painkillers should be made carefully. Painkillers should be used sparingly. They are a way to get through momentary periods of agony, but they can also lead us to vegetate into numbness if we are not careful. It is important to stay in touch with our body, because this is our contact with reality. Pain is our link to sensibility. Should our prognosis be good and the cause of the pain is being resolved, temporary pain-relief may provide a bridge to healing. Should we be lost in numbness, however, our incentive to resolve the issue will be decreased. Most health experts—even most pain doctors—agree that pain drugs should be used as minimally as possible. This is a conclusion made from observation of thousands of patients who have succumbed to addictions and psychological defects as a result of aggressive painkillers.

Incredibly intense and chronic pain is another thing altogether. This sort of pain is likely a natural signal for the inner self to transition out of the physical body. With intense pain, the inner self is forced by necessity to disassociate with the body. This disassociation process is perfectly natural, and is set up by the design of the Creator. Sometimes a person may die in their sleep, oblivious to the pain the body may be presenting.

Though the person appears to be asleep, the pain availed by the affliction will still work to further disassociate the inner self from the body—providing a process enabling a release from inner self.

This type of pain is not only natural, but also necessary for the inner self to experience. This is part of the learning experience of our physical journey. The message communicated in this experience is that this temporary physical body is not our true identity—and the physical environment is not our true home. The reason we experience pain in the first place is because we are in conflict with our identity. We are attempting to identify our self—the permanent emotional person—with a temporary vehicle. Acute chronic pain means the vehicle is becoming obsolete, through either injury or disease. We have become attached to it. This attachment manifests itself as pain. It is important that we become detached from our body somehow. Pain allows this to take place.

Some have proposed that pain is an imagination of the seer and not real. However, we understand that physical pain is very real. The body certainly undergoes damage, and during this damage, the nervous system communicates painful messages to the limbic system. These messages pulse onto the screen of the mind, allowing the inner self to experience it. The extent to which the inner self is attached to the body relates to the pain sensitivity. The messages from the body are real. The cause of the pain is real. Even a person not attached to the body will experience the pain. It is how these messages are responded to that matters. The attached person will focus on the pain. The detached person will first focus on how to solve the problem. Failing that, the detached person will transcend the pain with a focus on the philosophical lessons involved in the experience, and embrace learning those lessons. In many cases, chronic pain is an indication that we have not learned certain philosophical lessons about life. It may stimulate the realization that we may not have come to terms with our spiritual identity and our higher purpose for living. This realization would not be that different from the runner realizing the relationship between their pain and winning the race. In both cases, the person sees pain in relationship with a higher purpose, and therein lies an ability to transcend the pain.

Chapter Nine

A Time to Die

The goal of modern medicine—and subsequently most health advice—is to help avoid the death of the body at all costs. Should this be the ultimate goal, however? The operator in this question is the "all costs" clause. Society, chronic disease sufferers and medical doctors typically struggle with the consequential questions: Just how much effort should be made to avert death? What is the point when death has its natural place, and we should accept its arrival? Should we continue to mount excessive costs and countless hours of effort in a fruitless effort to try to prevent an eventuality? Does delaying death for a few days, weeks or months when there is little or no quality of life have any real value? Could it be a senseless and futile effort?

In June of 2006, the Centers for Disease Control released its annual report *Deaths: Preliminary Data for 2004*. This report showed a decrease in deaths in the United States by 3.9% from 2003. The 2003 report showed a decrease in deaths by 1.7% over 2002. This statistic is of course to be overlaid against the continued surging population of the United States during these years. In fact, this age-adjusted death statistic has been decreasing since 1900, with a few exceptions during disease outbreak years. This primarily means that over the past century, fewer babies die, and adults have been living longer in average years. In 2003, the average age of death was 77.5. Some records indicate that 49 was the average lifespan at the turn of the twentieth century.

Lifespan statistics are deceiving, however, because a hundred years ago there were significantly more stillborns and more infant deaths. This skews the lifespan statistics significantly. Many adults still lived to grand old ages, but the average between one stillborn and one *centenarian* (someone who lives to age 100) is close to 50 years old.

If we look closely at lifespan statistics, things look differently. Many of the longest lifespan statistics have been recorded among indigenous populations. When birth rates are removed—which is difficult to do retroactively—lifespan statistics can illustrate an opposite trend.

As far as diseases go, the number one cause of death in modern civilization has been heart disease, followed by cancer. Heart disease is a result of the modern diet. Over the past few years, cancer has overtaken heart disease as the leading killer. Higher cancer rates, of course, have been connected to the chemical revolution of the past fifty years. Due to the prevention education efforts and research focus of the American Heart Association and the American Cancer Society, death from these two diseases have been only slightly decreasing, while their occurrence appears to be continuing to increase. While this could be attributed to greater diagnosis, that would ignore the fact that Americans are also becoming more obese; eating too much fried foods, junk food and meat. We might attribute the lower death rates to further advances in cardiovascular surgery (stents and so on) and chemotherapy, in addition to earlier diagnosis.

Our medical institutions are remarkable in their ability to artificially extend privileged patients' lives through intervention. In some cases, these heroic efforts may add a few quality years to a person's lifespan. In many cases, however, the intervention merely temporarily delays the inevitable. Those extended years are often spent drugged, incapacitated and sometimes even unconscious.

Quite simply, death is a normal phase of the body's natural rhythms. It has the same importance to physical life that birth does. Death arrives at a time when the body is naturally becoming obsolete. As designed, the inner self exits when a significant portion of the body's major functions or organs break down. This is to our benefit. If we had to wait for all the parts of the body to break down before leaving, we would experience a greater amount of suffering. Instead, as soon as any of the major body parts—such as the heart, liver, kidneys, brain and so on—shuts down, the self is immediately escorted out of the body.

Every cell in the body has a programmed time to die. This genetic clock is subject to change according to our activities, however. Cellular death is called apoptosis. This can be programmed death driven either by an internal clock or by an external infliction that diseases the cell. Biologists have been investigating apoptosis' mysterious processes over the past few decades, and have determined that cell death can occur through a combination of several signaling circuits. One involves a programmed shutdown of the mitochondria (the energy production facilities of the cell), seemingly associated with the production of a signaling biochemical called the cytochrome-c. This signaling follows the development of a special signaling channel called the MAC (mitochondria apoptosis channel). The development of this special biocommunication channel appears mysterious. Still, we can surmise that this is simply part of the overall body's clockwork mechanism.

Scientists have also found that apoptosis also involves a complex process involving the internal self-destruct mechanism called tumor necrosis factor. The TNF mechanism was originally discovered in cancer research as the mechanism inhibiting the spread of a cancer. Researchers have since found that its process is related to several other mechanisms. These include the R1 and R2 receptor mechanisms. The R1 and R2 receptors receive signals from outside the cell to stimulate a process of shutting down the cell. The TNF signaling process instigates a cascading communication process called *death-induced signaling*. Here one signal to the R1 or R2 receptors stimulates a multi-instructional process that begins shutting down the cell. Part of this signaling process is transmitted through a genetic protein expression called the *p53 gene*. The p53 gene is a transcription protein affecting the process genetic copying. Researchers have discovered that many viruses and carcinogenic mutations are allowed to expand by disabling the p53 gene as well.

Another major signaling TNF mechanism is the *Fas-ligand* system. The Fas ligand is a specialized protein that signals to a receptor located on one of the chromosomes of the cell's DNA. This stimulation by the ligand—the signal-sending protein—seems to have its foundation in the T-cell immune system. As T-cells are activated, Fas ligands become more prolific, signaling the process of cell death. In many circumstances, this also initiates a halting of the process of mitosis—causing cells to die without replacements. In situations where a cell is infected by a virus or a carcinogenic mutation, halting of mitosis signaling can be inhibited by viral DNA mutations. By blocking the process of cell death, these viral mutations can multiply through cellular division. This of course allows the virus to replicate throughout the body.

The apoptosis signaling process is still not well understood by science. The body's master instructional mechanisms maintain that subtle programming feature scientists refer to as homeostasis. Homeostasis is sometimes used to describe cellular metabolism. Homeostasis also describes the body's ability to balance the number of cells that die with the number of new cells developed through cellular division or mitosis. This balancing act is a programming feature that is extremely complex. It cannot be unraveled by finding a few gene sequences. This process includes the expression of the p53 gene, the TNF process, various ligand-receptor mechanisms, and the overall mechanism of balancing the trillions of cells within the body. It becomes a macrocosm issue, and lies in the conscious epigenetic realm. The ability of the body to orchestrate particular activities among the trillions of cells simultaneously to achieve governance over the body's major functions can only lie within the domain of greater conscious intention—a master design by a Superior intelligence.

The overriding message of these death-signaling mechanisms is that the body maintains a rhythmic clock that times out the balance of cells. As time proceeds, dying cells outnumber dividing cells. As the body ages, this balance begins to weigh more heavily upon the dying cells. Living cells become less tolerant, and more prone to succumb to the challenges of our environment. At the same time, the immune system becomes more alert to challenged cells, responding quickly to eliminate cells that endanger the body during its remaining years.

These mechanisms all allow the self to proceed with its intentions of seeking fulfillment. We might compare this to the process of rationing. When a person knows that only so much food or water is left for a specific period of time, they will likely carefully divide up the available goods and measure out the intake each day. In the same way, the inner self always accommodates the limitations of the body and seeks more conservative goals with modified expectations. Logically, we could assess that the self could hardly expect fulfillment from reduced physical abilities. Surprisingly, despite this reduction, the self does not lose its expectation of fulfillment through the physical body.

This seems curious, but we know it to be true. We see it in its most obvious form during a *mid-life crisis.* Here the self realizes that the body is quickly moving beyond the point where we can maintain the hope that certain physical activities will be achieved. This presents a conflict of identity: The body is getting old but the inner self feels the same age. In a desperate attempt to reconcile this conflict, the misidentifying self may instigate a radical move. We have seen many examples of this. A person might purchase a motorcycle, re-enter a former sport, or attempt to date someone younger.

The more practical inner self operating the middle-aged body will accommodate these obvious physical changes by simply redirecting expectations. Instead of expecting fulfillment by winning a football game, the aging star will seek fulfillment by coaching a victorious team. In both efforts, the goal has not changed. The self seeks to gain the approval and love from others with the accomplishment. They simply redirect the body and mind towards what can be practically accomplished.

Later in life, as the body ages further, the self begins to lose the opportunities to accomplish anything significantly physical. We may then redirect our expectations for fulfillment in the physical world to the accomplishments of our children or grandchildren. As the elderly person sees it, when the child or grandchild succeeds, *they* succeed because of their body's initial seed donation. This proprietary mechanism is an extension of the false identification of the self with the physical body. We know this scientifically because we can observe not only successful young people remaining unfulfilled, but we also see successful adults continue to be unfulfilled, and successful parents and grandparents still plagued by loneliness, panic-attacks and a general lack of fulfillment despite their achievements and their family's collective achievements.

The Message of Death

The dying of the body has a clear message: It is time for us to exit. We have arrived at a point where the lessons of this lifetime should have been learned. Now it is time for a new journey. It is time for us to move on.

Death is like being shown the door. When we are visiting with friends at their house and our hosts suddenly get up off the sofa and begin to slowly walk towards the door, we know it is time to leave. It is time to move on, thank our host for the fun time, and say goodbye. It is not time to start up another conversation or go back and sit on the sofa. Should we do this, we will probably be accused of 'overstaying our welcome.' This is not too dissimilar to the scenario playing out in most hospitals today.

The natural body is simply not designed to live forever. Our western medical institutions tease us with notions of new technologies that can keep the body alive forever. We should know this will not be a reality, however. Nor is it a good use of our precious time while here. The laws of nature have a reason. We inhabit a physical body for a short time to learn specific lessons. It is a short-term vehicle. The body is not meant to house the living being forever. It is like putting on a spacesuit with a particular oxygen reserve. Once within the temporary spacesuit, a smart astronaut does not waste time debating about why there is not more oxygen in the tank. It is what it is, and the astronaut has a particular job to do before returning to the space ship.

The problem is that we begin to falsely identify with the physical body after a few years in it. This is also by design. Once this misidentification grabs us—which happens pretty early on in our lives in this body—we become connected to our body. We try to protect it at all costs. We scream when it becomes threatened. We raise our hackles when a life-threatening challenge presents itself.

We have discussed how the body, mind and self can be deceived by a misinterpretation of stress as a potentially life-threatening event. Our body can be pumping out emergency biochemicals and waveforms even when little is at stake. This misinterpretation can also be evident during a truly life-threatening situation. We have often seen situations where people become so anxious during a traumatic experience that they do not react appropriately. We might do the wrong thing under the circumstances. We might scream when in reality no one could hear us or help us. We might freeze like a deer in the headlights when we should be running from a threat. During the 9/11 disaster some people reacted calmly and intelligently during the disaster and evacuated orderly while helping others, while a significant number of people panicked and did not act appropriately. Most of us agree that an over-stimulated panic state can sometimes be a distraction or even a deterrent from dealing with an emergency. For this reason, most of us consider a state of panic with disdain. We also give respect to those who coolly and calmly react during a crisis.

Why do we respect those who calmly react appropriately in a crisis? This is because most of us see a state of panic as being disconnected from the reality of an emergency. An overstated panic response is often seen in groups. A panicking group of people can easily over-react and over-step the boundaries of what should take place. This is typically because these people are watching everyone else's response rather than assessing the situation directly. As a result, they are out of touch with the problem and tend to react as others do. Research has showed that in an emergency, crowds tend to immediately select a group leader or role model—often arbitrarily. As the inherited leaders of the group respond, the rest of the group is likely to respond similarly. Should these 'chosen ones' react inappropriately, the entire crowd responds in kind. Suddenly the situation becomes a crisis because an entire group or population of people responded inappropriately to a perceived threat. We might call this the *herd mentality*.

This is precisely the situation existing today amongst our medical institutions with regard to the process of death.

It is appropriate to respond to a patient who has been shot or injured. Attempts are made to extract the bullet or repair the injury. These are acceptable responses to a critical injury that may easily be healed with intervention. Heroic attempts to resuscitate an individual who has had a heart attack or someone who has had a stroke would be considered appropriate as well. There is a critical line, however, between these types of emergency interventions and unacceptable attempts to intervene in the natural process of death. The line becomes evident when the body is chronically malfunctioning and pain without medication is unbearable.

As we have discussed previously, tens of thousands of near-death experiences have documented real experiences after the clinical death of the body. Most documented clinical death experiences include the self first floating up over the body and looking down upon it. At this point, the self can observe the physical events taking place around the body. The self may observe the doctors and nurses operating or attempting resuscitation. Many have traveled into the hallways and into other rooms to observe other events. Thousands of these unembodied observations have been recalled following resuscitation and confirmed as accurate. This is physically impossible for a body lying in a bed unconscious. Many cases document the person able to travel to another location instantly (at the speed of thought). They might look upon a relative or spouse in an attempt to say goodbye. Again, resuscitation-accounts have accurately described the activities of this physically distant relative. Many have then reported entering a tunnel with a light at the other end. Many reported meeting with a spiritual personality. Many also reported being informed that it was "not their time yet," followed by an instant return to the body.

A significant number of clinical death patients have these sorts of experiences. Indeed, a significant majority of all revived patients reporting death experiences described an overall positive experience of "dying."

Note these studies of clinical death have been conducted with scientific scrutiny and peer review. Many were controlled to specifically address concerns made from previous clinical death studies. Some of the researchers—many of whom were medical doctors—were dubious regarding the reality of the after-death experience before their research began. Following their research, most became convinced of the possibility of life after death.

There is still some debate surrounding the meaning of these studies. The evidence is clear, however. The self separates from the body and somehow observes events surrounding them and outside their hospital room. The fact that their body was clinically dead at the time is important to remember. During clinical death, not only has the heart stopped and breathing stopped. Brainwaves have also stopped. There is little or no electrical activity in the body. If consciousness were part of the electrical activity of the brain as some contend, then the observations of the patient would have also stopped at the same time. Instead, those experiences continued for a significant percentage of clinically dead patients.

It should be pointed out that there were also some subjects in these studies who did not recall the death experience. Suicide and drug-overdose subjects, for example, typically had no recollection. For others, we would contend that an excess of painkillers, psychotic medications or simply an incoherent state of mind might have blocked the mental recollection of the experience upon awakening. This would be due to the mind and brain's inability to properly process the new information after the self returned to the body. This might be compared with Dr. Stevenson's research illustrating that many, but not all young children can remember their past lives, and this recollection typically fades after age seven.

Despite the clarity of these studies, some steadfast doubters have proposed that the clinical death experience is nothing but mental hallucination. This might be plausible if not for the fact that hallucinations are defined as seeing something that *did not happen.* Since the researchers confirmed a large majority of the physical observations made by the clinically dead were accurate (such as the doctors' and nurses' activities on the table, events down the hall, or remote relatives), hallucinations would not be a plausible explanation. Indeed, many have based their arguments on an assumption that thoughts originate in the physical brain. If the brain was electrically dead—as it was in many of these clinical death cases—then how could the person be hallucinating during that time?

The only logical explanation to be gained from this research and others we have covered is that we are not physical body. Rather, each of us has an identity transcendental to the body. The physical body we wear is merely a temporary vehicle. This is the truly scientific position, noting also that the body undergoes so many physical changes over a lifetime while we remain *ourselves.* The body is recycling cells and molecules while the personality within remains the same personality.

With these realities in mind, death is simply our leaving a worn-out vehicle and moving on to where ever our intended journey takes us. Where we go might be the appropriate conversation at this juncture. This is beyond the subject matter of this text, however. Besides, the knowledge of where we go after death is part of the personal learning experience each of us can choose to undergo during our physical lifetimes. What we can establish from the clinical death research is that the inner self lives on following the death of the physical body, and that experience is not necessarily a negative experience.

So we must now ask this important question: Knowing the body will inevitably become obsolete and will eventually die, and we will live beyond this death, why should we respond inappropriately to the prospect of death? Why should we unnaturally keep a person from the next step in their journey, and keep them in a state of suspension? Certainly, there is little quality of life in living out a few months in a hospital bed attached to life-support equipment, unable to conduct meaningful physical or mental activities.

Certainly, doctors are not feeling improper while they valiantly rescue a dying person. In many cases, they are not being improper either. However, we all know examples of situations where their efforts become ridiculous. Most of us have heard of cases where a person is kept on resuscitating equipment well past a reasonable period of time. The patient remains unconscious, and without the equipment the body would surely cease existing. At this point, the inner self is trapped within the body and not being let go. The self is stuck without the ability to communicate or request to be let go. This is simply not appropriate.

Note that we are not making a determination here of where the line should be drawn, or isolating which types of resuscitation are reasonable. This is a personal decision that should be made by each of us. Each of us is responsible for the efforts that others make on behalf of our body. Therefore each of us is responsible for making the determination for the limitation of heroic efforts, and making this clear (in writing) to our relatives and health professionals. In the absence of this, it will become the decision of our spouse or relatives. We should remember that this is a very difficult position to be in as a relative. Any caring spouse or family member will struggle with such a decision, because they do not want their mate or relative to leave them. They also will be presented with the appearance, possibly, of wanting to hasten the death of their spouse. Putting our spouse or relatives in this position is simply unfair. Sometimes, in the absence of clear instructions by the dying person, a court or legislative body will become involved in the decision of whether to disconnect the person from their life-support equipment. Why should we put others in this uncomfortable position? Why should we involve total strangers in the decision about whether we wish to be let go or not?

This is not to say that while we occupy the physical body we and others should not be working to keep our body in good condition as long as it is useful. Keeping the body in good condition will allow it to run efficiently and effectively. Certainly if we do not treat the body right, we will be condemned to dealing with the consequences of ill health. Ill health in this situation is also part of nature's design for learning. We get to learn lessons from our mistreatment and disrespect for the gift of this miraculous vehicle.

Nevertheless, once our bodies have played out their intended era, it is not the time to focus on attempts to avoid death at all costs. It is a time to embrace death as a natural progression of our physical journey. It is time for us to consider the meaning of life and death. It is a time to begin transcending the physical layers. It is time to achieve a higher understanding about our existence.

This is also the purpose of old age. We can no longer look towards any career advancement. We cannot achieve sexual prowess. We do not have the time to plan for our future retirement. We do not have the ability to train for winning a sporting event. We can certainly keep active through our elderly years. However, we must accept our elderly years as a period of weakened physical abilities for a reason. It is a time to focus on and prepare for our transition. Instead, our health care industry and society works to try to distract the elderly from this mission. For this reason, pharmaceutical drug use is rampant among the elderly. The elderly are often distracted in nursing homes with meaningless games, television and mind-altering drugs. Activity and social events may certainly have some positive attributes, but the importance of a clear mind to use for spiritual contemplation and reflection should not be downplayed.

Our artificial attempts to extend life are useless. Certainly, we have been able to extend the lifetime of people's bodies in some respects with our medical technologies. We have been able to transplant hearts, install stents and replace kidneys. What are the costs though? Are all these technologies really extending the quality of our lives? Is there a net gain after we consider the time spent on the effort? Some transplants like kidneys might be reasonable. Others, like heart transplants, are risky and often ultimately doomed for failure.

We might use a similar logic when deciding whether to drive or fly to a destination. We would compare the driving and stopping time to the airport waits, the flight, and the travel to and from the airport. Sometimes a drive might be faster than a flight, or the flight is cheaper than the drive after gas and meals are considered. The quality of our remaining life can be analyzed similarly. In measuring the cost of prolonging life, we have to net out how much time is taken by doctor's visits, hospitalization, surgery, recuperation, rehabilitation, various follow-up visits and of course the risks and side effects involved in treatment. This "process time" needs to be subtracted from the extra days or years gained from the treatment. We might also suggest we should subtract the time spent deciding on the process, researching the process and so on. All of this time spent avoiding death should be subtracted from the net conscious time gained in order to assess the value of the treatment. This relates directly to the quality of life achieved. If the process leaves us unable to return to our families and lifestyle in a reasonable amount of time then what good was all the effort?

Included in this consideration is that much of the effort of these doctors and hospitals could be spent on saving children who are dying of malaria, AIDS and other ailments. These children could well recover and have a significant quality of life remaining. We should consider in this evaluation the many billions of dollars and time resources spent by many researchers, doctors, professionals, hospitals, pharmaceutical companies and insurance providers; all aimed at attempting to add a few days, months or a year or two to lives that have already lasted 70 or 80 years. Is it worth all this effort? Currently the U.S. is number one in the world for per-capita spending on healthcare, yet ranked number fifty-eight for longevity. Obviously much of our spending and resources is going to waste anyway. What if we were to put all of the money, energy and resources we spend trying to unnaturally stay alive towards caring for childhood sickness and feeding hungry people around the world? We would probably live in a much kinder world, and be better prepared to leave it. We would probably also all live longer, as we would likely have less stress—a central cause of a majority of fatal diseases. The bottom line with this point is that a consciousness of kindness also makes our bodies healthier.

The United States' economy is drowning in medical costs. The current head of the Government Accounting Office admits that the cost of health care and pharmaceuticals in the United States will bankrupt Medicare and possibly the entire government within a decade or two. Most Americans know this situation from the rising cost of health care, but many do not realize that health care costs have risen from 4% of America's gross national product in 1950 to a whopping 16% in 2004.

Death by Institution

The research on the causes of this healthcare crisis reveals that the cost of new equipment and new pharmaceuticals are the leading causes. Increasingly new devices are being invented and manufactured. These are not only diagnostic tools, but also devices to artificially extend life. Many of these diagnostic tools are over-rated and sometimes not useful in the long run. One example is the breast mammogram. They exert about 1,000 times the radiation exposure as a chest x-ray, and yet research shows they provide little benefit in the way of early detection of cancer compared to manual breast examinations by physicians. They are also a contributing cause for breast cancer. A 2008 study out of Holland confirms this.

Much of the advances in technology have come in the way of various life-extension systems such as feeding tubes, ventilators, dialysis machines and heart-lung equipment. Today ones body can easily become a surrogate of one of these machines long after the intended time of death has past. Furthermore, the cost of putting someone on these extravagant machines bankrupts thousands of Americans every year.

Meanwhile, newer pharmaceuticals have been developed that chemically extend life by artificially reducing inflammation, pain and nervous issues. These efforts are certainly commendable, and the intentions of some researchers may be valiant. Still, these efforts come with a considerable price. Interestingly, many of these new technologies and medicines create as many early deaths as they may temporarily prevent. Over the past few decades, our medical industry has become the leading cause of death and injury in the United States. Carolyn Dean,

M.D., N.D., in her book *Death By Medicine* (2005), compiled the following statistics for 2005:

Hospital Adverse Reaction – 106,000 Deaths
Medical Error – 98,000 Deaths
Bedsores – 115,000 Deaths
Infection – 88,000 Deaths
Malnutrition – 108,800 Deaths
Outpatient Adverse Reaction – 199,000 Deaths
Unnecessary Procedures – 37,136 Deaths
Surgery-Related – 32,000 Deaths
Total Annual Deaths by Modern Medicine – 783,936

Think about this. This accounting of deaths out-numbers U.S. cardiovascular disease death rates and cancer death rates. In 2002 for example, 450,637 people died of heart disease and about 476,009 died of cancer.

The *Journal of the American Medical Association* (Lazarou *et al.* 1998) reported that in 1994, 2,216,000 Americans were either hospitalized, permanently disabled, or died as a result of pharmaceuticals. *The Nutrition Institute of America* reports that over 20 million unnecessary antibiotic prescriptions are prescribed. Over seven million medical and surgical procedures a year are unnecessary. Over eight million people are hospitalized without need. Our medical institution is quite simply suffocating in its own mismanagement.

According to a nationwide poll conducted by Louis Harris and Associates released in 1997 by the National Patient Safety Foundation and the American Medical Association, an estimated 100 million Americans experienced a medical mistake: 42% of those randomly surveyed. Misdiagnosis and wrong treatments accounted for 40% of those mistakes. Medical medication errors accounted for 28% of these, and medical procedure errors accounted for 22% of these (NPSF 1997).

In a study of four Boston adult primary care practices involving 1202 outpatients, 27% (95% confidence) of responders experienced adverse drug events (Gandhi *et al.* 2003).

In a 2004 interview with Dr. Lucian Leape, an expert in patient safety and an author of a number of studies, reported that over the past ten years since the 1997 NPSF studies were performed, improvements in our medical system have been inadequate. Barriers to improvement cited physician denial, hospital environment, lack of leadership and little system review (Leape 2004).

As we settle back into our seats after reading these startling facts, we should realize this means our medical institutions' supposed heroic endeavors for life extension actually cost more lives than they save. These efforts actually shorten more lives than they extend. To add insult to injury, the dramatically rising cost of medical care in our society also means less access to medical care for preventive care and non-critical treatment. In real terms, this means poorer people or the uninsured receive less healthcare, while preventive healthcare receives little attention.

Our medical institutions' supposed heroic effort to save lives is backfiring. Why? Because pharmaceutical and medical technology companies are madly pursuing profits while medical doctors are over-prescribing pharmaceuticals and over-applying diagnostic procedures in an attempt to avoid malpractice suits. The situation is not dissimilar to a large herd of confused animals recklessly stampeding, and mowing down anything in the way.

For those who believe America's advanced healthcare technologies are extending our lives, we only have to point to the statistics. The United States has one of the lowest life expectancies among the industrialized world, while leading the world in the application of the newest technologies and healthcare costs. Meanwhile we see people living very long lives in places like Okinawa and Tibet, where medical technology and advanced drugs are less available.

There have been many discussions about some of these traditional cultures. Many have focused on the specifics of their lifestyles in an attempt to find some magic *'fountain of youth.'* In reality, these people live longer lives because they are living their lives in tune with nature. Most of us living in industrialized society are faced with stress, processed foods and toxic environments, all of which shorten life span. We have traded in our blue skies for asbestos ceiling tiles and our sun for fluorescent lights. We traded air for soot and food for sugar and preservatives. The increases in life expectancy in the industrialized countries due primarily to increased live birth rates and childhood health dwarf the benefit of advanced medical technologies later in life.

There has been a major shift in the types of diseases modern man is faced with. Third world countries and traditional cultures are faced with death from infectious epidemics and birth deaths. Western society, however, is challenged by a myriad of autoimmune disorders, cancers, heart disease and nervous disorders. Modern medicine has valiantly challenged many infectious diseases with vaccination (a simple utilization of the body's own immune system) and antibiotics. The jury is still out, however, on whether these strategies will ultimately free us from infectious disease. With the rampant growth of antibiotic-resistant superbugs like methicillin resistant *Staphylococcus aureus* (MRSA) and antibiotic-resistant tuberculosis, our fight against infectious disease is far from over. As infectious organisms learn how to counteract our antibiotics, we are likely to contend with a host of new superbugs. This eliminates any expectation of dominance over infectious disease, and has effectively turned bacteria we used to have some immunity against into monsters with virtually little defense. We propose that while western medicine certainly has advanced with regard to birthing, surgery and emergency intervention, we have effectively opened up a Pandora's box of health issues like AIDS, autoimmune disease, cancer and superbugs in the meantime, creating pandemics that may rival if not outnumber deaths from past epidemics.

As a result of modern medicine's advancements, our doctors feel like superheroes when they extend the life of a person's body temporarily. This is regardless of the quality of life remaining with the patient. The quality of life of an elderly person undergoing multiple operations, medications, life-support equipment and severe chronic pain is obviously limited. Reduced to painkillers, heart-lung machines and ventilators, doctors are replacing the dignity of old age with zombied surrogates.

We must state clearly: *Old age is not a disease.*

These heroic efforts to 'save lives' by doctors are certainly valiant. Many activities in private medicine are motivated simply by profits, however. Pharmaceutical companies and healthcare organizations are generally multi-billion dollar enterprises built upon a mission of profitability. Their stockholders, directors, and management are thus focused upon making profitable decisions. Yet controlled research clearly indicates that herbal remedies are safe and effective over the long run with fewer side effects when dosed correctly and knowledgeably. The pharmaceutical giants are nevertheless using their influence to prevent people from nature's healing agencies, while they have isolated and patented many active constituents from medicinal plants. Why? It is all about profits.

Herbal medicine is simply not profitable for the pharmaceutical giants. Herbs are plants—and plants are living organisms. For the most part, plants cannot be patented. If we consider that hundreds of thousands of people die each year from medications, while very few if any die of herbal supplement use, the numbers simply do not imply a safety issue with herbs. Yet because they cannot be patented, they are not supported by the pharmaceutical and healthcare corporations built upon profitability and market dominance.

Again, Lazarou *et al.* calculated that over 2.2 million people in the U.S. either end up being hospitalized, permanently disabled, or fatally injured resulting from pharmaceutical use every year. That is over 2.2 million Americans annually with *reported* injuries from pharmaceuticals. The study, done at the University of Toronto, also showed that approximately 106,000 people die each year from taking *correctly prescribed* FDA-approved pharmaceuticals. This does not include the number of deaths resulting by overdose or by addiction to these same drugs. The U.S. FDA was sent 258,000 adverse drug events in 1999. Harvard researcher and associate professor of medicine Dr. David Bates told the *Los Angeles Times* in 2001 "*...these numbers translate to 36 million adverse drug events per year*" (Rappoport 2006). The plausibility of this number is confirmed in another study published in the *Journal of the American Medical Association* in 1995 (Bates *et al.*). This revealed that over a sixth month period, 12% of 4031 adult hospital admissions had either a confirmed adverse drug event or a potentially adverse drug event. If we extrapolate this rate using the population of 300 million Americans, we would arrive at the 36 million Rappoport calculated.

We might compare these horrific figures to effects of herbal medication usage—both prescribed and self-medicated. According to the FDA, a total of 184 deaths and 2621 adverse reactions resulted from consumer use of herbal supplements *over a five-year period.* Most of these deaths were associated with incorrect use of weight-loss formulas and subsequent cardiac events. Still, this is an average of 37 annual herbal deaths to 108,000 deaths among pharmaceuticals, and 524 adverse herbal reactions to possibly 36,000,000 adverse pharmaceutical reactions per year. For those who might think that these numbers reflect that pharmaceutical use is much greater than herbal use; herbal supplementation use in the U.S. ranged from 27% to 36% of the population during that period (Hirshon and Barrueto 2006). This nets out to about one-third of the population, which is higher than the range for prescription pharmaceutical use judging by elderly prescription rates as examined below.

For thousands of years, traditional doctors and scientists have carefully studied and documented particular botanicals associated with particular ailments. One of the earliest written records of herbal medicine is the *Pen Ts'ao,* written some 4500 years ago by a Chinese herbalist. The *Pen Ts'ao* recorded 366 different plant medicines and their specific uses. Ayurvedic texts—some even older—also document the use of hundreds of botanicals, as do the documents and spoken knowledge of the Greeks, the Romans, the Polynesians, the New Zealand Mauris, the Aborigines, the North American Indians, the Indonesians, the Mayans, the Egyptians, the Arabs, and the Northern Europeans. Herbal medications have thus been used safely by billions of people over thousands of years.

In comparison, a pharmaceutical drug might be approved based on a few studies of several hundred patients, often managed by researchers paid by the pharmaceutical company. This means we can compare billions of traditional users of herbs unconnected with their commercial value versus data on a few hundred users of a particular drug organized by someone being paid by the manufacturer.

Once a pharmaceutical company has designed new drug, it can receive patent protection for that chemical combination, giving them twenty years of potential exclusivity for selling that drug, at least in the United States. This means a guarantee of profits as long as doctors prescribe that drug. With a patent, there is protection from competition for 15-20 years, depending upon the speed of approval. Without the doctor prescribing the medication, there is no continual use. Thus, control must include both the patent and the doctor—or his or her licensure. For this reason, pharmaceutical giants focus their attention on a combination of drug research, patent protection, and regulation and marketing to physicians.

In our modern medical institutions, pathological documentation regarding diagnosis also accompanies the use of specific pharmaceutical drugs. The institution synchronizes with the pharmaceutical industry because of the tight relationships between pharmaceutical companies, medical schools, medical licensure and pathology documentation. Drug research by doctors—many of whom are also medical school professors—is typically funded by the pharmaceutical manufacturers. There is thus a built-in incentive for a successful outcome. As the cardiovascular and anti-inflammatory drug lawsuits have proved over the past few years, pharmaceutical manufacturers are often slow to disclose information that might damage the sales of their drugs.

Even if a pharmaceutical results in an improved condition for a particular ailment, there are often dangerous side effects. Some of these can be worse than the original ailment. In addition, most medications stress the liver and kidneys in one respect or another—shortening the lifespan of these critical organs. Some medications, like aminoglycoside antibiotics streptomycin, kanamycin, garamicin and others have been shown to cause kidney damage in as many as 15 percent of patients. Others, such as acetaminophen, carbamazepine, atenolol, cimetidine, phenylbutazone, acebutolol, piroxicam, mianserin, naproxen, sulindac, ranitidine, enflurane, halothane, valproic acid, phenobarbital, isoniazid and ketoconazole can cause acute dose-dependent liver damage. This is because the liver and the kidneys work together to process most chemicals out of the body. Together these organs break down and excrete the chemical byproducts of medications, resulting in their hopeful extraction from the body. With this chemical breakdown comes a number of dangerous residual chemical derivatives. The P450 liver enzyme process moves chemicals through the extraction pathway. This enzyme is effective in most healthy bodies for a few chemicals at a time. Yet multiple drugs can overwhelm and deplete this pathway. With the P450 extraction pathway overloaded by various chemicals, additional drugs can damage the body in a greater way. For this reason, a higher number of liver enzymes in a blood analysis is seen by doctors as a dangerous sign.

Sadly, multiple drug prescribing is commonplace among the elderly. In America, a large number of elderly persons (especially those who regularly see a doctor) are taking multiple medications. A 2004 Duke University study showed that 21% or 7 million Americans over the age of 65 take drugs classified as "dangerous." The over-65 population is 15% of the overall population, and this group is taking one-third of all drug prescriptions. Study researchers added that the study actually understated the problem, and that an elderly person taking at least ten to twelve prescription drugs is common.

What this translates to is an elderly population being drugged through their "golden years." Because doctors are prescribing multiple mood-altering drugs to this group of people, we are left with an aging population of drug-dependency. Suddenly drugs become necessary for sleep. Drugs become needed to eat. Drugs become needed to maintain composure. Drugs become needed to get through the day.

Why has our elderly become increasingly drug-dependent? Primarily because elderly people become vulnerable as they begin to face their many physical failings and pending death. After a lifetime of physical activity and an assumption that life was going to last forever, we become insecure about our identity and existence during old age. This is part of the lesson-plan. Impressed by the physician's credentials and the prolific advertising of the pharmaceutical industry, it is quite easy to be convinced of the necessity of taking these drugs. Drug advertising aimed at the elderly will typically show elderly people enjoying life, laughing and being active. This creates the message that the drug will help make us happy. Advertisers increasingly imply that drugs will create fulfillment and quality of life during a time meant for contemplation and introspection.

Dying and Healing

We must turn this equation around. At a time when a person needs to have clarity and purpose of mind, our medical institutions are drugging us and tempting us with unrealistic expectations. As we approach the crossroads of our physical journey—and begin our transition from this body to our next destination—we need to be prepared for the true healing event. What is the true healing event of our lives? This is the learning of the take-away points from a lifetime of lessons stemming from the challenges, growth, pain, laughter, love, relationships, losses, gains and finally the knowledge as we contemplate leaving it all behind. We thus need to utilize our faculties with clarity to navigate this important step in our experience.

In other words, we must preserve our awareness as we take this step.

There are several strategies we can execute to accomplish this. The first thing to consider putting in place is a *living will.* The living will can detail our wishes for how our body is maintained if we are no longer able to communicate those decisions directly. The living will can therefore contain detailed instructions on health care activities we would consider acceptable with regard to critical care and ambulatory resuscitation. For example, the living will may instruct whether life support equipment is to be connected in the event we become unconscious. It may also detail specific instructions, such as whether feeding tubes, blood transfusions, the heart-lung machine, ventilators, transplants and other care is acceptable to us, and if so, to what extent or for how long. It should be specific as to what types of medications are acceptable to us, and if so, how long those medications should be sustained. The living will should specify whatever our wishes regarding our health care are with the greatest of clarity and detail.

A critical part of the living will is the appointment of a *health care advocate.* The health care advocate is a person we trust to oversee our health care treatment should we become hospitalized or incapacitated. This person is also given the ability to make decisions on our behalf. Therefore, this person needs to be someone we trust implicitly to carry out our instructions as they are recorded in our living will.

Specific instructions regarding emergency medical treatment are often called *advance medical directives.* In such a situation where we are deemed unable to make our own decisions, these instructions must be followed. It is important that our health care advocate have a copy of this living will so that he or she can show it to doctors and hospital administrators in the case of a our need for emergency treatment. *(The comments above and below are not legal advice. Consult a legal professional for specific advice regarding the living will, advanced medical directives, health advocate and/or other solutions.)*

Without advance medical directives or such a living will, we could be given medications we cannot or do not want to physically, mentally, emotionally or spiritually tolerate for long periods of time. We may be given treatments that leave our bodies alive in suspended animation long after the body's intended death. Our bodies may end up being indefinitely hooked to life support equipment without our consent. In a suspended state, we may not be able to communicate our wishes to be let go. Frequently this issue stresses families, doctors and hospital administrators as they debate the costs and treatment of a *coma, permanent vegetative state* (PVS), or *minimally conscious state* (MCS).

Comas will often be temporary, from a few hours to days, weeks or months. The vegetative and minimally conscious states are typically permanent, however. Many MCS and PVS cases evolve from coma states. MCS is accompanied by cognitive ability, while PVS and the coma state leave observers with a question of whether the person is even there. MRI brain scans have illustrated that MCS patients can both recognize speech and respond—if not physically, through their brainwaves. Most coma and PVS patients appear to not be aware of their surroundings at all. The difference between a comatose and a PVS patient is simply that the PVS subject appears to be awake. This is deceptive, however, because there is still no apparent awareness in the PVS patient. All three states require life support systems—at least feeding tubes. MCS and PVS may only require a feeding tube, while PVS and coma states may also require ventilators.

People do wake up from comas, true. Yet waking up from PVS and MCS is rare. For this reason, the question of whether to maintain life through artificial means is quite controversial. Since the U.S. court system does not recognize coma, PVS or MCS as death, in the absence of specific instructions by the patient or their legal guardian, the hospital may keep these patients alive indefinitely. It is an ethical question that brings into focus the issue of what is death, and at what point should we let nature take its course?

Note that *euthanasia* or *mercy killing* is not being proposed here. Nor are we condoning suicide in any form, even its slower versions—namely alcoholism and drug abuse. Each of us has a designated time of death according to our consciousness and past behavior. No one has the right to interfere with our destiny. This would be fooling around with our most precious asset—time. Time in itself may not seem precious, but it represents the ability to learn. Every moment we dwell within these bodies is accompanied by learning experiences. Even the event of death itself—our leaving the body—is a part of our learning experience.

Each of us can and should make a personal decision of whether we want life support and if so, how long we want to be kept alive with life support should we become comatose, minimally conscious or vegetative.

We can decide for ourselves how long medication will be given if any, and if so, what types of medication types are to be given. We can also predetermine how much pain medication to be given as well. As we have discussed, pain is the rhythmic signaling process that helps escort the inner self out of the body at the intended time. Opioids may have their place during the healing of painful events. They can also block pain from doing its intended job—possibly keeping our bodies struggling with an affliction long after nature intended.

We can make our personal choices known with regard to coma, MCS or PVS in our living will. We can also have a clear conversation with our health advocate on how to oversee our decisions in case of our injury. The health advocate should be easily reachable in the case of our trauma or accident. Our nearest relative is suggested, but we might also consider that this nearest relative might have some conflict of interest in terms of letting go. A close-by attorney could also be appropriate. Our advocate would approve medications being prescribed according to our wishes. They also can check to make sure those medications match the prescriptions written by the attending physician to avoid hospital errors. Many drug mistakes are made by attendants who misread the doctor's script or mistake one medication for another. The doctor may also not realize a medication allergy exists, and the advocate can clarify this.

The advocate can also monitor whether we are receiving enough fluids and are receiving a good diet during our stay in a hospital or home. Hospitals are notorious for serving overly processed and overly sweetened foods, which can spike our blood sugar and cause a variety of metabolic problems. The advocate may request a special diet for us (hopefully plant-based foods with lots of fiber). They may also consider bringing bottled water, whole foods and supplements to us during their visits to the hospital. The doctor should be made aware of these, however.

Life-support systems may prove valuable in cases where a healthy body has been shot or involved in an accident. However, life-support systems used in enduring efforts to keep elderly people in their bodies past their appointed departure times could very well be classified as cruel and unusual punishment. When it is our time to leave the body, we need to be let go. Natural efforts to restart the heart using the palms or opening the esophagus with the *Heimlich maneuver* may be appropriate. However, the endeavor to put the body on a heart and lung machine or other such invasive methods for a significant duration merely enslaves the inner self to a dysfunctional body.

A visit to the intensive care unit of a local hospital will immediately illustrate this effect. We see unconscious surrogates lying in beds with various tubes and machines running their bodies, like some sort of ghoulish *Cocoon* (1985) scene. Their bodies are doped up, propped up and pumped up with synthetics to keep the blood moving and the brain cells minimally alive. This is not much different from lab scientists keeping cells alive in Petri dishes. The only problem is that leashed to each surrogate body is a poor inner self wanting to move on.

Should we allow the medical institution to manage our healthcare unbridled during critical care, they will generally continue treatment with every possible life-sustaining technology. This is their training. Hospital staff are usually very kind and caring. They may not be trained in the subject matter discussed here, however. Few will have studied ethics or have even read the *Classics*. The existence of the inner self and these sorts of ethical issues were profusely discussed in the *Classics* of Aristotle, Socrates, Plato and others. In addition, hospital staff are typically unaware of the body's absolute need for fresh air, sunlight, clean water and natural foods. Today's critical care institutions are set up to not only bring a body back from its natural death, but to ambulate the body for an indefinite period of time using drugs and unnatural restraints.

Our inner self is destined to leave the body at a particular time, determined by a combination of our current state of consciousness (our intentions) and our past activities. Many propose a person's death has been predetermined from birth. Empirical evidence shows that this certainly is not true, however. While a pre-arranged appointment with death might be coded into our body's DNA at birth, our activities throughout our life in the body alter these projections. Epigenetic research has illustrated that our DNA sequencing mutates with our ongoing choices and activities. This is evidenced also by the observation that people die from particular disorders caused by optional lifestyle decisions.

Each of us has a free will as to our intentions. We also have many options on how we exert those intentions as we direct the use of our physical vehicle. The better we care for the body, the longer it will last. This is fundamental to practically any vehicle. This alone does not guarantee a longer lifespan however. Our time of death is also determined by a complex combination of ongoing intentions and desires, associated with the results of our previous decisions and the evolution of our inner self. Our spiritual evolution is something we express directly with pure intention. Should we utilize this lifetime to grow and learn the lessons life presents us with, we will naturally evolve spiritually. This is the Almighty's design for nature's laws of cause and effect.

Our institutions need to support the rhythmic and intentional process of aging and dying—and not tease us with denial and a futile attempt to avoid death at all costs. We also need to care for the elderly while respecting their experience and knowledge. We need to allow the elderly to ponder the mysteries of existence during their final years without being drugged up and delirious. The world also needs to hear the wisdom of the elderly. The elderly must be able to communicate with the rest of us, to share their lifetime of learning. We need to aid and comfort without interfering with mental capacities and facilities. Sure, we can provide pain relief without sacrificing reality.

This same kind of respect needs to be given during the transition time of death. When a person is on his or her final deathbed, a time-honored intentional act is to bring to the bedside a spiritual advisor to offer final rites. This is an important process to assist the inner self in leaving the body while in a state of spiritual consciousness. Whatever our choice of spiritual practice is, gathering a religious guide or fellow worshiper by our bedside to proclaim and address the Almighty during our transition is a time-honored and blessed practice that expresses death with intentional dignity. Being surrounded by surgeons and nurses frantically struggling to keep the body alive despite the body's inability to function is far from dignified. This is dying with desperation.

Regardless of the circumstances of our death, it is the manner in which we lived our lives that ultimately determines our direction upon departure. Once we understand the reality of our identity as deeper than the changing physical body, we can have confidence that whatever intentions we lived with during our physical lives will project us towards our next destination. An intentional journey of learning, love and spiritual development during the life of this body simply continues its progression following our departure.

The healing of the 'real you' has nothing to do with preventing or curing cancer, colds, flu, arthritis, Crohn's, or any other disease. Face it: every body was designed to become diseased and at some point die. *No body makes it out alive.*

It is the healing of the deeper being—the real person inside of the temporary changing body—that is critical to our real health. It is the inner self, the same person who dwelled within the baby body, the teenage body, the adult body and the elderly body, who matters. Even as our bodies have changed, we each remain a distinct individual personality. This distinct individual—you—continues to exist after the body's death.

What will we take away from our life within this body? As the cells and molecules of our temporary body were gradually replaced by new cells and molecules, we took away the knowledge we gained from the experiences we had during those past physical endeavors. It was knowledge we took away. It was learning that we gained from those experiences. Not just the memories; but the lessons of love, giving, taking, and whatever spiritual realizations we've had that continue with us as we move on.

Therefore, healing and learning are synonymous. Healing is the utilization of the conscious anatomy for the purpose of learning. We must glean all the valuable lessons life teaches us each day and each moment. By learning, we grow. By growing, we become healed. Unlike the proposals of the sterile institutions that currently grip the agenda of today's biological and medical sciences, life is not purposeless. We are in fact here to learn and evolve. We are here to gain knowledge, understanding and hopefully the ability to truly love. Without this purpose, there is no logic or rationale for being conscious in the first place.

References and Bibliography

Abdou AM, Higashiguchi S, Horie K, Kim M, Hatta H, Yokogoshi H. Relaxation and immunity enhancement effects of gamma-aminobutyric acid GABA). *Biofactors.* 2006;26(3):201-8.

Abou-Seif MA. Blood antioxidant status and urine sulfate and thiocyanate levels in smokers. *J Biochem Toxicol.* 1996;11(3):133-138.

Ackerman D. *A Natural History of the Senses.* New York: Vintage, 1991.

Ackermann RT, Mulrow CD, Ramirez G, Gardner CD, Morbidoni L, Lawrence VA. Garlic shows promise for improving some cardiovascular risk factors. Arch Intern Med. 2001 Mar 26;161(6):813-24.

Airola P. *How to Get Well.* Phoenix, AZ: Health Plus, 1974.

Aissa J, Harran H, Rabeau M, Boucherie S, Brouilhet H, Benveniste J. Tissue levels of histamine, PAF-acether and lysopaf-acether in carrageenan-induced granuloma in rats. *Int Arch Allergy Immunol.* 1996 Jun;110(2):182-6.

Aissa J, Jurgens P, Litime M, Béhar I, Benveniste J. Electronic transmission of the cholinergic signal. *FASEB Jnl.* 1995;9: A683.

Aissa J, Litime M, Attias E, Allal A, Benveniste J. Transfer of molecular signals via electronic circuitry. *FASEB Jnl.* 1993;7: A602.

Aissa J, Litime MH, Attis E., Benveniste J. Molecular signalling at high dilution or by means of electronic circuitry. *J Immunol.* 1993;150:A146.

Aissa J, Nathan N, Arnoux B, Benveniste J. Biochemical and cellular effects of heparin-protamine injection in rabbits are partially inhibited by a PAF-acether receptor antagonist. *Eur J Pharmacol.* 1996 Apr 29;302(1-3):123-8.

Albrechtsen O. The influence of small atmospheric ions on human well-being and mental performance. *Intern. J. of Biometeorology.* 1978;22(4): 249-262.

Alexandre P, Darmanyan D, Yushen G, Jenks W, Burel L, Eloy D, Jardon P. Quenching of Singlet Oxygen by Oxygen- and Sulfur-Centered Radicals: Evidence for Energy Transfer to Peroxyl Radicals in Solution. *J. Am. Chem. Soc.,* 120 (2), 396 -403, 1998.

Allais G, Bussone G, De Lorenzo C, Castagnoli Gabellari I, Zonca M, Mana O, Borgogno P, Acuto G, Benedetto C. Naproxen sodium in short-term prophylaxis of pure menstrual migraine: pathophysiological and clinical considerations. *Neurol Sci.* 2007 May;28 Suppl 2:S225-8.

Allen SJ, Okoko B, Martinez E, Gregorio G, Dans LF. Probiotics for treating infectious diarrhea. The Cochrane Library. 2004;3. Chichester, UK: John Wiley & Sons, Ltd.

Amassian VE, Cracco RQ, Maccabee PJ. A sense of movement elicited in paralyzed distal arm by focal magnetic coil stimulation of human motor cortex. *Brain Res.* 1989 Feb 13;479(2):355-60.

American Dietetic Association; Dietitians of Canada. Position of the American Dietetic Association and Dietitians of Canada: vegetarian diets. *Can J Diet Pract Res.* 2003 Summer;64(2):62-81.

Ammor MS, Michaelidis C, Nychas GJ. Insights into the role of quorum sensing in food spoilage. *J Food Prot.* 2008 Jul;71(7):1510-25.

Anderson GC, Moore E, Hepworth J, Bergman N. Early skin-to-skin contact for mothers and their healthy newborn infants. *Cochrane Database Syst Rev.* 2003;(2):CD003519.

Anderson RC, Anderson JH. Acute toxic effects of fragrance products. *Arch Environ Health.* 1998 Mar-Apr;53(2):138-46.

Anderson RC, Anderson JH. Respiratory toxicity of fabric softener emissions. *J Toxicol Environ Health.* 2000 May 26;60(2):121-36.

Anderson RC, Anderson JH. Toxic effects of air freshener emissions. *Arch Environ Health.* 1997 Nov-Dec;52(6):433-41.

Anim-Nyame N, Sooranna SR, Johnson MR, Gamble J, Steer PJ. Garlic supplementation increases peripheral blood flow: a role for interleukin-6? J Nutr Biochem. 2004 Jan;15(1):30-6.

Anonymous. Cimetidine inhibits the hepatic hydroxylation of vitamin D. *Nutr Rev.* 1985;43:184-5.

Aoki T, Usuda Y, Miyakoshi H, Tamura K, Herberman RB. Low natural killer syndrome: clinical and immunologic features. *Nat Immun Cell Growth Regul.* 1987;6(3):116-28.

Appleman P ed. *Darwin: A Norton Critical Edition.* New York: Norton, 1970.

Armstrong BK. Absorption of vitamin B12 from the human colon. *Am J Clin Nutr.* 1968;21:298-9.

Aronne LJ, Thornton-Jones ZD. New targets for obesity pharmacotherapy. *Clin Pharmacol Ther.* 2007 May;81(5):748-52.

Asimov I. *The Chemicals of Life.* New York: Signet, 1954.

Askeland D. *The Science and Engineering of Materials.* Boston: PWS, 1994.

Aspect A, Grangier P, Roger G. Experimental Realization of Einstein-Podolsky-Rosen-Bohm Gedankenexperiment: A New Violation of Bell's Inequalities. *Physical Review Letters.* 1982;49(2): 91-94.

Aton SJ, Colwell CS, Harmar AJ, Waschek J, Herzog ED. Vasoactive intestinal polypeptide mediates circadian rhythmicity and synchrony in mammalian clock neurons. *Nat Neurosci.* 2005 Apr;8(4):476-83.

Atsumi T, Tonosaki K. Smelling lavender and rosemary increases free radical scavenging activity and decreases cortisol level in saliva. *Psychiatry Res.* 2007 Feb 28;150(1):89-96.

Avanzini G, Lopez L, Koelsch S, Majno M. The Neurosciences and Music II: From Perception to Performance. *Annals of the New York Academy of Sciences.* 2006 Mar;1060.

Aymard JP, Aymard B, Netter P, Bannwarth B, Trechot P, Streiff F. Haematological adverse effects of histamine H2-receptor antagonists. *Med Toxicol Adverse Drug Exp.* 1988 Nov-Dec;3(6):430-48.

Bach E. *Bach Flower Remedies.* New Canaan, CN: Keats, 1997.

Bach E. *Heal Thyself.* Saffron Walden: CW Daniel, 1931-2003.

Bache C. *Lifecycles: Reincarnation and the Web of Life.* New York: Paragon House, 1994.

Bachmann KA, Sullivan TJ, Jauregui L, Reese J, Miller K, Levine L. Drug interactions of H2-receptor antagonists. *Scand J Gastroenterol Suppl.* 1994;206:14-9.

Backster C. Primary *Perception: Biocommunication with Plants, Living Foods, and Human Cells.* Anza, CA: White Rose Millennium Press, 2003.

Bader J. The relative power of SNPs and haplotype as genetic markers for association tests. *Pharmacogenomics.* 2001;2:11-24.

Bai H, Yu P, Yu M. Effect of electroacununcture on sex hormone levels in patients with Sjogren's syndrome. *Zhen Ci Yan Jiu.* 2007;32(3):203-6.

Baker DW. An introduction to the theory and practice of German electroacupuncture and accompanying medications. *Am J Acupunct.* 1984;12:327-332.

Baker SM. *Detoxification and Healing.* Chicago: Contemporary Books, 2004.

Balch P, Balch J. *Prescription for Nutritional Healing.* New York: Avery, 2000.

Ballentine R. *Diet & Nutrition: A holistic approach.* Honesdale, PA: Himalayan Int., 1978.

Ballentine RM. *Radical Healing.* New York: Harmony Books, 1999.

Bannerjee H. *Americans Who Have Been Reincarnated.* New York: Macmillan, 1980.

Banyo T. The role of electrical neuromodulation in the therapy of chronic lower urinary tract dysfunction. *Ideggyogy Sz.* 2003 Jan 20;56(1-2):68-71.

Baranauskas G, Nistri A. Sensitization of pain pathways in the spinal cord: cellular mechanisms. *Prog Neurobiol.* 1998 Feb;54(3):349-65.

Barber CF. The use of music and colour theory as a behaviour modifier. *Br J Nurs.* 1999 Apr 8-21;8(7):443-8.

Barker A. *Scientific Method in Ptolemy's Harmonics.* Cambridge: Cambridge University Press, 2000.

Barron M. Light exposure, melatonin secretion, and menstrual cycle parameters: an integrative review. *Biol Res Nurs.* 2007 Jul;9(1):49-69.

Bastide M, Doucet-Jaboeuf M, Daurat V. Activity and chronopharmacology of very low doses of physiological immune inducers. *Immun Today.* 1985;6: 234-235.

Bastide M. Immunological examples on ultra high dilution research. In: Endler P, Schulte J (eds.): *Ultra High Dilution. Physiology and Physics.* Dordrech: Kluwer Academic Publishers, 1994:27-34.

Bates DW, Cullen DJ, Laird N, Petersen LA, Small SD, Servi D, Laffel G, Sweitzer BJ, Shea BF, Hallisey R, *et al.* Incidence of adverse drug events and potential adverse drug events. Implications for prevention. ADE Prevention Study Group. *JAMA.* 1995 Jul 5;274(1):29-34.

Batmangheilidj F. Neurotransmitter histamine: an alternative view point, *Science in Medicine Simplified.* Falls Church, VA: Foundation for the Simple in Medicine, 1990.

Batmanghelidj F. *Your Body's Many Cries for Water.* 2nd Ed. Vienna, VA: Global Health, 1992-1997.

Beauvais F, Bidet B, Descours B, Hieblot C, Burtin C, Benveniste J. Regulation of human basophil activation. I. Dissociation of cationic dye binding from histamine release in activated human basophils. *J Allergy Clin Immunol.* 1991 May;87(5):1020-8.

Beauvais F, Burtin C, Benveniste J. Voltage-dependent ion channels on human basophils: do they exist? *Immunol Lett.* 1995 May;46(1-2):81-3.

Beauvais F, Echasserieau K, Burtin C, Benveniste J. Regulation of human basophil activation; the role of Na+ and Ca2+ in IL-3-induced potentiation of IgE-mediated histamine release from human basophils. *Clin Exp Immunol.* 1994 Jan;95(1):191-4.

Beauvais F, Shimahara T, Inoue I, Hieblot C, Burtin C, Benveniste J. Regulation of human basophil activation. II. Histamine release is potentiated by K+ efflux and inhibited by Na+ influx.. *J Immunol.* 1992 Jan 1;148(1):149-54.

Becker R. *Cross Currents.* Los Angeles: Jeremy P. Tarcher, 1990.

Becker R. *The Body Electric.* New York: William Morrow, 1985.

Beckerman H, Becher J, Lankhorst GJ. The effectiveness of vibratory stimulation in anejaculatory men with spinal cord injury. *Paraplegia.* 1993 Nov;31(11):689-99.

Beeson, C. The moon and plant growth. *Nature.* 1946;158:572–3.

Bell B, Defouw R. Concerning a lunar modulation of geomagnetic activity. *J Geophys Res.* 1964;69:3169-3174.

Bell IR, Baldwin CM, Schwartz GE, Illness from low levels of environmental chemicals: relevance to chronic fatigue syndrome and fibromyalgia. *Am J Med.* 1998;105 (suppl 3A).:74-82. S.

Beloff J. Parapsychology and radical dualism. *J Rel & Psych Res.* 1985;8, 3-10.

Benatuil L, Apitz-Castro R, Romano E. Ajoene inhibits the activation of human endothelial cells induced by porcine cells: implications for xenotransplantation. *Xenotransplantation.* 2003 Jul;10(4):368-73.

Benedetti F, Radaelli D, Bernasconi A, Dallaspezia S, Falini A, Scotti G, Lorenzi C, Colombo C, Smeraldi E. Clock genes beyond the clock: CLOCK genotype biases neural correlates of moral valence decision in depressed patients. *Genes Brain Behav.* 2007 Mar 26.

Bengmark S. Curcumin, an atoxic antioxidant and natural NFkappaB, cyclooxygenase-2, lipooxygenase, and inducible nitric oxide synthase inhibitor: a shield against acute and chronic diseases. *JPEN J Parenter Enteral Nutr.* 2006 Jan-Feb;30(1):45-51.

Bennett GJ, Update on the neurophysiology of pain transmission and modulation: focus on the NMDA-receptor. *J Pain Symptom Manage.* 2000;19 (suppl 1):S.:2-6.

Benor D. Healing Research. Volume 1. Munich, Germany: Helix Verlag, 1992.

Bensky D, Gable A, Kaptchuk T (transl.). *Chinese Herbal Medicine Materia Medica.* Seattle: Eastland Press, 1986.

Bentley E. *Awareness: Biorhythms, Sleep and Dreaming.* London: Routledge, 2000

Benveniste J, Aïssa J, Guillonnet D. A simple and fast method for in vivo demonstration of electromagnetic molecular signaling (EMS) via high dilution or computer recording. *FASEB Jnl.* 1999;13: A163.

Benveniste J, Aïssa J, Guillonnet D. Digital Biology : Specificity of the digitized molecular signal. *FASEB Jnl.* 1998;12: A412.

Benveniste J, Aïssa J, Guillonnet D. The molecular signal is not functional in the absence of "informed" water. *FASEB Jnl.* 1999;13: A163.

Benveniste J, Aïssa J, Litime M, Tsangaris G, Thomas Y. Transfer of the molecular signal by electronic amplification. *FASEB J.* 1994;8:A398.

Benveniste J, Arnoux B, Hadji L. Highly dilute antigen increases coronary flow of isolated heart from immunized guinea-pigs. *FASEB J.* 1992;6:A1610.

Benveniste J, Davenas E, Ducot B, Spira A. Basophil achromasia by dilute ligand: a reappraisal. *FASEB Jnl.* 1991;5: A1008.

Benveniste J, Ducot B, Spira A. Memory of water revisited. *Nature.* 1994 Aug 4;370(6488):322.

Benveniste J, Guillonnet D. QED and digital biology. *Riv Biol.* 2004 Jan-Apr;97(1):169-72.

Benveniste J, Jurgens P, Aïssa J. Digital recording/transmission of the cholinergic signal. *FASEB Jnl.* 1996;10: A1479.

Benveniste J, Jurgens P, Hsueh W, Aïssa J. Transatlantic transfer of digitized antigen signal by telephone link. *Jnl Aller Clin Immun.* 1997;99: S175.

Benveniste J, Kahhak L, Guillonnet D. Specific remote detection of bacteria using an electromagnetic / digital procedure. *FASEB Jnl.* 1999;13: A852.

Benveniste J. Benveniste on Nature investigation. *Science.* 1988 Aug 26;241(4869):1028.

Benveniste J. Benveniste on the Benveniste affair. *Nature.* 1988 Oct 27;335(6193):759.

Benveniste J. Diagnosis of allergic diseases by basophil count and in vitro degranulation using manual and automated tests. *Nouv Presse Med.* 1981 Jan 24;10(3):165-9.

Benveniste J. Meta-analysis of homoeopathy trials. *Lancet.* 1998 Jan 31;351(9099):367.

Berg A, Konig D, Deibert P, Grathwohl D, Berg A, Baumstark MW, Franz IW. Effect of an oat bran enriched diet on the atherogenic lipid profile in patients with an increased coronary heart disease risk. A controlled randomized lifestyle intervention study. *Ann Nutr Metab.* 2003;47(6):306-11.

Bergner P. *The Healing Power of Garlic.* Prima Publishing, Rocklin CA 1996.

Berk M, Dodd S, Henry M. Do ambient electromagnetic fields affect behaviour? A demonstration of the relationship between geomagnetic storm activity and suicide. *Bioelectromagnetics.* 2006 Feb;27(2):151-5.

Berman S, Fein G, Jewett D, Ashford F. Luminance-controlled pupil size affects Landolt C task performance. *J Illumin Engng Soc.* 1993;22:150-165.

Berman S, Jewett D, Fein G, Saika G, Ashford F. Photopic luminance does not always predict perceived room brightness. *Light Resch and Techn.* 1990;22:37-41.

Bernardi D, Dini FL, Azzarelli A, Giaconi A, Volterrani C, Lunardi M. Sudden cardiac death rate in an area characterized by high incidence of coronary artery disease and low hardness of drinking water. *Angiology.* 1995;46:145-149.

Bertin G. *Spiral Structure in Galaxies: A Density Wave Theory.* Cambridge: MIT Press, 1996.

Bhandari U, Sharma JN, Zafar R. The protective action of ethanolic ginger (Zingiber officinale) extract in cholesterol fed rabbits. J Ethnopharmacol. 1998 Jun;61(2):167-71.

Bharani A, Ganguli A, Mathur LK, Jamra Y, Raman PG. Efficacy of Terminalia arjuna in chronic stable angina: a double-blind, placebo-controlled, crossover study comparing Terminalia arjuna with isosorbide mononitrate. Indian Heart J. 2002 Mar-Apr; 54(2):170-5.

Bharani A, Ganguly A, Bhargava KD. Salutary effect of Terminalia Arjuna in patients with severe refractory heart failure. Int J Cardiol. 1995 May;49(3):191-9.

Bhattacharjee C, Bradley P, Smith M, Scally A, Wilson B. Do animals bite more during a full moon? *BMJ.* 2000 December 23; 321(7276): 1559-1561.

Bishop B. Pain: its physiology and rationale for management. Part III. Consequences of current concepts of pain mechanisms related to pain management. *Phys Ther.* 1980 Jan;60(1):24-37.

Bishop, C. Moon influence in lettuce growth. *Astrol J.* 1977;10(1):13-15.

Bitbol M, Luisi PL. Autopoiesis with or without cognition: defining life at its edge. *J R Soc Interface.* 2004 Nov 22;1(1):99-107.

Blackmore SJ. Near-death experiences. J R Soc Med. 1996 Feb;89(2):73-6.

Bockemühl, J. *Towards a Phenomenology of the Etheric World.* New York: Anthroposophical Press, 1985.

Bodnar L, Simhan H. The prevalence of preterm birth varies by season of last menstrual period. *Am J Obst and Gyn.* 2003:195(6);S211-S211.

Boivin DB, Czeisler CA. Resetting of circadian melatonin and cortisol rhythms in humans by ordinary room light. *Neuroreport.* 1998 Mar 30;9(5):779-82.

Boivin DB, Duffy JF, Kronauer RE, Czeisler CA. Dose-response relationships for resetting of human circadian clock by light. *Nature.* 1996 Feb 8;379(6565):540-2.

Borchers AT, Hackman RM, Keen CL, Stern JS, Gershwin ME. Complementary medicine: a review of immunomodulatory effects of Chinese herbal medicines. *Am J Clin Nutr.* 1997 Dec;66(6):1303-12.

Borets VM, Lis MA, Pyrochkin VM, Kishkovich VP, Butkevich ND. Therapeutic efficacy of pantothenic acid preparations in ischemic heart disease patients. *Vopr Pitan.* 1987 Mar-Apr;(2):15-7.

Bose J. *Response in the Living and Non-Living.* New York: Longmans, Green & Co., 1902.

Bottorff JL. The use and meaning of touch in caring for patients with cancer. *Oncol Nurs Forum.* 1993 Nov-Dec;20(10):1531-8.

Bourgine P, Stewart J. Autopoiesis and cognition. *Artif Life.* 2004 Summer;10(3):327-45.

Bowler PJ. *The Eclipse of Darwinism: Antievolutionary Theories in the Decades Around 1900.* Baltimore: Johns Hopkins, 1983.

Brasseur JG, Nicosia MA, Pal A, Miller LS. Function of longitudinal vs circular muscle fibers in esophageal peristalsis, deduced with mathematical modeling. *World J Gastroenterol.* 2007 Mar 7;13(9):1335-46.

Braude S. *First Person Plural: Multiple Personality and the Philosophy of Mind.* Landham, MD: Rowman & Littlefield, 1995.

Braunstein G, Labat C, Brunelleschi S, Benveniste J, Marsac J, Brink C. Evidence that the histamine sensitivity and responsiveness of guinea-pig isolated trachea are modulated by epithelial prostaglandin E2 production. *Br J Pharmacol.* 1988 Sep;95(1):300-8.

Brighenti F, Valtueña S, Pellegrini N, Ardigò D, Del Rio D, Salvatore S, Piatti P, Serafini M, Zavaroni I. Total Antioxidant Capacity of the Diet Is Inversely and Independently Related to Plasma Concentration of High-Sensitivity C-Reactive Protein in Adult Italian Subjects. *Br J Nutr.* 2005;93(5):619-25.

Brinkhaus B, Witt CM, Jena S, Linde K, Streng A, Hummelsberger J, Irnich D, Hammes M, Pach D, Melchart D, Willich SN. Physician and treatment characteristics in a randomised multicentre trial of acupuncture in patients with osteoarthritis of the knee. *Complement Ther Med.* 2007 Sep;15(3):180-9.

Britt R. Hole Drilled to Bottom of Earth's Crust, Breakthrough to Mantle Looms. *LiveScience.* 2005. 07 Apr. http://www.livescience.com/ technology/050407_earth_drill.html. Acc. 2006 Nov.

Britton WB, Bootzin RR. Near-death experiences and the temporal lobe. Psychol Sci. 2004 Apr;15(4):254-8.

Brodeur P. Currents of Death. New York: Simon and Schuster, 1989.

Brody J. *Jane Brody's Nutrition Book.* New York: WW Norton, 1981.

Brosseau LU, Pelland LU, Casimiro LY, Robinson VI, Tugwell PE, Wells GE. Electrical stimulation for the treatment of rheumatoid arthritis. *Cochrane Database Syst Rev.* 2002;(2):CD003687.

Brown V. *The Amateur Naturalists Handbook.* Englewood Cliffs, NJ: Prentice-Hall, 1980.

Brown, F. & Chow, C.S. Lunar-correlated variations in water uptake by bean seeds. *Biolog Bull.* 1973;145:265-278.

Brown, F. The rhythmic nature of animals and plants. *Cycles.* 1960 Apr:81-92.

Brown, J. Stimulation-produced analgesia: acupuncture, TENS and alternative techniques. *Anaesthesia &intensive care medicine.* 2005 Feb;6(2):45-47.

Browne J. Developmental Care - Considerations for Touch and Massage in the Neonatal Intensive Care Unit. *Neonatatal Network.* 2000 Feb;19(1).

Brownstein D. *Salt: Your Way to Health.* West Bloomfield, MI: Medical Alternatives, 2006.

Brummer RJ, Geerling BJ, Stockbrugger RW. Initial and chronic gastric acid inhibition by lansoprazole and omeprazole in relation to meal administration. *Dig Dis Sci.* 1997;42:2132-7.

Buck L, Axel R. A novel multigene family may encode odorant receptors: A molecule basis for odor recognition. *Cell.* 1991;65(April 5):175-187.

Buckley NA, Whyte IM, Dawson AH. There are days ... and moons. Self-poisoning is not lunacy. *Med J Aust.* 1993 Dec 6-20;159(11-12):786-9.

Buijs RM, Scheer FA, Kreier F, Yi C, Bos N, Goncharuk VD, Kalsbeek A. Organization of circadian functions: interaction with the body. *Prog Brain Res.* 2006;153:341-60.

Bulsing PJ, Smeets MA, van den Hout MA. Positive Implicit Attitudes toward Odor Words. *Chem Senses.* 2007 May 7.

Burgess JF. Causative Factors in Eczema. *Can Med Assoc J.* 1930 Feb; 22(2): 207-211.

Burnham K, Andersson D. *Model Selection and Inference. A Practical Information-Theoretic Approach.* New York: Springer, 1998

Burr H, Hovland C. Bio-Electric Potential Gradients in the Chick. *Yale Journal of Biology & Medicine.* 1937;9:247-258

Burr H, Lane C, Nims L. A Vacuum Tube Microvoltmeter for the Measurement of Bioelectric Phenomena. *Yale Journal of Biology & Medicine.* 1936;10:65-76.

Burr H, Smith G, Strong L. Bio-electric Properties of Cancer-Resistant and Cancer-Susceptible Mice. *American Journal of Cancer.* 1938;32:240-248

Burr H. *The Fields of Life.* New York: Ballantine, 1972.

Buzsaki G. Theta rhythm of navigation: link between path integration and landmark navigation, episodic and semantic memory. *Hippocampus.* 2005;15(7):827-40.

Cajochen C, Jewett ME, Dijk DJ. Human circadian melatonin rhythm phase delay during a fixed sleep-wake schedule interspersed with nights of sleep deprivation. *J Pineal Res.* 2003 Oct;35(3):149-57.

Cajochen C, Zeitzer JM, Czeisler CA, Dijk DJ. Dose-response relationship for light intensity and ocular and electroencephalographic correlates of human alertness. *Behav Brain Res.* 2000 Oct;115(1):75-83.

Callender ST, Spray GH. Latent pernicious anemia. *Br J Haematol* 1962;8:230-240.

Calvin W. *The Handbook of Brain Theory and Neural Networks.* Boston: MIT Press, 1995.

Campbell A. The role of aluminum and copper on neuroinflammation and Alzheimer's disease. *J Alzheimers Dis.* 2006 Nov;10(2-3):165-72.

Capitani D, Yethiraj A, Burnell EE. Memory effects across surfactant mesophases. *Langmuir.* 2007 Mar 13;23(6):3036-48.

Carlsen E, Olsson C, Petersen JH, Andersson AM, Skakkebaek NE. Diurnal rhythm in serum levels of inhibin B in normal men: relation to testicular steroids and gonadotropins. *J Clin Endocrinol Metab.* 1999 May;84(5):1664-9.

Carlson DL, Hites RA. Polychlorinated biphenyls in salmon and salmon feed: global differences and bioaccumulation. *Environ Sci Technol.* 2005 Oct 1;39(19):7389-95.

Carroll D. *The Complete Book of Natural Medicines.* New York: Summit, 1980.

Cassileth B, Trevisan C, Gubili J. Complementary therapies for cancer pain. *Curr Pain Headache Rep.* 2007 Aug;11(4):265-9.

Cavalli-Sforza L, Feldman M. *Cultural Transmission and Evolution: A quantitative approach.* Princeton: Princeton UP, 1981.

Celec P, Ostatníková D, Hodosy J, Skoknová M, Putz Z, Kúdela M. Infradian rhythmic variations of salivary estradioland progesterone in healthy men. *Biol Res.* 2006;37(1): 37-44.

Celec P, Ostatníková D, Putz Z, Hodosy J, Burský P, Stárka L, Hampl R, Kúdela M. Circatrigintan Cycle of Salivary Testosterone in Human Male. *Biol Rhythm Res.* 2003;34(3): 305-315.

Celec P. Analysis of rhythmic variance - ANORVA. A new simple method for detecting rhythms in biological time series. *Biol Res.* 2004;37:777-782.

Cengel YA, *Heat Transfer: A Practical Approach.* Boston: McGraw-Hill, 1998.

Cesarone MR, Belcaro G, Nicolaides AN, Ricci A, Geroulakos G, Ippolito E, Brandolini R, Vinciguerra G, Dugall M, Griffin M, Ruffini I, Acerbi G, Corsi M, Riordan NH, Stuard S, Bavera P, Di Renzo A, Kenyon J, Errichi BM. Prevention of venous thrombosis in long-haul flights with Flite Tabs: the LONFLIT-FLITE randomized, controlled trial. *Angiology.* 2003 Sep-Oct;54(5):531-9.

Chaitow L, Trenev N. *ProBiotics.* New York: Thorsons, 1990.

Chaitow L. *Conquer Pain the Natural Way.* San Francisco: Chronicle Books, 2002.

Cham, B. Solasodine glycosides as anti-cancer agents: Pre-clinical and Clinical studies. *Asia Pac J Pharmac.* 1994;9: 113-118.

Chaney M, Ross M. *Nutrition.* New York: Houghton Mifflin, 1971.

Chao A, Thun MJ, Connell CJ, McCullough ML, Jacobs EJ, Flanders WD, Rodriguez C, Sinha R, Calle EE. Meat Consumption and Risk of Colorectal Cancer. *JAMA.* 2005 January 12: 172-182.

Chapat L, Chemin K, Dubois B, Bourdet-Sicard R, Kaiserlian D. Lactobacillus casei reduces CD8+ T cell-mediated skin inflammation. Eur J Immunol. 2004 Sep;34(9):2520-8.

Chapidze G, Kapanadze S, Dolidze N, Bachutashvili Z, Latsabidze N. Prevention of coronary atherosclerosis by the use of combination therapy with antioxidant coenzyme q10 and statins. Georgian Med News. 2005 Jan;(1):20-5.

Characterization and quantitation of Antioxidant Constituents of Sweet Pepper (*Capsicum annuum* - Cayenne). *J Agric Food Chem.* 2004 Jun 16;52(12):3861-9.

Chen HY, Shi Y, Ng CS, Chan SM, Yung KK, Zhang QL. Auricular acupuncture treatment for insomnia: a systematic review. *J Altern Complement Med.* 2007 Jul-Aug;13(6):669-76.

Chen-Goodspeed M, Cheng Chi Lee. Tumor suppression and circadian function. *J Biol Rhythms.* 2007 Aug;22(4):291-8.
Chilton F, Tucker L. *Win the War Within.* New York: Rodale, 2006.
Chirkova E. Mathematical methods of detection of biological and heliogeophysical rhythms in the light of developments in modern heliobiology: A platform for discussion. *Cybernet Sys.* 2000;31(6):903-918.
Chirkova EN, Suslov LS, Avramenko MM, Krivoruchko GE. Monthly and daily biorhythms of amylase in the blood of healthy men and their relation with the rhythms in the external environment. *Lab Delo.* 1990;(4):40-4.
Choi DW. Glutamate neurotoxicity and diseases of the nervous system. *Neuron.* 1988;1:623-34.
Chong AS, Boussy IA, Jiang XL, Lamas M, Graf LH Jr. CD54/ICAM-1 is acostimulator of NK cell-mediated cytotoxicity. *Cell Immunol.* 1994 Aug;157(1):92-105.
Chong NW, Codd V, Chan D, Samani NJ. Circadian clock genes cause activation of the human PAI-1 gene promoter with 4G/5G allelic preference. *FEBS Lett.* 2006 Aug 7;580(18):4469-72.
Christopher J. *School of Natural Healing.* Springville UT: Christopher Publ, 1976.
Christophersen, A. G., Jun, H., Jørgensen, K., and Skibsted, L. H. Photobleaching of astaxanthin and canthaxanthin: quantum-yields dependence of solvent, temperature, and wavelength of irradiation in relation to packageing and storage of carotenoid pigmented salmonoids. *Z. Lebensm. Unters. Forsch.*, 1991;192:433-439.
Chu Q, Wang L, Liu GZ. Clinical observation on acupuncture for treatment of diabetic nephropathy. *Zhongguo Zhen Jiu.* 2007 Jul;27(7):488-90.
Churchill G, Doerge R. Empirical threshold values for quantitative trait mapping. *Genetics* 1994;138:963-971.
Chwirot B, Kowalska M, Plóciennik N, Piwinski M, Michniewicz Z, Chwirot S. Variability of spectra of laser-induced fluorescence of colonic mucosa: Its significance for fluorescence detection of colonic neoplasia. *Indian J Exp. Biol.* 2003;41(5):500-510.
Chwirot WB, Popp F. White-light-induced luminescence and mitotic activity of yeast cells. *Folia Histochemica et Cytobiologica.* 1991;29(4):155.
Citro M, Endler PC, Pongratz W, Vinattieri C, Smith CW, Schulte J. Hormone effects by electronic transmission. *FASEB J.* 1995:Abstract 12161.
Citro M, Smith CW, Scott-Morley A, Pongratz W, Endler PC. Transfer of information from molecules by means of electronic amplification, in P.C. Endler, J. Schulte (eds.): *Ultra High Dilution. Physiology and Physics.* Dordrecht: Kluwer Academic Publishers. 1994;209-214.
Clark D. The use of electrical current in the treatment of nonunions. Vet Clin North Am Small Anim Pract. 1987 Jul;17(4):793-8.
Cocilovo A. Colored light therapy: overview of its history, theory, recent developments and clinical applications combined with acupuncture. *Am J Acupunct.* 1999;27(1-2):71-83.
Cohen S, Popp F. Biophoton emission of the human body. *J Photochem & Photobio.* 1997;B 40:187-189.
Cohen S, Popp F. Low-level luminescence of the human skin. *Skin Res Tech.* 1997;3:177-180.
Coles JA, Yamane S. Effects of adapting lights on the time course of the receptor potential of the anuran retinal rod. *J Physiol.* 1975 May;247(1):189-207.
Coll AP, Farooqi IS, O'Rahilly S. The hormonal control of food intake. *Cell.* 2007 Apr 20;129(2):251-62.
Conely J. Music and the Military. *Air University Review.* 1972 Mar-Ap.
Conquer JA, Holub BJ. Dietary docosahexaenoic acid as a source of eicosapentaenoic acid in vegetarians and omnivores. Lipids. 1997 Mar;32(3):341-5.
Contreras D, Steriade M. Cellular basis of EEG slow rhythms: a study of dynamic corticothalamic relationships. *J Neurosci.* 1995 Jan;15(1 Pt 2):604-22.
Cook J, The Therapeutic Use of Music. *Nursing Forum.* 1981;20:3: 253-66.
Cooper K. *The Aerobics Program for Total Well-Being.* New York: Evans, 1980.
Corkin S, Amaral DG, González RG, et al: H. M.'s medial temporal lobe lesion: findings from magnetic resonance imaging. *J Neurosci.* 1997;17:3964-3979.
Cox CB. Emory-led Study Links Metals to Alzheimer's and Other Neurodegenerative Diseases. *Emory Univ Mag.* 2007 Aug 10.
Craciunescu CN, Wu R, Zeisel SH. Diethanolamine alters neurogenesis and induces apoptosis in fetal mouse hippocampus. *FASEB J.* 2006 Aug;20(10):1635-40.
Crawley J. *The Biorhythm Book.* Boston: Journey Editions, 1996.
Creinin MD, Keverline S, Meyn LA. How regular is regular? An analysis of menstrual cycle regularity. *Contraception.* 2004 Oct;70(4):289-92.
Crick F. *Life Itself: Its Origin and Nature.* New York: Simon and Schuster, 1981.
Crofford LJ. Neuroendocrine abnormalities in fibromyalgia and related disorders. *Am J Med Sci.* 1998;315:359-66.

Cross ML. Immune-signalling by orally-delivered probiotic bacteria: effects on common mucosal immunoresponses and protection at distal mucosal sites. Int J Immunopathol Pharmacol. 2004 May-Aug;17(2):127-134.

Cruccu G, Aziz TZ, Garcia-Larrea L, Hansson P, Jensen TS, Lefaucheur JP, Simpson BA, Taylor RS. EFNS guidelines on neurostimulation therapy for neuropathic pain. *Eur J Neurol.* 2007 Sep;14(9):952-70.

Cummings DE, Overduin J. Gastrointestinal regulation of food intake. *J Clin Invest.* 2007 Jan;117(1):13-23.

Cummings M. *Human Heredity: Principles and Issues.* St. Paul, MN: West, 1988.

Curtis LH, Østbye T, Sendersky V, Hutchison S, Dans PE, Wright A, Woosley RL, Schulman KA. Inappropriate prescribing for elderly Americans in a large outpatient population. *Arch Intern Med.* 2004 Aug 9-23;164(15):1621-5.

Cuthbert SC, Goodheart GJ Jr. On the reliability and validity of manual muscle testing: a literature review. *Chiropr Osteopat.* 2007 Mar 6;15:4.

Dalmose A, Bjarkam C, Vuckovic A, Sorensen JC, Hansen J. Electrostimulation: a future treatment option for patients with neurogenic urodynamic disorders? *APMIS Suppl.* 2003;(109):45-51.

Darrow K. *The Renaissance of Physics.* New York: Macmillan, 1936.

Das UN. A defect in the activity of Delta6 and Delta5 desaturases may be a factor predisposing to the development of insulin resistance syndrome. *Prostagl Leukot Essent Fatty Acids.* 2005; May;72(5):343-50.

Davenas E, Beauvais F, Amara J, Oberbaum M, Robinzon B, Miadonna B, Tedeschi A, Pomeranz B, Fortner P, Belon P, Sainte-Laudy J, Poitevin B, Benveniste J. Human basophil degranulation triggered by very dilute antiserum against IgE. *Nature.* 1988;333: 816-818.

Davenas E, Poitevin B, Benveniste J. Effect on mouse peritoneal macrophages of orally administered very high dilutions of silica. *European Journal of Pharmacology.* 1987;135: 313-319.

Davidson T. *Rhinology: The Collected Writings of Maurice H. Cottle, M.D.* San Diego, CA: American Rhinologic Society, 1987.

DaVinci L. (Dickens E. ed.) *The Da Vinci Notebooks.* London: Profile, 2005.

Davis GE Jr, Lowell WE. Chaotic solar cycles modulate the incidence and severity of mental illness. *Med Hypotheses.* 2004;62(2):207-14.

Davis GE Jr, Lowell WE. Solar cycles and their relationship to human disease and adaptability. *Med Hypotheses.* 2006;67(3):447-61.

Davis GE Jr, Lowell WE. The Sun determines human longevity: teratogenic effects of chaotic solar radiation. *Med Hypotheses.* 2004;63(4):574-81.

Dawkins R. *Climbing Mount Improbable.* New York: Viking Press, 1996.

Dawkins R. *River out of Eden.* London: Weidenfeld and Nicholson, 1995.

Dawkins R. *The Blind Watchmaker.* Essex: Longman Scientific and Technical, 1986.

Dawkins R. *The Selfish Gene.* Oxford: Oxford UP, 1977 (1989 edition).

De Lucca AJ, Bland JM, Vigo CB, Cushion M, Selitrennikoff CP, Peter J, Walsh TJ. CAY-I, a fungicidal saponin from Capsicum sp. fruit. Med Mycol. 2002 Apr;40(2):131-7.

Dean C. *Death by Modern Medicine.* Belleville, ON: Matrix Verite-Media, 2005.

Dean E, Mihalasky J, Ostrander S, Schroeder L. *Executive ESP.* Englewood Cliffs, NJ: Prentice-Hall, 1974.

Dean E. Infrared measurements of healer-treated water. In: Roll W, Beloff J, White R (Eds.): *Research in parapsychology 1982.* Metuchen, NJ: Scarecrow Press, 1983:100-101.

Defrin R, Ohry A, Blumen N, Urca G. Sensory determinants of thermal pain. *Brain.* 2002 Mar;125(Pt 3):501-10.

Deitel M. Applications of electrical pacing in the body. *Obes Surg.* 2004 Sep;14 Suppl 1:S3-8.

Del Giudice E, Preparata G, Vitiello G. Water as a free electric dipole laser. *Phys Rev Lett.* 1988;61:1085-1088.

Del Giudice E. Is the 'memory of water' a physical impossibility?, in P.C. Endler, J. Schulte (eds.): *Ultra High Dilution. Physiology and Physics.* Dordrecht: Kluwer Academic Publishers, 1994:117-120.

Delcomyn F. *Foundations of Neurobiology.* New York: W.H. Freeman and Co., 1998.

Dement W, Vaughan C. *The Promise of Sleep.* New York: Dell, 1999.

Dennett D. *Brainstorms: Philosophical Essays on Mind & Psychology.* Cambridge: MIT Press., 1980.

Dennett D. *Consciousness Explained.* London: Little, Brown and Co., 1991.

Depue BE, Banich MT, Curran T. Suppression of emotional and nonemotional content in memory: effects of repetition on cognitive control. *Psychol Sci.* 2006 May;17(5):441-7.

Dere E, Kart-Teke E, Huston JP, De Souza Silva MA. The case for episodic memory in animals. *Neurosci Biobehav Rev.* 2006;30(8):1206-24.

Devaraj TL. *Speaking of Ayurvedic Remedies for Common Diseases.* New Delhi: Sterling, 1985.

Devulder J, Crombez E, Mortier E. Central pain: an overview. *Acta Neurol Belg.* 2002 Sep;102(3):97-103.

Dhond RP, Kettner N, Napadow V. Neuroimaging acupuncture effects in the human brain. *J Altern Complement Med.* 2007 Jul-Aug;13(6):603-16.

Dimitriadis GD, Raptis SA. Thyroid hormone excess and glucose intolerance. *Exp Clin Endocrinol Diabetes.* 2001;109 Suppl 2:S225-39.

Dobrowolski J, Ezzahir A, Knapik M. Possibilities of chemiluminescence application in comparative studies of animal and cancer cells with special attention to leucemic blood cells. In: Jezowska-Trzebiatowska, B., *et al.* (eds.). *Photon Emission from Biological Systems.* Singapore: World Scientific Publ, 1987:170-183.

Dolcos F, LaBar KS, Cabeza R. Interaction between the amygdala and the medial temporal lobe memory system predicts better memory for emotional events. *Neuron.* 2004 Jun 10;42(5):855-63.

Domonkos AN, Arnold HL, Odom RB. *Andrews' Diseases of the Skin: Clinical Dermatology.* 7th ed. Philadelphia, PA

Dong MH, Kaunitz JD. Gastroduodenal mucosal defense. *Curr Opin Gastroenterol.* 2006 Nov;22(6):599-606.

D'Orazio N, Ficoneri C, Riccioni G, Conti P, Theoharides TC, Bollea MR. Conjugated linoleic acid: a functional food? Int J Immunopathol Pharmacol. 2003 Sep-Dec;16(3):215-20.

Dotolo Institute. *The Study of Colon Hydrotherapy.* Pinellas Park, FL: Dotolo, 2003.

Drubaix I, Robert L, Maraval M, Robert AM. Synthesis of glycoconjugates by human diseased veins: modulation by procyanidolic oligomers. Int J Exp Pathol. 1997 Apr;78(2):117-21.

Dubrov, A. *Human Biorhythms and the Moon.* New York: Nova Science Publ., 1996.

Duke J. *The Green Pharmacy.* New York: St. Martins, 1997.

Duke M. *Acupuncture.* New York: Pyramid, 1973.

Dunlop KA, Carson DJ, Shields MD. Hypoglycemia due to adrenal suppression secondary to high-dose nebulized corticosteroid. *Pediatr Pulmonol.* 2002 Jul;34(1):85-6.

Dunne B, Jahn R, Nelson R. Precognitive Remote Perception. Princeton Engineering Anomalies *Res Lab Rep.* Princeton. 1983 Aug.

Dunstan JA, Roper J, Mitoulas L, Hartmann PE, Simmer K, Prescott SL. The effect of supplementation with fish oil during pregnancy on breast milk immunoglobulin A, soluble CD14, cytokine levels and fatty acid composition. *Clin Exp Allergy.* 2004 Aug;34(8):1237-42.

Durlach J, Bara M, Guiet-Bara A. Magnesium level in drinking water: its importance in cardiovascular risk. In: Itokawa Y, Durlach J: *Magnesium in Health and Disease.* London: J.Libbey, 1989:173-182.

Dwivedi S, Agarwal MP. Antianginal and cardioprotective effects of Terminalia arjuna, an indigenous drug, in coronary artery disease. *J Assoc Physicians India.* 1994 Apr;42(4):287-9.

Dwivedi S, Jauhari R. Beneficial effects of Terminalia arjuna in coronary artery disease. *Indian Heart J.* 1997 Sep-Oct;49(5):507-10.

Ebbesen F, Agati G, Pratesi R. Phototherapy with turquoise versus blue light. *Arch Dis Child Fetal Neonatal Ed.* 2003 Sep;88(5):F430-1.

Eden D, Feinstein D. *Energy Medicine.* New York: Penguin Putnam, 1998.

Edris AE. Pharmaceutical and therapeutic potentials of essential oils and their individual volatile constituents: a review. *Phytother Res.* 2007 Apr;21(4):308-23.

Edwards B. *Drawing on the Right Side of the Brain.* Los Angeles, CA: Tarcher, 1979.

Edwards R, Ibison M, Jessel-Kenyon J, Taylor R. Light emission from the human body. *Comple Med Res.* 1989;3(2): 16-19.

Edwards R, Ibison M, Jessel-Kenyon J, Taylor R. Measurements of human bioluminescence. *Acup Elect Res, Intl Jnl,* 1990;15: 85-94.

Edwards, L. *The Vortex of Life, Nature's Patterns in Space and Time.* Floris Press, 1993.

Egon G, Chartier-Kastler E, Denys P, Ruffion A. Spinal cord injury patient and Brindley neurostimulation. *Prog Urol.* 2007 May;17(3):535-9.

Electromagnetic fields: the biological evidence. *Science.* 1990;249: 1378-1381.

Electronic Evidence of Auras, Chakras in UCLA Study. *Brain/Mind Bulletin.* 1978;3:9 Mar 20.

Elias S, van Noord P, Peeters P, den Tonkelaar I, Kaaks R, Grobbee D. Menstruation during and after caloric restriction: The 1944-1945 Dutch famine. *Fertil Steril.* 2007 Jun 1.

Elwood PC. Epidemiology and trace elements. *Clin Endocrinol Metab.* 1985 Aug;14(3):617-28.

Endler PC, Pongratz W, Smith CW, Schulte J. Non-molecular information transfer from thyroxine to frogs with regard to 'homoeopathic' toxicology, *J Vet Hum Tox.* 1995:37:259-260.

Endler PC, Pongratz W, Van Wijk R, Kastberger G, Haidvogl M. Effects of highly diluted sucussed thyroxine on metamorphosis of highland frogs, *Berlin J Res Hom.* 1991;1:151-160.

Endler PC, Pongratz W, Van Wijk R, Waltl K, Hilgers H, Brandmaier R. Transmission of hormone information by non-molecular means, *FASEB J.* 1994;8:A400.

Endler PC, Pongratz W, Van Wijk R, Wiegant F, Waltl K, Gehrer M, Hilgers H. A zoological example on ultra high dilution research. In: Endler PC, Schulte J (eds.): *Ultra High Dilution. Physiology and Physics.* Dordrecht: Kluwer Academic Publishers. 1994:39-68.

Endler PC, Schulte, J. *Ultra High Dilution. Physiology and Physics.* Dordrecht: Kluwer Academic Publ, 1994.

Environmental Working Group. *Human Toxome Project.* 2007. http://www.ewg.org/sites/humantoxome/. Acc. 2007 Sep.

Erdelyi R. MHD waves and oscillations in the solar plasma. Introduction. *Philos Transact A Math Phys Eng Sci.* 2006 Feb 15;364(1839):289-96.

Ernst E. Herbal remedies for anxiety - a systematic review of controlled clinical trials. *Phytomedicine.* 2006 Feb;13(3):205-8.

Esch T, Stefano GB. The Neurobiology of Love. *Neuro Endocrinol Lett.* 2005 Jun;26(3):175-92.

Eschenhagen T, Zimmermann WH. Engineering myocardial tissue. *Circ Res.* 2005 Dec 9;97(12):1220-31.

Evans P, Forte D, Jacobs C, Fredhoi C, Aitchison E, Hucklebridge F, Clow A. Cortisol secretory activity in older people in relation to positive and negative well-being. *Psychoneuroendocrinology.* 2007 Aug 7

Exley C. Aluminium and iron, but neither copper nor zinc, are key to the precipitation of beta-sheets of Abeta in senile plaque cores in Alzheimer's disease. *J Alzheimers Dis.* 2006 Nov;10(2-3):173-7.

Ezzo JM, Richardson MA, Vickers A, Allen C, Dibble SL, Issell BF, Lao L, Pearl M, Ramirez G, Roscoe J, Shen J, Shivnan JC, Streitberger K, Treish I, Zhang G. Acupuncture-point stimulation for chemotherapy-induced nausea or vomiting. *Cochrane Database Syst Rev.* 2006 Apr 19;(2):CD002285.

Falcon CT. *Happiness and Personal Problems.* Lafayette, LA: Sensible Psychology, 1992.

Fallen EL, Kamath MV, Tougas G, Upton A. Afferent vagal modulation. Clinical studies of visceral sensory input. *Auton Neurosci.* 2001 Jul 20;90(1-2):35-40.

Fan X, Zhang D, Zheng J, Gu N, Ding A, Jia X, Qing H, Jin L, Wan M, Li Q. Preparation and characterization of magnetic nano-particles with radiofrequency-induced hyperthermia for cancer treatment. *Sheng Wu Yi Xue Gong Cheng Xue Za Zhi.* 2006 Aug;23(4):809-13.

FAO/WHO Expert Committee. Fats and Oils in Human Nutrition. Food and Nutrition Paper. 1994;(57).

Fecher LA, Cummings SD, Keefe MJ, Alani RM. Toward a molecular classification of melanoma. *J Clin Oncol.* 2007 Apr 20;25(12):1606-20.

Fehring RJ, Schneider M, Raviele K. Variability in the phases of the menstrual cycle. J Obstet Gynecol Neonatal Nurs. 2006 May-Jun;35(3):376-84.

Feleszko W, Jaworska J, Rha RD, Steinhausen S, Avagyan A, Jaudszus A, Ahrens B, Groneberg DA, Wahn U, Hamelmann E. Probiotic-induced suppression of allergic sensitization and airway inflammation is associated with an increase of T regulatory-dependent mechanisms in a murine model of asthma. *Clin Exp Allergy.* 2007 Apr;37(4):498-505.

Felton GE. Fibrinolytic and antithrombotic action of bromelain may eliminate thrombosis in heart patients. *Med Hypotheses.* 1980 Nov;6(11):1123-33.

Ferrari R, Merli E, Cicchitelli G, Mele D, Fucili A, Ceconi C. Therapeutic effects of L-carnitine and propionyl-L-carnitine on cardiovascular diseases: a review. Ann N Y Acad Sci. 2004 Nov;1033:79-91.

Feskanich D, Willett W, Colditz G. Calcium, vitamin D, milk consumption, and hip fractures: a prospective study among postmenopausal women. *Am J Clin Nutr.* 2003 Feb;77(2): 504-511.

Fischer JL, Mihelc EM, Pollok KE, Smith ML. Chemotherapeutic selectivity conferred by selenium: a role for p53-dependent DNA repair. *Mol Cancer Ther.* 2007 Jan;6(1):355-61.

Flandrin, J, Montanari M(eds.). *Food: A Culinary History from Antiquity to the Present.* New York: Penguin Books, 1999.

Forget-Dubois N, Boivin M, Dionne G, Pierce T, Tremblay RE, Perusse D. A longitudinal twin study of the genetic and environmental etiology of maternal hostile-reactive behavior during infancy and toddlerhood. *Infant Behav Dev.* 2007 Aug;30(3):453-65.

Fox RD, *Algoculture.* Doctorate Disseration, 1983 Jul.

Fraga CG. Relevance, essentiality and toxicity of trace elements in human health. Mol Aspects Med. 2005 Aug-Oct;26(4-5):235-44.

Frawley D, Lad V. *The Yoga of Herbs.* Sante Fe: Lotus Press, 1986.

Freeman W. *The Physiology of Perception. Sci. Am.* 1991 Feb.

Frey A. Electromagnetic field interactions with biological systems. *FASEB Jnl.* 1993;7: 272-28.

Fu XH. Observation on therapeutic effect of acupuncture on early peripheral facial paralysis. *Zhongguo Zhen Jiu.* 2007 Jul;27(7):494-6.

Fuhrman B, Rosenblat M, Hayek T, Coleman R, Aviram M. Ginger extract consumption reduces plasma cholesterol, inhibits LDL oxidation and attenuates development of atherosclerosis in atherosclerotic, apolipoprotein E-deficient mice. J Nutr. 2000 May;130(5):1124-31.

Fukada Y, Okano T. Circadian clock system in the pineal gland. *Mol Neurobiol.* 2002 Feb;25(1):19-30.

Fuster JM. Prefrontal neurons in networks of executive memory. *Brain Res Bull.* 2000 Jul 15;52(5):331-6.

Gabriel S, Schaffner S, Nguyen H, Moore J, Roy J. The structure of haplotype blocks in the human genome. *Science.* 2002;296:2225-2229.

Galaev, YM. The Measuring of Ether-Drift Velocity and Kinematic Ether Viscosity within Optical Wave Bands. *Spacetime & Substance.* 2002;3(5): 207-224.

Gambini JP, Velluti RA, Pedemonte M. Hippocampal theta rhythm synchronizes visual neurons in sleep and waking. *Brain Res.* 2002 Feb 1;926(1-2):137-41.

Gandhi T, Weingart S, Borus J, Seger A, Peterson J, Burdick E, Seger D, Shu K, Federico F, Leape L, Bates D. Adverse drug events in ambulatory care. *N Engl J Med.* 2003 Apr 17;348(16):1556-64.

Garcia Gomez LJ, Sanchez-Muniz FJ. Review: cardiovascular effect of garlic (Allium sativum). Arch Latinoam Nutr. 2000 Sep;50(3):219-29.
Garcia-Lazaro JA, Ahmed B, Schnupp JW. Tuning to natural stimulus dynamics in primary auditory cortex. *Curr Biol.* 2006 Feb 7;16(3):264-71.
Gardner CD, Fortmann SP, Krauss RM. Association of small low-density lipoprotein particles with the incidence of coronary artery disease in men and women. JAMA. 1996 Sep 18;276(11):875-81.
Gau SS, Soong WT, Merikangas KR. Correlates of sleep-wake patterns among children and young adolescents in Taiwan. Sleep. 2004 May 1;27(3):512-9.
Gehr P, Im Hof V, Geiser M, Schurch S. The mucociliary system of the lung—role of surfactants. *Schweiz Med Wochenschr.* 2000 May 13;130(19):691-8.
Gerber R. *Vibrational Healing.* Sante Fe: Bear, 1988.
Ghayur MN, Gilani AH. Ginger lowers blood pressure through blockade of voltage-dependent calcium Channels acting as a cardiotonic pump activator in mice, rabbit and dogs. J Cardiovasc Pharmacol. 2005 Jan;45(1):74-80.
Gibbons E. *Stalking the Healthful Herbs.* New York: David McKay, 1966.
Gibson RA. Docosa-hexaenoic acid (DHA) accumulation is regulated by the polyunsaturated fat content of the diet: Is it synthesis or is it incorporation? Asia Pac J Clin Nutr. 2004;13(Suppl):S78.
Gionchetti P, Rizzello F, Helwig U, Venturi A, Lammers KM, Brigidi P, Vitali B, Poggioli G, Miglioli M, Campieri M. Prophylaxis of pouchitis onset with probiotic therapy: a double-blind, placebo-controlled trial. Gastroenterology. 2003 May;124:1202-9.
Gisler GC, Diaz J, Duran N. Observations on Blood Plasma Chemiluminescence in Normal Subjects and Cancer Patients. *Arq Biol Tecnol.* 1983;26(3):345-352.
Gittleman AL. *Guess What Came to Dinner.* New York: Avery, 2001.
Glover J. *The Philosophy of Mind.* Oxford University Press, 1976.
Glück U, Gebbers J. Ingested probiotics reduce nasal colonization with pathogenic bacteria (Staphylococcus aureus, Streptococcus pneumoniae, and b-hemolytic streptococci. *Am J. Clin. Nutr.* 2003;77:517-520.
Goff DC Jr, D'Agostino RB Jr, Haffner SM, Otvos JD. Insulin resistance and adiposity influence lipoprotein size and subclass concentrations. Results from the Insulin Resistance Atherosclerosis Study. *Metabolism.* 2005 Feb;54(2):264-70.
Gohil K, Packer L. Bioflavonoid-Rich Botanical Extracts Show Antioxidant and Gene Regulatory Activity. *Ann N Y Acad Sci.* 2002:957:70-7.
Goldberg B. *Past Lives, Future Lives.* New York: Ballantine, 1982.
Golub E. *The Limits of Medicine.* New York: Times Books, 1994.
Gomes A, Fernandes E, Lima JL. Fluorescence probes used for detection of reactive oxygen species. *J Biochem Biophys Methods.* 2005 Dec 31;65(2-3):45-80.
Gomez-Abellan P, Hernandez-Morante JJ, Lujan JA, Madrid JA, Garaulet M. Clock genes are implicated in the human metabolic syndrome. *Int J Obes.* 2007 Jul 24.
González ME, Alarcón B, Carrasco L. Polysaccharides as antiviral agents: antiviral activity of carrageenan. *Antimicrob Agents Chemother.* 1987 Sep;31(9):1388-93.
Gould SJ. *Eight Little Piggies.* New York: Norton, 1993.
Gould SJ. *Wonderful Life: The Burgess Shale and the nature of history.* New York: Penguin Books, 1989.
Govindarajan VS, Sathyanarayana MN. Capsicum-production, technology, chemistry, and quality. Part V. Impact on physiology, pharmacology, nutrition, and metabolism; structure, pungency, pain, and desensitization sequences. Crit Rev Food Sci Nutr. 1991;29(6):435-74.
Govindarajan VS, Sathyanarayana MN. Capsicum-production, technology, chemistry, and quality. Part V. Impact on physiology, pharmacology, nutrition, and metabolism; structure, pungency, pain, and desensitization sequences. Crit Rev Food Sci Nutr. 1991;29(6):435-74.
Grad B, Dean E. Independent confirmation of infrared healer effects. In: White R, Broughton R (Eds.): *Research in parapsychology 1983.* Metuchen, NJ: Scarecrow Press, 1984:81-83.
Grad B. A Telekinetic Effect on Plant Growth. *Intl Jnl Parapsy.* 1964;6: 473.
Grad B. The 'Laying on of Hands': Implications for Psychotherapy, Gentling, and the Placebo Effect. *Jnl Amer Soc for Psych Res.* 1967 Oct;61(4): 286-305.
Grad, B. A telekinetic effect on plant growth: II. Experiments involving treatment of saline in stoppered bottles. *Internl J Parapsychol.* 1964;6:473-478, 484-488.
Grady D, Herrington D, Bittner V, Blumenthal R, Davidson M, Hlatky M, Hsia J, Hulley S, Herd A, Khan S, Newby LK, Waters D, Vittinghoff E, Wenger N. Cardiovascular disease outcomes during 6.8 years of hormone therapy: Heart and Estrogen/progestin Replacement Study follow-up (HERS II). *JAMA.* 2002 Jul 3;288(1):49-57.
Grasmuller S, Irnich D. Acupuncture in pain therapy. *MMW Fortschr Med.* 2007 Jun 21;149(25-26):37-9.
Grasso F, Grillo C, Musumeci F, Triglia A, Rodolico G, Cammisuli F, Rinzivillo C, Fragati G, Santuccio A, Rodolico M. Photon emission from normal and tumour human tissues. *Experientia.* 1992;48:10-13.

Grasso F, Musumeci F, Triglia A, Rodolico G, Cammisuli F, Rinzivillo C, Fragati G, Santuccio A, Rodolico M. In Stanley P, Kricka L (ed). *Ultraweak Luminescence from Cancer Tissues. In Bioluminescence and Chemiluminescence - Current Status.* New York: J Wiley & Sons. 1991:277-280.

Grasso F, Musumeci F, Triglia A. Yanbastiev M. Borisova, S. Self-irradiation effect on yeast cells. *Photochemistry and Photobiology.* 1991;54(1):147-149.

Gray-Davison F. *Ayurvedic Healing.* New York: Keats, 2002.

Greger M. Bird Flu: Virus of Our Own Hatching. *Mother Earth.* 2007 Dec-Jan:103-109.

Grissom C. Magnetic field effects in biology: A survey of possible mechanisms with emphasis on radical pair recombination. *Chem. Rev.* 1995;95: 3-24.

Grobstein P. Directed movement in the frog: motor choice, spatial representation, free will? *Neurobiology of motor programme selection.* Pergamon Press, 1992.

Groneberg DA, Wahn U, Hamelmann E. Probiotic-induced suppression of allergic sensitization and airway inflammation is associated with an increase of T regulatory-dependent mechanisms in a murine model of asthma. *Clin Exp Allergy.* 2007 Apr;37(4):498-505.

Gronfier C, Wright KP Jr, Kronauer RE, Czeisler CA. Entrainment of the human circadian pacemaker to longer-than-24-h days. *Proc Natl Acad Sci USA.* 2007 May 22;104(21):9081-6.

Grzanna R, Lindmark L, Frondoza CG. Ginger—an herbal medicinal product with broad anti-inflammatory actions. *J Med Food.* 2005 Summer;8(2):125-32.

Guo J. Chronic fatigue syndrome treated by acupuncture and moxibustion in combination with psychological approaches in 310 cases. *J Tradit Chin Med.* 2007 Jun;27(2):92-5.

Gupta A, Rash GS, Somia NN, Wachowiak MP, Jones J, Desoky A. The motion path of the digits. J Hand *Surg.* 1998; 23A:1038-1042.

Gupta R, Singhal S, Goyle A, Sharma VN. Antioxidant and hypocholesterolaemic effects of Terminalia arjuna tree-bark powder: a randomised placebo-controlled trial. J Assoc Physicians India. 2001 Feb;49:231-5.

Gupta YK, Gupta M, Kohli K. Neuroprotective role of melatonin in oxidative stress vulnerable brain. *Indian J Physiol Pharmacol.* 2003 Oct;47(4):373-86.

Gutmanis J. *Hawaiian Herbal Medicine.* Waipahu, HI: Island Heritage, 2001.

Haas M, Cooperstein R, Peterson D. Disentangling manual muscle testing and Applied Kinesiology: critique and reinterpretation of a literature review. Chiropr Osteopat. 2007 Aug 23;15:11.

Hadji L, Arnoux B, Benveniste J. Effect of dilute histamine on coronary flow of guinea-pig isolated heart. Inhibition by a magnetic field. *FASEB Jnl.* 1991;5: A1583.

Hagins WA, Penn RD, Yoshikami S. Dark current and photocurrent in retinal rods. *Biophys J.* 1970 May;10(5):380-412.

Hagins WA, Robinson WE, Yoshikami S. Ionic aspects of excitation in rod outer segments. *Ciba Found Symp.* 1975;(31):169-89.

Hagins WA, Yoshikami S. Ionic mechanisms in excitation of photoreceptors. *Ann N Y Acad Sci.* 1975 Dec 30;264:314-25.

Hagins WA, Yoshikami S. Proceedings: A role for Ca2+ in excitation of retinal rods and cones. *Exp Eye Res.* 1974 Mar;18(3):299-305.

Hagins WA. The visual process: Excitatory mechanisms in the primary receptor cells. *Annu Rev Biophys Bioeng.* 1972;1:131-58.

Halliday GM, Agar NS, Barnetson RS, Ananthaswamy HN, Jones AM. UV-A fingerprint mutations in human skin cancer. *Photochem Photobiol.* 2005 Jan-Feb;81(1):3-8.

Halpern G, Miller A. *Medicinal Mushrooms.* New York: M. Evans, 2002.

Halpern S. *Tuning the Human Instrument.* Palo Alto, CA: Spectrum Research Institute, 1978.

Hamel P. *Through Music to the Self: How to Appreciate and Experience Music.* Boulder: Shambala, 1979.

Hameroff SR, Penrose R. Conscious events as orchestrated spacetime selections. *J Consc Studies.* 1996;3(1):36-53.

Hameroff SR, Penrose R. Orchestrated reduction of quantum coherence in brain microtubules: A model for consciousness. In: Hameroff SN, Kaszniak A, Scott AC (eds.): *Toward a Science of Consciousness - The First Tucson Discussions and Debates.* Cambridge: MIT Press, 1996.

Hameroff SR, Smith, S, Watt.R. Nonlinear electrodynamics in cytoskeletal protein lattices. In: Adey W, Lawrence A (eds.), *Nonlinear Electrodynamics in Biological Systems.* 1984:567-583.

Hameroff SR, Watt, R. Information processing in microtubules. *J Theor Biology.* 1982;98:549-561.

Hameroff SR. Coherence in the cytoskeleton: Implications for biological information processing. In: Fröhlich H. (ed.): *Biological Coherence and Response to External Stimuli.* Springer, Berlin-New York 1988, pp.242-264.

Hameroff SR. Light is heavy: Wave mechanics in proteins - A microtubule hologram model of consciousness. *Proceedings 2nd. International Congress on Psychotronic Research.* Monte Carlo, 1975:168-169.

Hameroff SR. *Ultimate Biocomputing - Biomolecular Consciousness and Nanotechnology.* Amsterdam: Elsevier, 1987.

Hameroff, SR. Ch'i: A neural hologram? Microtubules, bioholography and acupuncture. *Am J Chin Med.* 1974;2(2):163-170.

Hamilton-Miller JM. Probiotics and prebiotics in the elderly. London: Department of Medical Microbiology, Royal Free and University College Medical School, 2004.

Hammond BG, Mayhew DA, Kier LD, Mast RW, Sander WJ. Safety assessment of DHA-rich microalgae from *Schizochytrium* sp. *Regul Toxicol Pharmacol.* 2002;35(2 Pt 1):255-65.

Handwerk B. Lobsters Navigate by Magnetism, Study Says. *Natl Geogr News.* 2003 Jan 6.

Hannoun AB, Nassar AH, Usta IM, Zreik TG, Abu Musa AA. Effect of war on the menstrual cycle. *Obstet Gynecol.* 2007 Apr;109(4):929-32.

Hans J. *The Structure and Dynamics of Waves and Vibrations.* New York:.Schocken and Co., 1975.

Hantusch B, Knittelfelder R, Wallmann J, Krieger S, Szalai K, Untersmayr E, Vogel M, Stadler BM, Scheiner O, Boltz-Nitulescu G, Jensen-Jarolim E. Internal images: human anti-idiotypic Fab antibodies mimic the IgE epitopes of grass pollen allergen Phl p 5a. *Mol Immunol.* 2006 Jul;43(14):2180-7.

Hardin P. Transcription regulation within the circadian clock: the E-box and beyond. *J Biol Rhythms.* 2004 Oct;19(5):348-60.

Harlow HF, Dodsworth RO, Harlow MK. Total social isolation in monkeys. *Proc Natl Acad Sci U S A.* 1965.

Harlow HF. Development of affection in primates. In Bliss E (ed): *Roots of Behavior.* New York: Harper, 1962: 157-166.

Harlow HF. Early social deprivation and later behavior in the monkey. In: Abrams A, Gurner H, Tomal J (eds): *Unfinished tasks in the behavioral sciences.* Baltimore: Williams & Wilkins. 1964: 154-173.

Hauschild M, Theintz G. Severe chronic anemia and endocrine disorders in children. *Rev Med Suisse.* 2007 Apr 18;3(107):988-91.

Haye-Legrand I, Norel X, Labat C, Benveniste J, Brink C. Antigenic contraction of guinea pig tracheal preparations passively sensitized with monoclonal IgE: pharmacological modulation. *Int Arch Allergy Appl Immunol.* 1988;87(4):342-8.

Heart Disease. New York State Department of Health. Oct. 2004.

Heckman JD, Ingram AJ, Loyd RD, Luck JV Jr, Mayer PW. Nonunion treatment with pulsed electromagnetic fields. *Clin Orthop Relat Res.* 1981 Nov-Dec;(161):58-66.

Hectorne KJ, Fransway AF. Diazolidinyl urea: incidence of sensitivity, patterns of cross-reactivity and clinical relevance. *Contact Dermatitis.* 1994 Jan;30(1):16-9.

Heinrich H. Assessment of non-sinusoidal, pulsed, or intermittent exposure to low frequency electric and magnetic fields. *Health Phys.* 2007 Jun;92(6):541-6.

Helms JA, Farnham PJ, Segal E, Chang HY. Functional demarcation of active and silent chromatin domains in human HOX loci by noncoding RNAs. *Cell.* 2007 Jun 29;129(7):1311-23.

Hendel B, Ferreira P. *Water & Salt: The Essence of Life.* Gaithersburg: Natural Resources, 2003.

Herbert V. Vitamin B12: Plant sources, requirements, and assay. *Am J Clin Nutr.* 1988;48:852-858.

Hernandez Avila M, Walker AM, Jick H. Use of replacement estrogens and the risk of myocardial infarction. *Epidemiology.* 1990 Mar;1(2):128-33.

Heyers D, Manns M, Luksch H, Gu¨ ntu¨ rku¨n O, Mouritsen H. A Visual Pathway Links Brain Structures Active during Magnetic Compass Orientation in Migratory Birds. *PLoS One.* 2007;2(9): e937. 2007.

Hillecke T, Nickel A, Bolay HV. Scientific perspectives on music therapy. *Ann N Y Acad Sci.* 2005 Dec;1060:271-82.

Ho MW. Assessing Food Quality by Its After-Glow. *Inst. Sci in Society.* Press release. 2004 May 1.

Ho SE, Ide N, Lau BH. S-allyl cysteine reduces oxidant load in cells involved in the atherogenic process. *Phytomedicine.* 2001 Jan;8(1):39-46.

Hobbs C. *Medicinal Mushrooms.* Summertown, TN: Botanica Press, 1986.

Hobbs C. *Stress & Natural Healing.* Loveland, CO: Interweave Press, 1997.

Hoffmann D. *Holistic Herbal.* London: Thorsons, 1983-2002.

Hollfoth K. Effect of color therapy on health and wellbeing: colors are more than just physics. *Pflege Z.* 2000 Feb;53(2):111-2.

Hollwich F, Dieckhues B. Effect of light on the eye on metabolism and hormones. *Klinische Monatsblatter fur Augenheilkunde.* 1989;195(5):284-90.

Hollwich F. Hartmann C. Influence of light through the eyes on metabolism and hormones. Ophtalmologie. 1990;4(4):385-9.

Hollwich F. *The influence of ocular light perception on metabolism in man and in animal.* New York: Springer-Verlag, 1979.

Holmquist G. Susumo Ohno left us January 13, 2000, at the age of 71. *Cytogenet and Cell Genet.* 2000;88:171-172.

Hope M. *The Psychology of Healing.* Longmead UK: Element Books, 1989.

Hoskin M.(ed.). *The Cambridge Illustrated History of Astronomy.* Cambridge: Cambridge Press, 1997.

Hoyle F. *Evolution from Space.* Londong: JM Dent, 1981.

Hu FB, Willett WC. Optimal diets for prevention of coronary heart disease. *JAMA.* 2002 Nov 27;288(20):2569-78.

Hu X, Wu B, Wang P. Displaying of meridian courses travelling over human body surface under natural conditions. *Zhen Ci Yan Jiu.* 1993;18(2):83-9.

Huang D, Ou B, Prior RL. The chemistry behind antioxidant capacity assays. *J Agric Food Chem.* 2005 Mar 23;53(6):1841-56.

Huffman C. Archytas of Tarentum: *Pythagorean, philosopher and Mathematician King.* Cambridge: Cambridge University Press, 2005.

Hull D. *Science as a Process: An evolutionary account of the social and conceptual development of science.* Chicago: Univ Chicago Press, 1988.

Hunt V. *Infinite Mind: Science of the Human Vibrations of Consciousness.* Malibu: Malibu Publ. 2000.

Hur YM, Rushton JP. Genetic and environmental contributions to prosocial behaviour in 2- to 9-year-old South Korean twins. *Biol Lett.* 2007 Aug 28.

Ide N, Lau BH. Garlic compounds minimize intracellular oxidative stress and inhibit nuclear factor-kappa b activation. *J Nutr.* 2001 Mar;131(3s):1020S-6S.

Igarashi T, Izumi H, Uchiumi T, Nishio K, Arao T, Tanabe M, Uramoto H, Sugio K, Yasumoto K, Sasaguri Y, Wang KY, Otsuji Y, Kohno K. Clock and ATF4 transcription system regulates drug resistance in human cancer cell lines. *Oncogene.* 2007 Jul 19;26(33):4749-60.

Iizuka C. at al. Extract of Basidomycetes especially Lentinus edodes, for treatment of human immunodeficiency virus (HIV). *Patent Application by Shokin Kogyo Co.* 1990: EP 370,673.

Ikonomov OC, Stoynev AG. Gene expression in suprachiasmatic nucleus and circadian rhythms. *Neurosci Biobehav Rev.* 1994 Fall;18(3):305-12.

Inaba H. INABA Biophoton. Exploratory Research for Advanced Technology. *Japan Science and Technology Agency.* 1991. http://www.jst.go.jp/erato/project/isf_P/isf_P.html. Acc. 2006 Nov.

Innis SM, Hansen JW. Plasma fatty acid responses, metabolic effects, and safety of microalgal and fungal oils rich in arachidonic and docosahexaenoic acids in adults. Am J Clin Nutr. 1996 Aug;64(2):159-67.

International HapMap Consortium. The international HapMap project. *Nature.* 2003;426:789-794.

Itokawa Y. Magnesium intake and cardiovascular disease. *Clin Calcium.* 2005 Feb;15(2):154-9.

Ivanovic-Zuvic F, de la Vega R, Ivanovic-Zuvic N, Renteria P. Affective disorders and solar activity. *Actas Esp Psiquiatr.* 2005 Jan-Feb;33(1):7-12.

Iwase T, Kajimura N, Uchiyama M, Ebisawa T, Yoshimura K, Kamei Y, Shibui K, Kim K, Kudo Y, Katoh M, Watanabe T, Nakajima T, Ozeki Y, Sugishita M, Hori T, Ikeda M, Toyoshima R, Inoue Y, Yamada N, Mishima K, Nomura M, Ozaki N, Okawa M, Takahashi K, Yamauchi T. Mutation screening of the human Clock gene in circadian rhythm sleep disorders. *Psychiatry Res.* 2002 Mar 15;109(2):121-8.

Jagetia G, Aggarwal B. "Spicing up" of the immune system by curcumin. *J Clin Immunol.* 2007 Jan;27(1):19-35.

Jagetia GC, Aggarwal BB. "Spicing up" of the immune system by curcumin. *J Clin Immunol.* 2007 Jan;27(1):19-35.

Jahn R, Dunne, B. *Margins of Reality: the Role of Consciousness in the Physical World.* New York: Harcourt Brace Jovanovich, 1987.

Janelle KC, Barr SI. Nutrient intakes and eating behavior scores of vegetarian and nonvegetarian women. *J Am Diet Assoc.* 1995 Feb;95(2):180-6, 189, quiz 187-8.

Janssens D, Delaive E, Houbion A, Eliaers F, Remacle J, Michiels C. Effect of venotropic drugs on the respiratory activity of isolated mitochondria and in endothelial cells. *Br J Pharmacol.* 2000 Aug;130(7):1513-24.

Jarvis DC. *Folk Medicine.* Greenwich, CN: Fawcett, 1958.

Jensen B. *Foods that Heal.* Garden City Park, NY: Avery Publ, 1988, 1993.

Jensen B. *Nature Has a Remedy.* Los Angeles: Keats, 2001.

Jensen HK. The molecular genetic basis and diagnosis of familial hypercholesterolemia in Denmark. *Dan Med Bull.* 2002 Nov;49(4):318-45.

Jensen R, Lammi-Keefe C, Henderson R, Bush V, Ferris A.M. Effect of dietary intake of n-6 and n-3 fatty acids on the fatty acid composition of human milk in North America. J Pediatr. 1992;120:S87-92.

Jhon MS. *The Water Puzzle and the Hexagonal Key.* Uplifting, 2004.

Ji Y, Liu YB, Zheng LY, Zhang XQ. Survey of studies on tissue structures and biological characteristics of channel lines. *Zhongguo Zhen Jiu.* 2007 Jun;27(6):427-32.

Jin CN, Zhang TS, Ji LX, Tian YF. Survey of studies on mechanisms of acupuncture and moxibustion in decreasing blood pressure. *Zhongguo Zhen Jiu.* 2007 Jun;27(6):467-70.

Johari H. *Ayurvedic Massage: Traditional Indian Techniques for Balancing Body and Mind.* Rochester, VT: Healing Arts, 1996.

Johari H. *Chakras.* Rochester, VT: Destiny, 1987.

Johnston A. A spatial property of the retino-cortical mapping. *Spatial Vision.* 1986;1(4):319-331.

Johnston RE. Pheromones, the vomeronasal system, and communication. From hormonal responses to individual recognition. *Ann N Y Acad Sci.* 1998 Nov 30;855:333-48.
Jovanovic-Ignjatic Z, Rakovic D. A review of current research in microwave resonance therapy: novel opportunities in medical treatment. *Acupunct Electrother Res.* 1999; 24:105-125.
Jovanovic-Ignjatic Z. Microwave Resonant Therapy: Novel Opportunities in Medical Treatment. *Acup. & Electro-Therap. Res., The Int. J.* 1999;24(2):105-125.
Kahhak L, Roche A, Dubray C, Arnoux C, Benveniste J. Decrease of ciliary beat frequency by platelet activating factor: protective effect of ketotifen. *Inflamm Res.* 1996 May;45(5):234-8.
Kalmijn S, Launer LJ, Ott A, Witteman JC, Hofman A, Breteler MM. Dietary fat intake and the risk of incident dementia in the Rotterdam Study. *Ann of Neurol.* 1997;42(5):776-782.
Kalsbeek A, Perreau-Lenz S, Buijs RM. A network of (autonomic) clock outputs. *Chronobiol Int.* 2006;23(1-2):201-15.
Kamide Y. We reside in the sun's atmosphere. *Biomed Pharmacother.* 2005 Oct;59 Suppl 1:S1-4.
Kandel E, Siegelbaum S, Schwartz J. *Synaptic transmission. Principles of Neural Science.* New York: Elsevier, 1991.
Kang Y, Li M, Yan W, Li X, Kang J, Zhang Y. Electroacupuncture alters the expression of genes associated with lipid metabolism and immune reaction in liver of hypercholesterolemia mice. *Biotechnol Lett.* 2007 Aug 18.
Kaptchuk TJ. The placebo effect in alternative medicine: can the performance of a healing ritual have clinical significance? *Ann Intern Med.* 2002 Jun 4;136(11):817-25.
Karis TE, Jhon MS. Flow-induced anisotropy in the susceptibility of a particle suspension. *Proc Natl Acad Sci USA.* 1986 Jul;83(14):4973-4977.
Karnstedt J. Ions and Consciousness. *Whole Self.* 1991 Spring.
Kataoka M, Tsumura H, Kaku N, Torisu T. Toxic effects of povidone-iodine on synovial cell and articular cartilage. *Clin Rheumatol.* 2006 Sep;25(5):632-8.
Kato Y, Kawamoto T, Honda KK. Circadian rhythms in cartilage. *Clin Calcium.* 2006 May;16(5):838-45.
Keil J, Stevenson I. Do cases of the reincarnation type show similar features over many years? A study of Turkish cases. *J. Sci. Exploration.* 1999;13(2) 189-198.
Keil J. New cases in Burma, Thailand, and Turkey: A limited field study replication of some aspects of Ian Stevenson's work. *J. Sci. Exploration.* 1991;5(1):27-59.
Kelder P. *Ancient Secret of the Fountain of Youth: Book 1.* New York: Doubleday, 1998.
Kelley GA, Kelley KS, Tran ZV. Aerobic exercise and lipids and lipoproteins in women: a meta-analysis of randomized controlled trials. *J Womens Health.* 2004 Dec;13(10):1148-64.
Kennedy KL, Steidle CP, Letizia TM. Urinary incontinence: the basics. *Ostomy Wound Manage.* 1995 Aug;41(7):16-8, 20, 22 passim; quiz 33-4.
Keogh JB, Grieger JA, Noakes M, Clifton PM. Flow-Mediated Dilatation Is Impaired by a High-Saturated Fat Diet but Not by a High-Carbohydrate Diet. *Arterioscler Thromb Vasc Biol.* 2005 Mar 17
Kerckhoffs DA, Brouns F, Hornstra G, Mensink RP. Effects on the human serum lipoprotein profile of beta-glucan, soy protein and isoflavones, plant sterols and stanols, garlic and tocotrienols. *J Nutr.* 2002 Sep;132(9):2494-505.
Kerr CC, Rennie CJ, Robinson PA. Physiology-based modeling of cortical auditory evoked potentials. *Biol Cybern.* 2008 Feb;98(2):171-84.
Keville K, Green M. *Aromatherapy: A Complete Guide to the Healing Art.* Freedom, CA: Crossing Press, 1995.
Key T, Appleby P, Davey G, Allen N, Spencer E, Travis R. Mortality in British vegetarians: review and preliminary results from EPIC-Oxford. *Amer. Jour. Clin. Nutr. Suppl.* 2003;78(3): 533S-538S.
Kiecolt-Glaser JK, Graham JE, Malarkey WB, Porter K, Lemeshow S, Glaser R. Olfactory influences on mood and autonomic, endocrine, and immune function. *Psychoneuroendocrinology.* 2008 Apr;33(3):328-39.
Kim JT, Ren CJ, Fielding GA, Pitti A, Kasumi T, Wajda M, Lebovits A, Bekker A. Treatment with lavender aromatherapy in the post-anesthesia care unit reduces opioid requirements of morbidly obese patients undergoing laparoscopic adjustable gastric banding. *Obes Surg.* 2007 Jul;17(7):920-5.
Kinoshameg SA, Persinger MA. Suppression of experimental allergic encephalomyelitis in rats by 50-nT, 7-Hz amplitude-modulated nocturnal magnetic fields depends on when after inoculation the fields are applied. *J Neulet.*.2004;08:18.
Kirlian SD, Kirlian V, Photography and Visual Observation by Means of High-Frequency Currents. *J Sci Appl Photog.* 1963;6(6).
Klatz RM, Goldman RM, Cebula C. *Infection Protection.* New York: HarperResource, 2002.
Klaus M. Mother and infant: early emotional ties. *Pediatrics.* 1998 Nov;102(5 Suppl E):1244-6.
Klein E, Smith D, Laxminarayan R. Trends in Hospitalizations and Deaths in the United States Associated with Infections Caused by *Staphylococcus aureus* and MRSA, 1999-2004. *Emerging Infectious Diseases.* University of Florida Press Release. 2007 Dec 3.
Klein R, Landau MG. *Healing: The Body Betrayed.* Minneapolis: DCI:Chronimed, 1992.

Klima H, Haas O, Roschger P. Photon emission from blood cells and its possible role in immune system regulation. In: Jezowska-Trzebiatowska B., *et al.* (eds.): *Photon Emission from Biological Systems.* Singapore: World Scientific, 1987:153-169.

Kloss J. *Back to Eden.* Twin Oaks, WI: Lotus Press, 1939-1999.

Kniazeva TA, Kuznetsova LN, Otto MP, Nikiforova TI. Efficacy of chromotherapy in patients with hypertension. *Vopr Kurortol Fizioter Lech Fiz Kult.* 2006 Jan-Feb;(1):11-3.

Kobayashi M, Shoji N, Ohizumi Y. Gingerol, a novel cardiotonic agent, activates the Ca2+-pumping ATPase in skeletal and cardiac sarcoplasmic reticulum. *Biochim Biophys Acta.* 1987 Sep 18;903(1):96-102.

Koch C. Debunking the Digital Brain. *Sci. Am.* 1997 Feb.

Kollerstrom N, Staudenmaier G. Evidence for Lunar-Sidereal Rhythms in Crop Yield: A Review. *Biolog Agri & Hort.* 2001;19:247–259

Kollerstrom N, Steffert B. Sex difference in response to stress by lunar month: a pilot study of four years' crisis-call frequency. *BMC Psychiatry.* 2003 Dec 10;3:20.

Koo KL, Ammit AJ, Tran VH, Duke CC, Roufogalis BD. Gingerols and related analogues inhibit arachidonic acid-induced human platelet serotonin release and aggregation. *Thromb Res.* 2001 Sep 1;103(5):387-97.

Koop H, Bachem MG. Serum iron, ferritin, and vitamin B12 during prolonged omeprazole therapy. *J Clin Gastroenterol.* 1992;14:288-92.

Koszowski B, Goniewicz M, Czogala J. Alternative methods of nicotine dependence treatment. *Przegl Lek.* 2005;62(10):1176-9.

Kotani S, Sakaguchi E, Warashina S, Matsukawa N, Ishikura Y, Kiso Y, Sakakibara M, Yoshimoto T, Guo J, Yamashima T. Dietary supplementation of arachidonic and docosahexaenoic acids improves cognitive dysfunction. *Neurosci Res.* 2006 Oct;56(2):159-64.

Krause R, Buhring M, Hopfenmuller W, Holick MF, Sharma AM. Ultraviolet B and blood pressure. *Lancet.* 1998 Aug 29;352(9129):709-10.

Kräutler B. Colorless Tetrapyrrolic Chlorophyll Catabolites in Ripening Fruit Are Effective Antioxidants. *Angewandte Chemie International Edition.* 2007;46;8699-8702.

Krebs K. The spiritual aspect of caring—an integral part of health and healing. *Nurs Adm Q.* 2001 Spring;25(3):55-60.

Kreig M. *Black Market Medicine.* New York: Bantam, 1968.

Kris-Etherton PM, Pearson TA, Wan Y, Hargrove RL, Moriarty K, Fishell V, Etherton TD. High-monounsaturated Fatty Acid Diets Lower Both Plasma Cholesterol and Triacylglycerol Concentrations. *Am J Clin Nutr.* 1999;70:1009-15

Krsnich-Shriwise S. Fibromyalgia syndrome: an overview. *Phys Ther.* 1997;77:68-75.

Kubler-Ross E. *On Life After Death.* Berkeley, CA: Celestial Arts, 1991.

Kubo I, Fujita K, Kubo A, Nihei K, Ogura T. Antibacterial activity of coriander volatile compounds against Salmonella choleraesuis. *J Agric Food Chem.* 2004 Jun 2;52(11):3329-32.

Kullo IJ, Ballantyne CM. Conditional risk factors for atherosclerosis. *Mayo Clin Proc.* 2005 Feb;80(2):219-30.

Kumar PU, Adhikari P, Pereira P, Bhat P. Safety and efficacy of Hartone in stable angina pectoris-an open comparative trial. *J Assoc Physicians India.* 1999 Jul;47(7):685-9.

Kuo FF, Kuo JJ. *Recent Advances in Acupuncture Research, Institute for Adnanced Research in Asian Science and Medicine.* Garden City, New York. 1979.

Kuuler R, Ballal S, Laike T Mikellides B, Tonello G. The impact of light and colour on psychological mood: a cross-cultural study of indoor work environments. *Ergonomics.* 2006 Nov 15;49(14):1496.

Kwang Y, Cha , Daniel P, Wirth J, Lobo R. Does Prayer Influence the Success of *in Vitro.* Fertilization–Embryo Transfer? Report of a Masked, Randomized Trial. *J Reproductive Med.* 2001;46(9).

Laaksonen M, Karkkainen M, Outila T, Vanninen T, Ray C, Lamberg-Allardt C. Vitamin D receptor gene BsmI-polymorphism in Finnish premenopausal and postmenopausal women: its association with bone mineral density, markers of bone turnover, and intestinal calcium absorption, with adjustment for lifestyle factors. *J Bone Miner Metab.* 2002;20(6):383-90.

Lad V. *Ayurveda: The Science of Self-Healing.* Twin Lakes, WI: Lotus Press.

Lafrenière, G. The material Universe is made purely out of Aether. *Matter is made of Waves.* 2002. http://www.glafreniere.com/matter.htm. Acc. 2007 June.

Lakin-Thomas PL. Transcriptional feedback oscillators: maybe, maybe not. *J Biol Rhythms.* 2006 Apr;21(2):83-92.

Lam F, Jr, Tsuei JJ, Zhao Z. Studies on the bioenergetic measurement of acupuncture points for determination of correct dosage of allopathic or homeopathic medicine in the treatment of diabetes mellitus. *Am J Acupunct.* 1990;18:127-33.

Lambing K. Biophoton Measurement as a Supplement to the Conventional Consideration of Food Quality. In: Popp F, Li K, Gu Q (eds.). *Recent Advances in Biophoton Research.* Singapore: World Scientific Publ. 1992:393-413.

Landmark K, Reikvam A. Do vitamins C and E protect against the development of carotid stenosis and cardiovascular disease? *Tidsskr Nor Laegeforen.* 2005 Jan 20;125(2):159-62.

Langhinrichsen-Rohling J, Palarea RE, Cohen J, Rohling ML. Breaking up is hard to do: unwanted pursuit behaviors following the dissolution of a romantic relationship. *Violence Vict.* 2000 Spring;15(1):73-90.

Lappe FM. *Diet for a Small Planet.* New York: Ballantine, 1971.

Latour E. Functional electrostimulation and its using in neurorehabilitation. *Ortop Traumatol Rehabil.* 2006 Dec 29;8(6):593-601.

Laura AG, Armas, B, Heaney H, Heaney R. Vitamin D_2 Is Much Less Effective than Vitamin D_3 in Humans. *J Clin Endocr & Metab.* 2004;89(11):5387-5391.

LaValle JB. *The Cox-2 Connection.* Rochester, VT: Healing Arts, 2001.

Lazarou J, Pomeranz BH, Corey PN. Incidence of adverse drug reactions in hospitalized patients: a meta-analysis of prospective studies. *JAMA.* 1998 Apr.

Lean G. US study links more than 200 diseases to pollution. *London Independent.* 2004 Nov 14.

Leape L. Lucian Leape on patient safety in U.S. hospitals. Interview by Peter I Buerhaus. *J Nurs Scholarsh.* 2004;36(4):366-70.

Leary, PC. Rock as a critical-point system and the inherent implausibility of reliable earthquake prediction. *Geophysical Journal International.* 1997;131(3):451-466. doi:10.1111/j.1365-246X.1997.

Leder D. Spooky actions at a distance: physics, psi, and distant healing. *J Altern Complement Med.* 2005 Oct;11(5):923-30.

Lefort J, Sedivy P, Desquand S, Randon J, Coeffier E, Maridonneau-Parini I, Floch A, Benveniste J, Vargaftig BB. Pharmacological profile of 48740 R.P., a PAF-acether antagonist. *Eur J Pharmacol.* 1988 Jun 10;150(3):257-68.

Lehmann B. The vitamin D3 pathway in human skin and its role for regulation of biological processes. *Photochem Photobiol.* 2005 Nov-Dec;81(6):1246-51.

Leitzmann C. Vegetarian diets: what are the advantages? *Forum Nutr.* 2005;(57):147-56.

Lennihan B. Homeopathy: natural mind-body healing. *J Psychosoc Nurs Ment Health Serv.* 2004 Jul;42(7):30-40.

Lewis A. Rescue remedy. *Nurs Times.* 1999 May 26-Jun 1;95(21):27.

Lewis WH, Elvin-Lewis MPF. *Medical Botany: Plants Affecting Man's Health.* New York: Wiley, 1977.

Lewontin R. *The Genetic Basis of Evolutionary Change.* New York: Columbia Univ Press, 1974.

Leyel CF. *Culpeper's English Physician & Complete Herbal.* Hollywood, CA: Wilshire, 1971.

Li KH. Bioluminescence and stimulated coherent radiation. *Laser und Elektrooptik 3.* 1981:32-35.

Li N, Wang DL, Wang CW, Wu B. Discussion on randomized controlled trials about clinical researches of acupuncture and moxibustion medicine. *Zhongguo Zhen Jiu.* 2007 Jul;27(7):529-32.

Liao H, Xi P, Chen Q, Yi L, Zhao Y. Clinical study on acupuncture, moxibustion, acupuncture plus moxibustion at Weiwanxiashu (EX-B3) for treatment of diabetes. *Zhongguo Zhen Jiu.* 2007 Jul;27(7):482-4.

Lieber AL. Human aggression and the lunar synodic cycle. *J Clin Psychiatry.* 1978 May;39(5):385-92.

Lin PW, Chan WC, Ng BF, Lam LC. Efficacy of aromatherapy (Lavandula angustifolia) as an intervention for agitated behaviours in Chinese older persons with dementia: a cross-over randomized trial. *Int J Geriatr Psychiatry.* 2007 May;22(5):405-10.

Lininger S, Gaby A, Austin S, Brown D, Wright J, Duncan A. *The Natural Pharmacy.* New York: Three Rivers, 1999.

Lipkind M. Can the vitalistic Entelechia principle be a working instrument ? (The theory of the biological field of Alexander G.Gurvich). In: Popp F, Li K, Gu Q (eds.). *Recent Advances in Biophoton Research.* Singapore: World Sci Publ, 1992:469-494.

Lipkind M. Registration of spontaneous photon emission from virus-infected cell cultures: development of experimental system. *Indian J Exp Biol.* 2003 May;41(5):457-72.

Lipski E. *Digestive Wellness.* Los Angeles, CA: Keats, 2000.

Litime M, Aïssa J, Benveniste J. Antigen signaling at high dilution. *FASEB Jnl.* 1993;7: A602.

Litscher G. Bioengineering assessment of acupuncture, part 5: cerebral near-infrared spectroscopy. *Crit Rev Biomed Eng.* 2006;34(6):439-57.

Liukkonen-Lilja H, Piepponen S. Leaching of aluminium from aluminium dishes and packages. *Food Addit Contam.* 1992 May-Jun;9(3):213-23.

Livanova L, Levshina I, Nozdracheva L, Elbakidze MG, Airapetiants MG. The protective action of negative air ions in acute stress in rats with different typological behavioral characteristics. *Zh Vyssh Nerv Deiat Im I P Pavlova.* 1998 May-Jun;48(3):554-7.

Lloyd D and Murray D. Redox rhythmicity: clocks at the core of temporal coherence. *BioEssays.* 2007;29(5): 465-473.

Lloyd JU. *American Materia Medica, Therapeutics and Pharmacognosy.* Portland, OR: Eclectic Medical Publications, 1989-1983.

Lopez-Garcia E, Schulze MB, Meigs JB, Manson JE, Rifai N, Stampfer MJ, Willett WC, Hu FB. Consumption of trans fatty acids is related to plasma biomarkers of inflammation and endothelial dysfunction. *J Nutr.* 2005 Mar;135(3):562-6.

Lorenz I, Schneider EM, Stolz P, Brack A, Strube J. Sensitive flow cytometric method to test basophil activation influenced by homeopathic histamine dilutions. *Forsch Komplementarmed Klass Naturheilkd.* 2003 Dec;10(6):316-24.

Lovejoy S, Pecknold S, Schertzer D. Stratified multifractal magnetization and surface geomagnetic fields-I. Spectral analysis and modeling. *Geophysical Journal International.* 2001 145(1):112-126.

Lovelock, J. *Gaia: A New Look at Life on Earth.* Oxford: Oxford Press, 1979.

Lovely RH. Recent studies in the behavioral toxicology of ELF electric and magnetic fields. *Prog Clin Biol Res.* 1988;257:327-47.

Lu J, Cui Y, Shi R. *A Practical English-Chinese Library of Traditional Chinese Medicine: Chinese Acupuncture and Moxibustion.* Shanghai: Publishing House of the Shanghai College of Traditional Chinese Medicine, 1988.

Lucas A, Morley R, Cole T, Lister G, Leeson-Payne C. Breast milk and subsequent intelligence quotient in children born premature. Lancet. 1992;339:261-264.

Lucas WB (ed). *Regression Therapy: A Handbook for Professionals. Past-Life Therapy.* Crest Park, CA: Deep Forest Press, 1993.

Lydic R, Schoene WC, Czeisler CA, Moore-Ede MC. Suprachiasmatic region of the human hypothalamus: homolog to the primate circadian pacemaker? *Sleep.* 1980;2(3):355-61.

Lynch M, Walsh B. *Genetics and Analysis of Quantitative Traits.* Sunderland, MA: Sinauer, 1998

Lythgoe JN. Visual pigments and environmental light. *Vision Res.* 1984;24(11):1539-50.

Lytle CD, Sagripanti JL. Predicted inactivation of viruses of relevance to biodefense by solar radiation. *J Virol.* 2005 Nov;79(22):14244-52.

Maas J, Jayson, J. K.. & Kleiber, D. A. Effects of spectral differences in illumination on fatigue. *J Appl Psychol.* 1974;59:524-526.

Mabey R, ed. *The New Age Herbalist.* New York: Simon & Schuster, 1941.

Maccabee PJ, Amassian VE, Cracco RQ, Cracco JB, Eberle L, Rudell A. Stimulation of the human nervous system using the magnetic coil. *J Clin Neurophysiol.* 1991 Jan;8(1):38-55.

Macdessi JS, Randell TL, Donaghue KC, Ambler GR, van Asperen PP, Mellis CM. Adrenal crises in children treated with high-dose inhaled corticosteroids for asthma. *Med J Aust.* 2003 Mar 3;178(5):214-6.

MacDougall D. The Soul: Hypothesis Concerning Soul Substance Together with Experimental Evidence of The Existence of Such Substance. *J Am Soc Psych Res.* 1907 May.

Machado RF, Laskowski D, Deffenderfer O, Burch T, Zheng S, Mazzone PJ, Mekhail T, Jennings C, Stoller JK, Pyle J, Duncan J, Dweik RA, Erzurum SC. Detection of lung cancer by sensor array analyses of exhaled breath. *Am J Respir Crit Care Med.* 2005 Jun 1;171(11):1286-91.

MacKay D. *Science, Chance, and Providence.* Oxford: Oxford Univ Press, 1978.

MacKay D. *The Open Mind and Other Essays.* Downer's Grove, IL: Inter-Varsity Press, 1988.

Maes HH, Silberg JL, Neale MC, Eaves LJ. Genetic and cultural transmission of antisocial behavior: an extended twin parent model. *Twin Res Hum Genet.* 2007 Feb;10(1):136-50.

Magni P, Motta M, Martini L. Leptin: a possible link between food intake, energy expenditure, and reproductive function. *Regul Pept.* 2000 Aug 25;92(1-3):51-6.

Magnusson A, Stefansson JG. Prevalence of seasonal affective disorder in Iceland. *Arch Gen Psychiatry.* 1993 Dec;50(12):941-6.

Mahachoklertwattana P, Sudkronrayudh K, Direkwattanachai C, Choubtum L, Okascharoen C. Decreased cortisol response to insulin induced hypoglycaemia in asthmatics treated with inhaled fluticasone propionate. *Arch Dis Child.* 2004 Nov;89(11):1055-8.

Makomaski Illing EM, Kaiserman MJ. Mortality attributable to tobacco use in Canada and its regions, 1998. *Can J Public Health.* 2004;95(1):38-44.

Makrides M, Neumann M, Byard R, Simmer K, Gibson R. Fatty acid composition of brain, retina, and erythrocytes in breast- and formula-fed infants. Am J Clin Nutr. 1994;60:189-94.

Makrides M, Neumann M, Gibson R. Effect of maternal docosahexaenoic acid (DHA) supplementation on breast milk composition. *Europ Jrnl of Clin Nutr.* 1996;50:352-357.

Manson JE, *et al.* Estrogen plus progestin and the risk of coronary heart disease. *NE J Med.* 2003; 349(6):523–534.

Mansour HA, Monk TH, Nimgaonkar VL. Circadian genes and bipolar disorder. *Ann Med.* 2005;37(3):196-205.

Marasanov SB, Matveev II. Correlation between protracted premedication and complication in cancer patients operated on during intense solar activity. *Vopr Onkol.* 2007;53(1):96-9.

Marcuard SP, Albernaz L, Khazanie PG. Omeprazole therapy causes malabsorption of cyanocobalamin (Vitamin B12). *Ann Intern Med.* 1994;120:211-5.

Marie PJ. Optimizing bone metabolism in osteoporosis: insight into the pharmacologic profile of strontium ranelate. *Osteoporos Int.* 2003;14 Suppl 3:S9-12.
Marie PJ. Strontium ranelate: a physiological approach for optimizing bone formation and resorption. *Bone.* 2006 Feb;38(2 Suppl 1):S10-4.
Marks C. *Commissurotomy, Consciousness, and Unity of Mind.* Cambridge: MIT Press, 1981.
Marks L. *The Unity of the Senses: Interrelations among the Modalities.* New York: Academic Press, 1978.
Martinez M. Docosahexaenoic acid therapy in docosahexaenoic acid-deficient patients with disorders of peroxisomal biogenesis. *Versicherungsmedizin.* 1996;31 Suppl:145-152
Mason D, Moore J, Green S, Liggett S. A gain-of-function polymorphism in a G-protein coupling domain of the human β1-adrenergic receptor. *J. Biol. Chem.* 1999;274:12670-12674.
Mastorakos G, Pavlatou M. Exercise as a stress model and the interplay between the hypothalamus-pituitary-adrenal and the hypothalamus-pituitary-thyroid axes. *Horm Metab Res.* 2005 Sep;37(9):577-84.
Mattix KD, Winchester PD, Scherer LR. Incidence of abdominal wall defects is related to surface water atrazine and nitrate levels. *J Pediatr Surg.* 2007 Jun;42(6):947-9.
Matutinovic Z, Galic M. Relative magnetic hearing threshold. *Laryngol Rhinol Otol.* 1982 Jan;61(1):38-41.
Maurer HR. Bromelain: biochemistry, pharmacology and medical use. *Cell Mol Life Sci.* 2001 Aug;58(9):1234-45.
Mayr E. *Toward a New Philosophy of Biology: Observations of an evolutionist.* Boston: Belknap Press, 1988.
Mayron L, Ott J, Nations R, Mayron E. Light, radiation and academic behaviour: Initial studies on the effects of full-spectrum lighting and radiation shielding on behaviour and academic performance of school children. *Acad Ther.* 1974;10, 33-47.
McCauley B. 2005. *Achieving Great Health.* Spartan, Lansing, MI.
McConnaughey E. *Sea Vegetables.* Happy Camp, CA: Naturegraph, 1985.
McConnel JV, Cornwell PR, Clay M. An apparatus for conditioning Planaria. *Am J Psychol.* 1960 Dec;73:618-22.
McCulloch M, Jezierski T, Broffman M, Hubbard A, Turner K, Janecki T. Diagnostic accuracy of canine scent detection in early- and late-stage lung and breast cancers. *Integr Cancer Ther.* 2006 Mar;5(1):30-9.
McDougall J, McDougall M. *The McDougal Plan.* Clinton, NJ: New Win, 1983.
McTaggart L. *The Field.* New York: Quill, 2003.
Meinecke FW. Sequelae and rehabilitation of spinal cord injuries. *Curr Opin Neurol Neurosurg.* 1991 Oct;4(5):714-9.
Melzack R, Coderre TJ, Katz J, Vaccarino AL. Central neuroplasticity and pathological pain. *Ann N Y Acad Sci.* 2001 Mar;933:157-74.
Melzack R, Wall PD. Pain mechanisms: a new theory. *Science.* 1965 Nov 19;150(699):971-9.
Melzack R. Evolution of the neuromatrix theory of pain. The prithvi raj lecture: presented at the third world congress of world institute of pain, barcelona 2004. *Pain Pract.* 2005 Jun;5(2):85-94.
Melzack R. Pain: past, present and future. *Can J Exp Psychol.* 1993 Dec;47(4):615-29.
Melzack R. Pain—an overview. *Acta Anaesthesiol Scand.* 1999 Oct;43(9):880-4.
Mendoza J. Circadian clocks: setting time by food. *J Neuroendocrinol.* 2007 Feb;19(2):127-37.
Meyer A, Kirsch H, Domergue F, Abbadi A, Sperling P, Bauer J, Cirpus P, Zank TK, Moreau H, Roscoe TJ, Zahringer U, Heinz E. Novel fatty acid elongases and their use for the reconstitution of docosahexaenoic acid biosynthesis. *J Lipid Res.* 2004 Oct;45(10):1899-909.
Milke Garcia Mdel P. Ghrelin: beyond hunger regulation. *Rev Gastroenterol Mex.* 2005 Oct-Dec;70(4):465-74.
Miller GT. *Living in the Environment.* Belmont, CA: Wadsworth, 1996.
Miller JD, Morin LP, Schwartz WJ, Moore RY. New insights into the mammalian circadian clock. *Sleep.* 1996 Oct;19(8):641-67.
Miller K. Cholesterol and In-Hospital Mortality in Elderly Patients. Am Family Phys. 2004 May.
Mills A. A replication study: Three cases of children in northern India who are said to remember a previous life," *J. Sci. Explor.* 1989;3(2):133-184.
Mills A. Moslem cases of the reincarnation type in northern India: A test of the hypothesis of imposed identification, Part I: Analysis of 26 cases. *J. Sci. Exploration.* 1990;4(2):171-188.
Mindell E, Hopkins V. *Prescription Alternatives.* New Canaan CT: Keats, 1998.
Mineev VN, Bulatova NI, Fedoseev GB. Erythrocyte insulin-reactive system and carbohydrate metabolism in bronchial asthma. *Ter Arkh.* 2002;74(3):14-7.
Mishkin M, Appenzeller T. The Anatomy of Memory. *Sci. Am.* 1987 June.
Mishkin M. Memory in monkeys severely impaired by combined but not by separate removal of amygdala and hippocampus. *Nature.* 1978;273: 297-298.
Mitchell JL. *Out-of-Body Experiences: A Handbook.* New York: Ballantine Books, 1981.
Miu AC, Benga O. Aluminum and Alzheimer's disease: a new look. *J Alzheimers Dis.* 2006 Nov;10(2-3):179-201.
Modern Biology. Austin: Harcourt Brace, 1993.

Moini H, Packer L, Saris NE. Antioxidant and Prooxidant Activities of Alpha-Lipoic Acid and Dihydrolipoic Acid. *Toxicol Appl Pharmacol.* 2002;182(1):84-90.
Monod J. *Chance and Necessity.* New York: Vintage, 1972.
Monroe R. *Far Journeys.* Garden City, NY: Doubleday & Co., 1985.
Monroe R. *Journeys Out of the Body.* Garden City, NY: Anchor Press, 1977.
Montanes P, Goldblum MC, Boller F. The naming impairment of living and nonliving items in Alzheimer's disease. *J Int Neuropsychol Soc.* 1995 Jan;1(1):39-48.
Moody R. *Coming Back: A Psychiatrist Explores Past-Life Journeys.* New York: Bantam Books, 1991.
Moody R. *Life After Life.* New York: Bantam, 1975.
Moody, R. *Reflections on Lfe After Life: More Important Discoveries In The Ongoing Investigation Of Survival Of Life After Bodily Death.* New York: Bantam, 1977.
Moore KH. Conservative management for urinary incontinence. *Baillieres Best Pract Res Clin Obstet Gynaecol.* 2000 Apr;14(2):251-89.
Moore R. Circadian Rhythms: A Clock for the Ages. *Science* 1999 June 25;284(5423):2102 – 2103.
Moore RY, Speh JC. Serotonin innervation of the primate suprachiasmatic nucleus. *Brain Res.* 2004 Jun 4;1010(1-2):169-73.
Moore RY. Neural control of the pineal gland. *Behav Brain Res.* 1996;73(1-2):125-30.
Moore RY. Organization and function of a central nervous system circadian oscillator: the suprachiasmatic hypothalamic nucleus. *Fed Proc.* 1983 Aug;42(11):2783-9.
Morick H. *Introduction to the Philosophy of Mind: Readings from Descartes to Strawson.* Glenview, Ill: Scott Foresman, 1970.
Morse M. *Closer to the Light.* New York: Ivy Books, 1990.
Morton C. *Velocity Alters Electric Field.* www.amasci.com/ freenrg/ morton1.html. Accessed 2007 July.
Morton G. Hypothalamic Leptin Regulation of Energy Homeostasis and Glucose Metabolism. *J Physiol.* 2007 Jun 21.
Moshe M. Method and apparatus for predicting the occurrence of an earthquake by identifying electromagnetic precursors. US Patent Issued on May 28, 1996. Number 5521508.
Motoyama H. Acupuncture Meridians. *Science & Medicine.* 1999 July/August.
Motoyama H. Before Polarization Current and the Acupuncture Meridians. *Journal of Holistic Medicine.* 1986;8(1&2).
Motoyama H. Deficient/ Excessive Patterns Found in Meridian Functioning in Cases of Liver Disease. *Subtle Energy & Energy Medicine.* 2000; 11(2).
Motoyama H. Energetic Medicine: new science of healing: An interview with A. Jackson. www.shareintl.org/archives/health-healing/hh_adjenergetic.html. Acc. 2007 Oct.
Motoyama H. Smith, W. Harada T. Pre-Polarization Resistance of the Skin as Determined by the Single Square Voltage Pulse. *Psychophysiology.* 1984;21(5).
Mozafar A. Enrichment of some B-vitamin in plants with application of organic fertilizers. *Plant and Soil.* 1994;167:305-11.
Mozafar A. Is there vitamin B12 in plants or not? A plant nutritionist's view. *Vegetarian Nutrition: An International Journal.* 1997;1/2:50-52.
Müller JP, Steinegger A, Schlatter C. Contribution of aluminum from packaging materials and cooking utensils to the daily aluminum intake. *Z Lebensm Unters Forsch.* 1993 Oct;197(4):332-41.
Muhlack S, Lemmer W, Klotz P, Muller T, Lehmann E, Klieser E. Anxiolytic effect of rescue remedy for psychiatric patients: a double-blind, placebo-controlled, randomized trial. *J Clin Psychopharmacol.* 2006 Oct;26(5):541-2.
Muller H, Lindman AS, Blomfeldt A, Seljeflot I, Pedersen JI. A diet rich in coconut oil reduces diurnal postprandial variations in circulating tissue plasminogen activator antigen and fasting lipoprotein (a) compared with a diet rich in unsaturated fat in women. *J Nutr.* 2003 Nov;133(11):3422-7.
Mumby DG, Wood ER, Pinel J. Object-recognition memory is only mildly impaired in rats with lesions of the hippocampus and amygdala. *Psychobio.* 1992;20: 18-27.
Municino A, Nicolino A, Milanese M, Gronda E, Andreuzzi B, Oliva F, Chiarella F, Cardio-HKT Study Group. Hydrotherapy in advanced heart failure: the cardio-HKT pilot study. *Monaldi Arch Chest Dis.* 2006 Dec;66(4):247-54.
Murchie G. *The Seven Mysteries of Life.* Boston: Houghton Mifflin Company, 1978.
Murphy R. *Organon Philosophy Workbook.* Blacksburg, VA: HANA, 1994.
Murray M and Pizzorno J. *Encyclopedia of Natural Medicine.* 2nd Edition. Roseville, CA: Prima Publishing, 1998.
Musaev AV, Nasrullaeva SN, Zeinalov RG. Effects of solar activity on some demographic indices and morbidity in Azerbaijan with reference to A. L. Chizhevsky's theory. *Vopr Kurortol Fizioter Lech Fiz Kult.* 2007 May-Jun;(3):38-42.
Muzzarelli L, Force M, Sebold M. Aromatherapy and reducing preprocedural anxiety: A controlled prospective study. *Gastroenterol Nurs.* 2006 Nov-Dec;29(6):466-71.

Myss C. *Anatomy of the Spirit.* New York: Harmony, 1996.
Nadkarni AK, Nadkarni KM. *Indian Materia Medica.* (Vols 1 and 2). Bombay, India: Popular Pradashan, 1908, 1976.
Nakamura K, Urayama K, Hoshino Y. Lumbar cerebrospinal fluid pulse wave rising from pulsations of both the spinal cord and the brain in humans. *Spinal Cord.* 1997 Nov;35(11):735-9.
Nakamura MT, Nara TY. Structure, function, and dietary regulation of delta6, delta5, and delta9 desaturases. *Ann Rev Nutr.* 2004;24:345-76.
Nakatani K, Yau KW. Calcium and light adaptation in retinal rods and cones. *Nature.* 1988 Jul 7;334(6177):69-71.
Napoli N, Thompson J, Civitelli R, Armamento-Villareal R. Effects of dietary calcium compared with calcium supplements on estrogen metabolism and bone mineral density. *Am J Clin Nutr.* 2007;85(5): 1428-1433.
Naruszewicz M, Daniewski M, Nowicka G, Kozlowska-Wojciechowska M. Trans-unsaturated fatty acids and acrylamide in food as potential atherosclerosis progression factors. Based on own studies. *Acta Microbiol Pol.* 2003;52 Suppl:75-81.
Natarajan E, Grissom C. The Origin of Magnetic Field Dependent Recombination in Alkylcobalamin Radical Pairs. *Photochem Photobiol.* 1996;64: 286-295.
Navarro Silvera SA, Rohan TE. Trace elements and cancer risk: a review of the epidemiologic evidence. *Cancer Causes Control.* 2007 Feb;18(1):7-27.
Neeck G, Riedel W. Hormonal perturbations in fibromyalgia syndrome. *Ann N Y Acad Sci.* 1999;876:325-38.
Nestel PJ. Adulthood - prevention: Cardiovascular disease. *Med J Aust.* 2002 Jun 3;176(11 Suppl):S118-9.
Nestor PJ, Graham KS, Bozeat S, Simons JS, Hodges JR. Memory consolidation and the hippocampus: further evidence from studies of autobiographical memory in semantic dementia and frontal variant frontotemporal dementia. *Neuropsychologia.* 2002;40(6):633-54.
Netheron M. *Past Lives Therapy.* New York: Morrow, 1978.Wambach H. *Reliving Past Lives.* New York: Bantam, 1978.Fiore E. *You Have Been Here Before.* New York: Ballantine, 1978.
Newmark T, Schulick P. *Beyond Aspirin.* Prescott, AZ: Holm, 2000.
Newton M. *Destiny of Souls: New Case Studies of Life between Lives.* St. Paul: Llewellyn Publications, 2000.
Newton M. *Journey of Souls: Case Studies of Life between Lives.* St. Paul: Llewellyn Publications, 1994.
Newton PE. The Effect of Sound on Plant Growth. *JAES.* 1971 Mar;19(3): 202-205.
Niculescu MD, Wu R, Guo Z, da Costa KA, Zeisel SH. Diethanolamine alters proliferation and choline metabolism in mouse neural precursor cells. *Toxicol Sci.* 2007 Apr;96(2):321-6.
Nievergelt CM, Kripke DF, Remick RA, Sadovnick AD, McElroy SL, Keck PE Jr, Kelsoe JR. Examination of the clock gene Cryptochrome 1 in bipolar disorder: mutational analysis and absence of evidence for linkage or association. *Psychiatr Genet.* 2005 Mar;15(1):45-52.
Niggli H. Temperature dependence of ultraweak photon emission in fibroblastic differentiation after irradiation with artificial sunlight. *Indian J Exp Biol.* 2003 May;41:419-423.
Nishigori C, Hattori Y, Toyokuni S. Role of reactive oxygen species in skin carcinogenesis. *Antioxid Redox Signal.* 2004 Jun;6(3):561-70.
Noone EJ, Roche HM, Nugent AP, Gibney MJ. The effect of dietary supplementation using isomeric blends of conjugated linoleic acid on lipid metabolism in healthy human subjects. *Br J Nutr.* 2002 Sep;88(3):243-51.
North J. *The Fontana History of Astronomy and Cosmology.* London: Fontana Press, 1994.
O'Dwyer JJ. *College Physics.* Pacific Grove, CA: Brooks/Cole, 1990.
O'Brien SJ, Shannon JE, Gail MH. A molecular approach to the identification and individualization of human and animal cells in culture: isozyme and allozyme genetic signatures. *In Vitro.* 1980 Feb;16(2):119-35.
O'Connell OF, Ryan L, O'Brien N. Xanthophyll carotenoids are more bioaccessible from fruits than dark green vegetables. *Nutr Res.* 2007;27(5):258-264.
O'Connor J., Bensky D. (ed). *Shanghai College of Traditional Chinese Medicine: Acupuncture: A Comprehensive Text.* Seattle: Eastland Press, 1981.
Oehme FW (ed.). *Toxicity of heavy metals in the environment. Part 1.* New York: M.Dekker, 1979.
Oh CK, Lücker PW, Wetzelsberger N, Kuhlmann F. The determination of magnesium, calcium, sodium and potassium in assorted foods with special attention to the loss of electrolytes after various forms of food preparations. *Mag.-Bull.* 1986;8:297-302.
Okamura H. Clock genes in cell clocks: roles, actions, and mysteries. *J Biol Rhythms.* 2004 Oct;19(5):388-99.
Okayama Y, Begishvili TB, Church MK. Comparison of mechanisms of IL-3 induced histamine release and IL-3 priming effect on human basophils. *Clin Exp Allergy.* 1993 Nov;23(11):901-10.
Ole D. Rughede, On the Theory and Physics of the Aether. *Progress in Physics.* 2006; (1).
O'Leary KD, Rosenbaum A, Hughes PC. Fluorescent lighting: a purported source of hyperactive behavior. *J Abnorm Child Psychol.* 1978 Sep;6(3):285-9.

Olney JW, Farber NB, Spitznagel E, Robins LN. Increasing brain tumor rates: is there a link to aspartame? *J Neuropathol Exp Neurol.* 1996;55:1115-23.

Olney JW. Excitotoxins in foods. *Neurotoxicology.* 1994;15:535-44.

Onder G, Landi F, Volpato S, Fellin R, Carbonin P, Gambassi G, Bernabei R. Serum cholesterol levels and in-hospital mortality in the elderly. *Am J Med.* 2003 Sept;115:265-71

One Hundred Million Americans See Medical Mistakes Directly Touching Them as Patients, Friends, Relatives. *National Patient Safety Foundation. Press Release.* 1997 Oct 9. http://npsf.org/pr/pressrel/finalsur.htm. Acc. 2007 Mar.

Oosterga M, ten Vaarwerk IA, DeJongste MJ, Staal MJ. Spinal cord stimulation in refractory angina pectoris—clinical results and mechanisms. *Z Kardiol.* 1997;86 Suppl 1:107-13.

Ostrander S, Schroeder L, Ostrander N. *Super-Learning.* New York: Delta, 1979.

Otani S. Memory trace in prefrontal cortex: theory for the cognitive switch. *Biol Rev Camb Philos Soc.* 2002 Nov;77(4):563-77.

Otsu A, Chinami M, Morgenthale S, Kaneko Y, Fujita D, Shirakawa T. Correlations for number of sunspots, unemployment rate, and suicide mortality in Japan. *Percept Mot Skills.* 2006 Apr;102(2):603-8.

Ott J. Color and Light: Their Effects on Plants, Animals, and People (Series of seven articles in seven issues). *Internl J Biosoc Res.* 1985-1991.

Ott J. *Health and Light: The Effects of Natural and Artificial Light on Man and Other Living Things.* Self published, 1973,

Otto SJ, van Houwelingen AC, Hornstra G. The effect of supplementation with docosahexaenoic and arachidonic acid derived from single cell oils on plasma and erythrocyte fatty acids of pregnant women in the second trimester. *Prost Leuk Essent Fatty Acids.* 2000 Nov;63(5):323-8.

Ou CC, Tsao SM, Lin MC, Yin MC. Protective action on human LDL against oxidation and glycation by four organosulfur compounds derived from garlic. *Lipids.* 2003 Mar;38(3):219-24.

Packard CC. *Pocket Guide to Ayurvedic Healing.* Freedom, CA: Crossing Press, 1996.

Park AE, Fernandez JJ, Schmedders K, Cohen MS. The Fibonacci sequence: relationship to the human hand. *J Hand Surg.* 2003 Jan;28(1):157-60.

Partonen T, Haukka J, Nevanlinna H, Lonnqvist J. Analysis of the seasonal pattern in suicide. *J Affect Disord.* 2004 Aug;81(2):133-9.

Pasricha S. Cases of the reincarnation type in northern India with birthmarks and birth defects. *J. Sci. Exploration.* 1998;12(2) 259-293.

Pasricha S. *Claims of reincarnation: An Empirical Study of Cases in India.* New Delhi: Harman, 1990.

Patwardhan B, Gautam M. Botanical immunodrugs: scope and opportunities. *Drug Discov Today.* 2005 Apr 1;10(7):495-502.

Physicians' Desk Reference. Montvale, NJ: Thomson, 2003.

Pehowich DJ, Gomes AV, Barnes JA. Fatty acid composition and possible health effects of coconut constituents. West Indian Med J. 2000 Jun;49(2):128-33.

Pendell D. *Plant Powers, Poisons, and Herbcraft.* San Francisco: Mercury House, 1995.

Penn RD, Hagins WA. Kinetics of the photocurrent of retinal rods. *Biophys J.* 1972 Aug;12(8):1073-94.

Penn RD, Hagins WA. Signal transmission along retinal rods and the origin of the electroretinographic a-wave. *Nature.* 1969 Jul 12;223(5202):201-4.

Penson RT, Kyriakou H, Zuckerman D, Chabner BA, Lynch TJ Jr. Teams: communication in multidisciplinary care. *Oncologist.* 2006 May;11(5):520-6.

Perez-Galvez A, Martin HD, Sies H, Stahl W. Incorporation of carotenoids from paprika oleoresin into human chylomicrons. *Br J Nutr.* 2003 Jun;89(6):787-93.

Perl DP, Moalem S. Aluminum and Alzheimer's disease, a personal perspective after 25 years. *J Alzheimers Dis.* 2006;9(3 Suppl):291-300.

Peroxisomes from pepper fruits (Capsicum annuum L.): purification, characterisation and antioxidant activity. *J Plant Physiol.* 2003 Dec;160(12):1507-16.

Perreau-Lenz S, Kalsbeek A, Van Der Vliet J, Pevet P, Buijs RM. In vivo evidence for a controlled offset of melatonin synthesis at dawn by the suprachiasmatic nucleus in the rat. *Neuroscience.* 2005;130(3):797-803.

Perry J. *A Dialogue on Personal Identity and Immortality.* Indianapolis, IN: Hackett, 1978.

Perry J. *Personal Identity.* Berkeley: University of California Press, 1975.

Persson R, Orbaek P, Kecklund G, Akerstedt T. Impact of an 84-hour workweek on biomarkers for stress, metabolic processes and diurnal rhythm. *Scand J Work Environ Health.* 2006 Oct;32(5):349-58.

Persinger M.A., Krippner S. Dream ESP experiments and geomagnetic activity. *Journal of the American Society of Psychical Research.* 1989;83:101- 106.

Persinger M.A. Psi phenomena and temporal lobe activity: The geomagnetic factor. In L.A. Henkel & R.E. Berger (Eds.), *Research in parapsychology.* (121- 156). Metuchen, NJ: Scarecrow Press, 1989.

Pert C. *Molecules of Emotion.* New York: Scribner, 1997.

Petiot JF, Sainte-Laudy J, Benveniste J. Interpretation of results on a human basophil degranulation test. *Ann Biol Clin (Paris).* 1981;39(6):355-9.

Phillips M, Cataneo RN, Cummin AR, Gagliardi AJ, Gleeson K, Greenberg J, Maxfield RA, Rom WN. Detection of lung cancer with volatile markers in the breath. *Chest.* 2003 Jun;123(6):2115-23.

Piggins HD. Human clock genes. *Ann Med.* 2002;34(5):394-400.

Piluso LG, Moffatt-Smith C. Disinfection using ultraviolet radiation as an antimicrobial agent: a review and synthesis of mechanisms and concerns. *PDA J Pharm Sci Technol.* 2006 Jan-Feb;60(1):1-16.

Piolino P, Desgranges B, Belliard S, Matuszewski V, Lalevee C, De la Sayette V, Eustache F. Autobiographical memory and autonoetic consciousness: triple dissociation in neurodegenerative diseases. *Brain.* 2003 Oct;126(Pt 10):2203-19.

Piper PW. Yeast superoxide dismutase mutants reveal a pro-oxidant action of weak organic acid food preservatives. *Free Radic Biol Med.* 1999 Dec;27(11-12):1219-27.

Pitt-Rivers R, Trotter WR. *The Thyroid Gland.* London: Butterworth Publisher, 1954.

Plaut T, Jones T. *Asthma Guide for People of All Ages.* Amherst MA: Pedipress, 1999.

Plotkin H. *Darwin Machines and the Nature of Knowledge: Concerning adaptations, instinct and the evolution of intelligence.* New York: Penguin, 1994.

Plotnikoff G, Quigley J. Prevalence of Severe Hypovitaminosis D in Patients With Persistent, Nonspecific Musculoskeletal Pain. *Mayo Clin Proc.* 2003;78:1463-1470.

Poitevin B, Davenas E, Benveniste J. In vitro immunological degranulation of human basophils is modulated by lung histamine and Apis mellifica. *Br J Clin Pharmacol.* 1988 Apr;25(4):439-44.

Polkinghorne J. *Science and Providence.* Boston: Shambhala Publications, 1989.

Pongratz W, Endler PC, Poitevin B, Kartnig T. Effect of extremely diluted plant hormone on cell culture, *Proc. 1995 AAAS Ann. Meeting*, Atlanta, 1995.

Pool R. Is there an EMF-Cancer connection? *Science.* 1990;249: 1096-1098.

Popp F Chang J. Mechanism of interaction between electromagnetic fields and living organisms. *Science in China.* 2000 Series C;43(5):507-518.

Popp F, Chang J, Herzog A, Yan Z, Yan Y. Evidence of non-classical (squeezed) light in biological systems. *Physics Lett.* 2002;293:98-102.

Popp F, Yan Y. Delayed luminescence of biological systems in terms of coherent states. *Phys.Lett.* 2000;293:91-97.

Popp F. Properties of biophotons and their theoretical implications. *Indian J Exper Biology.* 2003 May;41:391-402.

Popp F. Molecular Aspects of Carcinogenesis. In Deutsch E, Moser K, Rainer H, Stacher A (eds.). *Molecular Base of Malignancy.* Stuttgart: G.Thieme, 1976:47-55.

Popper KR, Eccles, JC. *The Self and Its Brain.* London: Routledge, 1983.

Postlethwait EM. Scavenger receptors clear the air. *J Clin Invest.* 2007 Mar;117(3):601-4.

Poulos LM, Toelle BG, Marks GB. The burden of asthma in children: an Australian perspective. *Paediatr Respir Rev.* 2005 Mar;6(1):20-7.

Prescott J. Alienation of Affection. *Psych Today.* 1979 Dec.

Prescott J. The Origins of Human Love and Violence. *Pre- and Perinatal Psych J.* 1996;10(3):143-188.

Pribram K. *Brain and perception: holonomy and structure in figural processing.* Hillsdale, N. J.: Lawrence Erlbaum Assoc., 1991.

Pronina TS. Circadian and infradian rhythms of testosterone and aldosterone excretion in children. *Probl Endokrinol.* 1992 Sep-Oct;38(5):38-42.

Protheroe WM, Captiotti ER, Newsom GH. *Exploring the Universe.* Columbus, OH: Merrill, 1989,

Provalova NV, Suslov NI, Skurikhin EG, Dygaĭ AM. Local mechanisms of the regulatory action of Scutellaria baicalensis and ginseng extracts on the erythropoiesis after paradoxical sleep deprivation. *Eksp Klin Farmakol.* 2006 Sep-Oct;69(5):31-5.

Puthoff H, Targ R, May E. Experimental Psi Research: Implication for Physics. AAAS Proceedings of the 1979 Symposium on the Role of Consciousness in the Physical World. 1981.

Puthoff H, Targ R. A Perceptual Channel for Information Transfer Over Kilometer distances: Historical Perspective and Recent Research. Proc. *IEEE.* 1976;64(3):329-254.

Radin D. *The Conscious Universe.* San Francisco: HarperEdge, 1997.

Rahman K. Garlic and aging: new insights into an old remedy. *Ageing Res Rev.* 2003 Jan;2(1):39-56.

Raiten DJ, Talbot JM, Fisher KD, eds. Life Sciences Research Office Report. Executive summary from the report. Analysis of adverse reactions to monosodium glutamate (MSG). *J Nutr.* 1995;125 (suppl).:2892-906.

Raloff J. Ill Winds. *Science News:* 2001;160(14):218.

Rapley G. Keeping mothers and babies together—breastfeeding and bonding. *RCM Midwives.* 2002 Oct;5(10):332-4.

Rappoport J. Both sides of the pharmaceutical death coin. *Townsend Letter for Doctors and Patients.* 2006 Oct.

Rauma A. Antioxidant status in vegetarians versus omnivores. *Nutrition.* 2003;16(2): 111-119.
Rawlings M. *Beyond Death's Door.* New York: Bantam, 1979.
Reger D, Goode S, Mercer E. *Chemistry: Principles & Practice.* Fort Worth, TX: Harcourt Brace, 1993.
Regis E. *Virus Ground Zero.* New York: Pocket, 1996.
Reiffenberger DH, Amundson LH. Fibromyalgia syndrome: a review. *Am Fam Physician.* 1996;53:1698-704.
Reilly T, Taylor M, McSharry C, Aitchison T. Is homoeopathy a placebo response? Controlled trial of homoeopathic potency, with pollen in hayfever as model. *Lancet.* 1986;II: 881-886.
Reiter RJ, Garcia JJ, Pie J. Oxidative toxicity in models of neurodegeneration: responses to melatonin. *Restor Neurol Neurosci.* 1998 Jun;12(2-3):135-42.
Reiter RJ, Tan DX, Manchester LC, Qi W. Biochemical reactivity of melatonin with reactive oxygen and nitrogen species: a review of the evidence. *Cell Biochem Biophys.* 2001;34(2):237-56.
Renaud S, Lanzmann-Petithory D. Dietary fats and coronary heart disease pathogenesis. *Curr Atheroscler Rep.* 2002;4(6):419-24.
Renault S, De Lucca AJ, Boue S, Bland JM, Vigo CB, Selitrennikoff CP. CAY-1, a novel antifungal compound from cayenne pepper. *Med Mycol.* 2003 Feb;41(1):75-81.
Retallack D. *The Sound of Music and Plants.* Marina Del Rey, CA: Devorss, 1973.
Richards R. *Darwin and the Emergence of Evolutionary Theories of Mind and Behavior.* Chicago: Univ Chicago Press, 1987.
Rieder M. *Mission to Millboro.* Nevada City, CA: Blue Dolphin, 1995.
Rieder M. *Return to Millboro: The Reincarnation Drama Continues.* Nevada City, CA: Blue Dolphin, 1995.
Rietbrock N, Hamel M, Hempel B, Mitrovic V, Schmidt T, Wolf GK. Actions of standardized extracts of Crataegus berries on exercise tolerance and quality of life in patients with congestive heart failure. *Arzneimittelforschung.* 2001 Oct;51(10):793-8.
Rindos D. *The Origins of Agriculture: An evolutionary perspective.* Burlington, MA: Academic Press, 1984.
Ring K. *Life at Death: A Scientific Investigation of the Near-Death Experience.* New York: Quill, 1982.
Roach M. *Stiff: The Curious Lives of Human Cadavers.* New York: W.W. Norton, 2003.
Robert AM, Groult N, Six C, Robert L. The effect of procyanidolic oligomers on mesenchymal cells in culture II-Attachment of elastic fibers to the cells. *Pathol Biol.* 1990 Jun;38(6):601-7.
Robert AM, Tixier JM, Robert L, Legeais JM, Renard G. Effect of procyanidolic oligomers on the permeability of the blood-brain barrier. *Pathol Biol.* 2001 May;49(4):298-304.
Roberts JE. Light and immunomodulation. *Ann N Y Acad Sci.* 2000;917:435-45.
Robilliard DL, Archer SN, Arendt J, Lockley SW, Hack LM, English J, Leger D, Smits MG, Williams A, Skene DJ, Von Schantz M. The 3111 Clock gene polymorphism is not associated with sleep and circadian rhythmicity in phenotypically characterized human subjects. *J Sleep Res.* 2002 Dec;11(4):305-12.
Rodale R. *Our Next Frontier.* Emmaus, PA: Rodale, 1981.
Rodermel SR, Smith-Sonneborn J. Age-correlated changes in expression of micronuclear damage and repair in Paramecium tetraurelia. *Genetics.* 1977 Oct;87(2):259-74.
Rodgers JT, Puigserver P. Fasting-dependent glucose and lipid metabolic response through hepatic sirtuin 1. *Proc Natl Acad Sci USA.* 2007 Jul 31;104(31):12861-6.
Rosenfeldt V, Benfeldt E, Nielsen SD, Michaelsen KF, Jeppesen DL, Valerius NH, Paerregaard A. Effect of probiotic Lactobacillus strains in children with atopic dermatitis. *J Allergy Clin Immunol.* 2003 Feb;111(2):389-95.
Rosenlund M, Picciotto S, Forastiere F, Stafoggia M, Perucci CA. Traffic-related air pollution in relation to incidence and prognosis of coronary heart disease. *Epidemiology.* 2008 Jan;19(1):121-8.
Rosenthal N, Blehar M (Eds.). *Seasonal affective disorders and phototherapy.* New York: Guildford Press, 1989.
Rossouw JE, Prentice RL, Manson JE, Wu L, Barad D, Barnabei VM, Ko M, LaCroix AZ, Margolis KL, Stefanick ML. Postmenopausal hormone therapy and risk of cardiovascular disease by age and years since menopause. *JAMA.* 2007 Apr 4;297(13):1465-77.
Routasalo P, Isola A. The right to touch and be touched. *Nurs Ethics.* 1996 Jun;3(2):165-76.
Rowland AS, Baird DD, Long S, Wegienka G, Harlow SD, Alavanja M, Sandler DP. Influence of medical conditions and lifestyle factors on the menstrual cycle. *Epidemiology.* 2002 Nov;13(6):668-74.
Roy M, Kirschbaum C, Steptoe A. Intraindividual variation in recent stress exposure as a moderator of cortisol and testosterone levels. Ann Behav Med. 2003 Dec;26(3):194-200.
Roybal K, Theobold D, Graham A, DiNieri JA, Russo SJ, Krishnan V, Chakravarty S, Peevey J, Oehrlein N, Birnbaum S, Vitaterna MH, Orsulak P, Takahashi JS, Nestler EJ, Carlezon WA Jr, McClung CA. Mania-like behavior induced by disruption of CLOCK. *Proc Natl Acad Sci USA.* 2007 Apr 10;104(15):6406-11.
Rubenowitz E, Molin I, Axelsson G, Rylander R. (2000) Magnesium in drinking water in relation to morbidity and mortality from acute myocardial infarction. *Epidemiology.* 2000;11:416-421.
Rubin E and Farber J. *Pathology 3rd Edition.* Lippincott-Raven, Philadelphia, PA, 1999.

Russ MJ, Clark WC, Cross LW, Kemperman I, Kakuma T, Harrison K. Pain and self-injury in borderline patients: sensory decision theory, coping strategies, and locus of control. *Psychiatry Res.* 1996 Jun 26;63(1):57-65.

Russek LG, Schwartz GE. Narrative descriptions of parental love and caring predict health status in midlife: a 35-year follow-up of the Harvard Mastery of Stress Study. *Altern Ther Health Med.* 1996 Nov;2(6):55-62.

Russell IJ. Advances in fibromyalgia: possible role for central neurochemicals. *Am J Med Sci.* 1998;315:377-84.

Russell RM, Golner BB, Krasinski SD, Sadowski JA, Suter PM, Braun CL. Effect of antacid and H2 receptor antagonists on the intestinal absorption of folic acid. *J Lab Clin Med.* 1988;112:458-63.

Russo PA, Halliday GM. Inhibition of nitric oxide and reactive oxygen species production improves the ability of a sunscreen to protect from sunburn, immunosuppression and photocarcinogenesis. *Br J Dermatol.* 2006 Aug;155(2):408-15.

Saarijarvi S, Lauerma H, Helenius H, Saarilehto S. Seasonal affective disorders among rural Finns and Lapps. *Acta Psychiatr Scand.* 1999 Feb;99(2):95-101.

Sabom M. *Light and Death: One Doctor's Fascinating Account of Near Death Experiences.* Grand Rapids, MI: Zondervan Publishing, 1998.

Sabom M. *Recollections of Death: A Medical Investigation.* New York: Harper and Row, 1982.

Sacks O. *The Man Who Mistook his Wife for a Hat and Other Clinical Tales.* New York: Simon & Schuster, 1998.

Sahlin C, Pettersson FE, Nilsson LN, Lannfelt L, Johansson AS. Docosahexaenoic acid stimulates non-amyloidogenic APP processing resulting in reduced Abeta levels in cellular models of Alzheimer's disease. *Eur J Neurosci.* 2007 Aug;26(4):882-9.

Sainte-Laudy J, Belon P. Analysis of immunosuppressive activity of serial dilutions of histamine on human basophil activation by flow cytometry. *Inflam Rsrch.* 1996 Suppl. 1: S33-S34.

Sakugawa H, Cape JN. Harmful effects of atmospheric nitrous acid on the physiological status of

Salem N, Wegher B, Mena P, Uauy R. Arachidonic and docosahexaenoic acids are biosynthesized from their 18-carbon precursors in human infants. *Proc Natl Acad Sci.* 1996;93:49-54.

Salom IL, Silvis SE, Doscherholmen A. Effect of cimetidine on the absorption of vitamin B12. *Scand J Gastroenterol.* 1982;17:129-31.

Sanders R. Slow brain waves play key role in coordinating complex activity. *UC Berkeley News.* 2006 Sep 14.

Sarah Janssen S, Solomon G, Schettler T. Chemical Contaminants and Human Disease:A Summary of Evidence. *The Collaborative on Health and the Environment.* 2006. http://www.healthandenvironment.org. Acc. 2007 Jul.

Saran, S., Gopalan, S. and Krishna, T. P. Use of fermented foods to combat stunting and failure to thrive. *Nutrition.* 2002;8:393-396.

Sarveiya V, Risk S, Benson HA. Liquid chromatographic assay for common sunscreen agents: application to in vivo assessment of skin penetration and systemic absorption in human volunteers. *J Chromatogr B Analyt Technol Biomed Life Sci.* 2004 Apr 25;803(2):225-31.

Sato TK, Yamada RG, Ukai H, Baggs JE, Miraglia LJ, Kobayashi TJ, Welsh DK, Kay SA, Ueda HR, Hogenesch JB. Feedback repression is required for mammalian circadian clock function. *Nat Genet.* 2006 Mar;38(3):312-9.

Satyanarayana S, Sushruta K, Sarma GS, Srinivas N, Subba Raju GV. Antioxidant activity of the aqueous extracts of spicy food additives-evaluation and comparison with ascorbic acid in in-vitro systems. *J Herb Pharmacother.* 2004;4(2):1-10.

Sauvant M, Pepin D. Drinking water and cardiovascular disease. *Food Chem Toxicol.* 2002;40:1311-1325.

Schenk BE, Festen HP, Kuipers EJ, Klinkenberg-Knol EC, Meuwissen SG. Effect of short-and long-term treatment with omeprazole on the absorption and serum levels of cobalamin. *Aliment Pharmacol Ther.* 1996;10:541-5.

Schirber M. Earth as a Giant Pinball Machine. *LiveScience.* 2004; 19 Nov 19. http://www.livescience.com/environment/041119_earth_layers.html. Acc. 2006 Nov.

Schlebusch KP, Maric-Oehler W, Popp FA. Biophotonics in the infrared spectral range reveal acupuncture meridian structure of the body. *J Altern Complement Med.* 2005 Feb;11(1):171-3.

Schlumpf M, Cotton B, Conscience M, Haller V, Steinmann B, Lichtensteiger W. In vitro and in vivo estrogenicity of UV screens. *Environ Health Perspect.* 2001 Mar;109(3):239-44.

Schmidt H, Quantum processes predicted? *New Sci.* 1969 Oct 16.

Schmitt B, Frölich L. Creative therapy options for patients with dementia—a systematic review. *Fortschr Neurol Psychiatr.* 2007 Dec;75(12):699-707.

Schonberger B. Bladder dysfunction and surgery in the small pelvis. Therapeutic possibilities. *Urologe A.* 2003 Dec;42(12):1569-75.

Schulz T, Zarse K, Voigt A, Urban N, Birringer M, Ristow M. Glucose Restriction Extends Caenorhabditis elegans Life Span by Inducing Mitochondrial Respiration and Increasing Oxidative Stress. *Cell Metabolism.* 2007 Oct 3;6:280-293.

Schumacher P. *Biophysical Therapy Of Allergies.* Stuttgart: Thieme, 2005.

Schwartz GG, Skinner HG. Vitamin D status and cancer: new insights. *Curr Opin Clin Nutr Metab Care.* 2007 Jan;10(1):6-11.

Schwartz S, De Mattei R, Brame E, Spottiswoode S. Infrared spectra alteration in water proximate to the palms of therapeutic practitioners. In: Wiener D, Nelson R (Eds.): *Research in parapsychology 1986.* Metuchen, NJ: Scarecrow Press, 1987:24-29.

Schwellenbach LJ, Olson KL. McConnell KJ, Stolepart RS, Nash JD, Merenich JA. The triglyceride-lowering effects of a modest dose of docosahexaenoic acid alone versus in combination with low dose eicosapentaenoic acid in patients with coronary artery disease and elevated triglycerides. *J Am Coll Nutr.* 2006;25(6):480-485.

Scoville WB, Milner B. Loss of recent memory after bilateral hippocampal lesions. *J Neurol Neurosurg Psychiatry.* 1957;20:11-21.

Semenza C. Retrieval pathways for common and proper names. *Cortex.* 2006 Aug;42(6):884-91.

Senekowitsch F, Endler PC, Pongratz W, Smith CW. Hormone effects by CD record /replay. *FASEB J.* 1995:A12025.

Senior F. Fallout. *New York Mag.* 2003 Fall.

Seo K, Jung S, Park M, Song Y, Choung S. Effects of leucocyanidines on activities of metabolizing enzymes and antioxidant enzymes. *Biol Pharm Bull.* 2001 May;24(5):592-3.

Serra-Valls A. Electromagnetic Industrion and the Conservation of Momentum in the Spiral Paradox. *Cornell University Library.* http://arxiv.org/ftp/physics/papers/0012/0012009.pdf. Acc. 2007 Jul.

Serway R. *Physicis For Scientists & Engineers.* Philadelphia: Harcourt Brace, 1992.

Shaffer D. *Developmental Psychology: Theory, Research and Applications.* Monterey, CA: Brooks/Cole, 1985.

Shafik A. Role of warm-water bath in anorectal conditions. The "thermosphincteric reflex". *J Clin Gastroenterol.* 1993 Jun;16(4):304-8.

Shankar R. *My Music, My Life.* New York: Simon & Schuster, 1968.

Sharp KC. *After the Light.* New York: William Morrow & Co., 1995.

Shearman LP, Zylka MJ, Weaver DR, Kolakowski LF Jr, Reppert SM. Two period homologs: circadian expression and photic regulation in the suprachiasmatic nuclei. *Neuron.* 1997 Dec;19(6):1261-9.

Shen YF, Goddard G. The short-term effects of acupuncture on myofascial pain patients after clenching. *Pain Pract.* 2007 Sep;7(3):256-64.

Shevelev IA, Kostelianetz NB, Kamenkovich VM, Sharaev GA. EEG alpha-wave in the visual cortex: check of the hypothesis of the scanning process. *Int J Psychophysiol.* 1991 Aug;11(2):195-201.

Shupak NM, Prato FS, Thomas AW. Human exposure to a specific pulsed magnetic field: effects on thermal sensory and pain thresholds. *Neurosci Lett.* 2004 Jun 10;363(2):157-62.

Shutov AA, Panasiuk IIa. Efficacy of rehabilitation of patients with chronic primary low back pain at the spa Klyuchi using balneopelotherapy and transcranial electrostimulation. *Vopr Kurortol Fizioter Lech Fiz Kult.* 2007 Mar-Apr;(2):16-8.

Sicher F, Targ E, Moore D, Smith H. A Randomized Double-Blind Study of the Effect of Distant Healing in a Population With Advanced AIDS. Western Journal of Medicine. 1998;169 Dec::356-363.

Siegfried J. Electrostimulation and neurosurgical measures in cancer pain. *Recent Results Cancer Res.* 1988;108:28-32.

Simpson G. *The Major Features of Evolution.* New York: Columbia Univ Press, 1953.

Sin DD, Man J, Sharpe H, Gan WQ, Man SF. Pharmacological management to reduce exacerbations in adults with asthma: a systematic review and meta-analysis. *JAMA.* 2004 Jul 21;292(3):367-76.

Skoczylas A, Wiecek A. Ghrelin, a new hormone involved not only in the regulation of appetite. *Wiad Lek.* 2006;59(9-10):697-701.

Skwerer RG, Jacobsen FM, Duncan CC, Kelly KA, Sack DA, Tamarkin L, Gaist PA, Kasper S, Rosenthal NE. Neurobiology of Seasonal Affective Disorder and Phototherapy. *J Biolog Rhyth.* 1988;3(2):135-154.

Sloan F and Gelband (ed). Cancer Control Opportunities in Low- and Middle-Income Countries. Committee on Cancer Control in Low- and Middle-Income Countries. 2007.

Smith CW. Coherence in living biological systems. *Neural Network World.* 1994:4(3):379-388.

Smith MJ. "Effect of Magnetic Fields on Enzyme Reactivity" in Barnothy M.(ed.), *Biological Effects of Magnetic Fields.* New York: Plenum Press, 1969.

Smith MJ. *The Influence on Enzyme Growth By the 'Laying on of Hands: Dimenensions of Healing.* Los Altos, California: Academy of Parapsychology and Medicine, 1973.

Smith T. *Homeopathic Medicine: A Doctor's Guide.* Rochester, VT: Healing Arts, 1989.

Smith-Sonneborn J. Age-correlated effects of caffeine on non-irradiated and UV-irradiated Paramecium Aurelia. *J Gerontol.* 1974 May;29(3):256-60.

Smith-Sonneborn J. DNA repair and longevity assurance in Paramecium tetraurelia. *Science.* 1979 Mar 16;203(4385):1115-7.

Snyder K. Researchers Produce Firsts with Bursts of Light: Team generates most energetic terahertz pulses yet, observes useful optical phenomena. *Press Release: Brookhaven National Laboratory.* 2007 July 24.

Soler M, Chandra S, Ruiz D, Davidson E, Hendrickson D, Christou G. A third isolated oxidation state for the Mn12 family of singl molecule magnets. *ChemComm;* 2000; Nov 22.

Soni MG, Carabin IG, Burdock GA. Safety assessment of esters of p-hydroxybenzoic acid (parabens). *Food Chem Toxicol.* 2005 Jul;43(7):985-1015.

Soul Has Weight, Physician Thinks. *The New York Times.* 1907 March 11:5.

Southgate, D. Nature and variability of human food consumption. *Philosophical Transactions of the Royal Society of London.* 1991;*B*(334): 281-288.

Spanagel R, Rosenwasser AM, Schumann G, Sarkar DK. Alcohol consumption and the body's biological clock. *Alcohol Clin Exp Res.* 2005 Aug;29(8):1550-7.

Speed Of Light May Not Be Constant, Physicist Suggests. *Science Daily.* 1999 Oct 6. www.sciencedaily.com/releases/1999/10/991005114024.htm. Acc. 2007 Jun.

Spence A. *Basic Human Anatomy.* Menlo Park, CA: Benjamin/Commings, 1986.

Spetner L. *Not By Chance! -Shattering The Modern Theory of Evolution.* New York: The Judaica Press, 1997.

Spillane M. Good Vibrations, A Sound 'Diet' for Plants. *The Growing Edge.* 1991 Spring.

Spiller G. *The Super Pyramid.* New York: HRS Press, 1993.

Squire LR, Zola-Morgan S. The medial temporal lobe memory system. *Science.* 1991;253(5026):1380-1386.

St Hilaire MA, Klerman EB, Khalsa SB, Wright KP Jr, Czeisler CA, Kronauer RE. Addition of a non-photic component to a light-based mathematical model of the human circadian pacemaker. *J Theor Biol.* 2007 Aug 21;247(4):583-99.

Stachowska E, Dolegowska B, Chlubek D, Wesolowska T, Ciechanowski K, Gutowski P, Szumilowicz H, Turowski R. Dietary trans fatty acids and composition of human atheromatous plaques. *Eur J Nutr.* 2004 Oct;43(5):313-8.

Stahler C. 1994. How many vegetarians are there?" *Veget Jnl.* 1994: July/August.

Stamets P. *Mycelium Running.* Berkeley, CA: Ten Speed Press, 2005.

Stampfer MJ, Willett WC, Colditz GA, Rosner B, Speizer FE, Hennekens CH. A prospective study of postmenopausal estrogen therapy and coronary heart disease. *N Engl J Med.* 1985 Oct 24;313(17):1044-9.

Stanford, C. B. The hunting ecology of wild chimpanzees: Implications for the evolutionary ecology of Pliocene hominids. *American Anthropologist.* 1996;98: 96-113.

Steck B. Effects of optical radiation on man. *Light Resch Techn.* 1982;14:130-141.

Steiner R. *Agriculture.* Kimberton, PA: Bio-Dynamic Farming, 1924-1993.

Stevenson I, Samararatne G. Three new cases of the reincarnation type in Sri Lanka with written records made before verification. *J. Sci. Exploration.* 1988;2(2): 217-238.

Stevenson I. American children who claim to remember previous lives. *J. Nervous and Mental Disease.* 1983;171:742-748.

Stevenson I. *Cases of the Reincarnation Type.* Charlottesville, VA: Univ Virginia Press. Vol. 1: *Ten Cases in India,* 1975. Vol. 2: *Ten Cases in Sri Lanka,* 1977. Vol. 3: *Twelve Cases in Lebanon and Turkey,* 1980. Vol. 4: *Twelve Cases in Thailand and Burma,* 1983.

Stevenson I. *Children Who Remember Previous Lives: A Question of Reincarnation.* Charlottesville, VA: Univ Virginia Press, 1987.

Stevenson I. *European Cases of the Reincarnation Type.* Jefferson, NC: McFarland and Co., 2003.

Stevenson I. *Reincarnation and Biology: A Contribution to the Etiology of Birthmarks and Birth Defects.* (2 volumes). Westport, CN: Praeger Publishers, 1997.

Stevenson I. *Twenty Cases Suggestive of Reincarnation.* New York: American Society for Psychical Research, 1967.

Stevenson I. *Where Reincarnation and Biology Intersect.* Westport, CN: Praeger, 1997.

Stojanovic MP, Abdi S. Spinal cord stimulation. *Pain Physician.* 2002 Apr;5(2):156-66.

Stoupel E, Babyev E, Mustafa F, Abramson E, Israelevich P, Sulkes J. Acute myocardial infarction occurrence: Environmental links - Baku 2003-2005 data. *Med Sci Monit.* 2007 Aug;13(8):BR175-179.

Stoupel E, Kalediene R, Petrauskiene J, Gaizauskiene A, Israelevich P, Abramson E, Sulkes J. Monthly number of newborns and environmental physical activity. *Medicina Kaunas.* 2006;42(3):238-41.

Stoupel E, Monselise Y, Lahav J. Changes in autoimmune markers of the anti-cardiolipin syndrome on days of extreme geomamagnetic activity. *J Basic Clin Physiol Pharmacol.* 2006;17(4):269-78.

Stoupel EG, Frimer H, Appelman Z, Ben-Neriah Z, Dar H, Fejgin MD, Gershoni-Baruch R, Manor E, Barkai G, Shalev S, Gelman-Kohan Z, Reish O, Lev D, Davidov B, Goldman B, Shohat M. Chromosome aberration and environmental physical activity: Down syndrome and solar and cosmic ray activity, Israel, 1990-2000. *Int J Biometeorol.* 2005 Sep;50(1):1-5.

Strange BA, Dolan RJ. Anterior medial temporal lobe in human cognition: memory for fear and the unexpected. *Cognit Neuropsychiatry.* 2006 May;11(3):198-218.

Streitberger K, Ezzo J, Schneider A. Acupuncture for nausea and vomiting: an update of clinical and experimental studies. *Auton Neurosci.* 2006 Oct 30;129(1-2):107-17.

Sulman FG, Levy D, Lunkan L, Pfeifer Y, Tal E. New methods in the treatment of weather sensitivity. *Fortschr Med.* 1977 Mar 17;95(11):746-52.

Sulman FG. Migraine and headache due to weather and allied causes and its specific treatment. *Ups J Med Sci Suppl.* 1980;31:41-4.

Suppes P, Han B, Epelboim J, Lu ZL. Invariance of brain-wave representations of simple visual images and their names. *Proc Natl Acad Sci Psych-BS.* 1999;96(25):14658-14663.

Suzuki Y, Kondo K, Ichise H, Tsukamoto Y, Urano T, Umemura K. Dietary supplementation with fermented soybeans suppresses intimal thickening. *Nutrition.* 2003 Mar;19(3):261-4.

Szyf M, McGowan P, Meaney MJ. The social environment and the epigenome. *Environ Mol Mutagen.* 2008 Jan;49(1):46-60.

Tan DX, Manchester LC, Reiter RJ, Qi WB, Karbownik M, Calvo JR. Significance of melatonin in antioxidative defense system: reactions and products. *Biol Signals Recept.* 2000 May-Aug;9(3-4):137-59.

Tanagho EA. Principles and indications of electrostimulation of the urinary bladder. *Urologe A.* 1990 Jul;29(4):185-90.

Tang G, Serfaty-Lacronsniere C, Camilo ME, Russell RM. Gastric acidity influences the blood response to a beta-carotene dose in humans. *Am J Clin Nutr.* 1996;64:622-6.

Taoka S, Padmakumar R, Grissom C, Banerjee R. Magnetic Field Effects on Coenzyme B-12 Dependent Enzymes: Validation of Ethanolamine Ammonia Lyase Results and Extension to Human Methylmalonyl CoA Mutase. *Bioelectromagnetics.* 1997;18: 506-513.

Tapiero H, Ba GN, Couvreur P, Tew KD. Polyunsaturated fatty acids (PUFA) and eicosanoids in human health and pathologies. *Biomed Pharmacother.* 2002 Jul;56(5):215-22.

Tapsell LC, Hemphill I, Cobiac L, Patch CS, Sullivan DR, Fenech M, Roodenrys S, Keogh JB, Clifton PM, Williams PG, Fazio VA, Inge KE. Health benefits of herbs and spices: the past, the present, the future. *Med J Aust.* 2006 Aug 21;185(4 Suppl):S4-24.

Taraban M, Leshina T, Anderson M, Grissom C. Magnetic Field Dependence and the Role of electron spin in Heme Enzymes: Horseradish Peroxidase. *J. Am. Chem. Soc.* 1997;119: 5768-5769.

Targ R, Katra J, Brown D, Wiegand W. Viewing the future: A pilot study with an error-detecting protocol. *J Sci Expl.* 9:3:367-380, 1995.

Targ R, Puthoff H. Information transfer under conditions of sensory shielding. *Nature.* 1975;251:602-607.

Tassone F, Broglio F, Gianotti L, Arvat E, Ghigo E, Maccario M. Ghrelin and other gastrointestinal peptides involved in the control of food intake. *Mini Rev Med Chem.* 2007 Jan;7(1):47-53.

Tauchert M. Efficacy and safety of crataegus extract WS 1442 in comparison with placebo in patients with chronic stable New York Heart Association class-III heart failure. *Am Heart J.* 2002 May;143(5):910-5.

Taussig SJ, Batkin S. Bromelain, the enzyme complex of pineapple (Ananas comosus) and its clinical application. An update. *J Ethnopharmacol.* 1988 Feb-Mar;22(2):191-203.

Taylor A. *Soul Traveler: A Guide to Out-of-Body Experiences and the Wonders Beyond.* New York: Penguin, 2000.

Teitelbaum J. *From Fatigue to Fantastic.* New York: Avery, 2001.

Termanini B, Gibril F, Sutliff VE, Yu F, Venzon DJ, Jensen RT. Effect of long-term gastric acid suppressive therapy on serum vitamin B12 levels in patients with Zollinger-Ellison syndrome. *Am J Med.* 1998 May;104(5):422-30.

Tevini M, ed. *UV-B Radiation and Ozone Depletion: Effects on humans, animals, plants, microorganisms and materials.* Boca Raton: Lewis Pub, 1993.

Thakur CP, Sharma D. Full moon and crime. *Br Med J.* 1984 December 22; 289(6460): 1789-1791.

Thaut MH. The future of music in therapy and medicine. *Ann N Y Acad Sci.* 2005 Dec;1060:303-8.

The Mystery of Smell. Howard Hughes Medical Instit. http://www.hhmi.org/senses/d110.html. Acc. 2007 Jul.

The Timechart Company. *Timetables of Medicine.* New York: Black Dog & Leventhal, 2000.

Thie J. *Touch for Health.* Marina del Rey, CA: Devorss Publications, 1973-1994.

Thomas MK, Lloyd-Jones DM, Thadhani RI, Shaw AC, Deraska DJ, Kitch BT, Vamvakas EC, Dick IM, Prince RL, Finkelstein JS. Hypovitaminosis D in medical inpatients. *N Engl J Med.* 1998 Mar 19;338(12):777-83

Thomas Y, Litime H, Benveniste J. Modulation of human neutrophil activation by "electronic" phorbol myristate acetate (PMA). *FASEB Jnl.* 1996;10: A1479.

Thomas Y, Schiff M, Belkadi L, Jurgens P, Kahhak L, Benveniste J. Activation of human neutrophils by electronically transmitted phorbol-myristate acetate. *Med Hypoth.* 2000;54: 33-39.

Thomas Y, Schiff M, Litime M, Belkadi L, Benveniste J. Direct transmission to cells of a molecular signal (phorbol myristate acetate, PMA) via an electronic device. *FASEB Jnl.* 1995;9: A227.

Thomas-Anterion C, Jacquin K, Laurent B. Differential mechanisms of impairment of remote memory in Alzheimer's and frontotemporal dementia. *Dement Geriatr Cogn Disord.* 2000 Mar-Apr;11(2):100-6.

Thompson D. *On Growth and Form.* Cambridge: Cambridge University Press, 1992.

Thorogood M, Mann J, Appleby P, McPherson K. Risk of death from cancer and ischaemic heart disease in meat and non-meat eaters. *BMJ.* 1994 June 25;308:1667-1670.

Threlkeld DS, ed. Central Nervous System Drugs, Analeptics, Caffeine. *Facts and Comparisons Drug Information.* St. Louis, MO: Facts and Comparisons. 1998 Feb: 230-d.

Threlkeld DS, ed. Gastrointestinal Drugs, Proton Pump Inhibitors. *Facts and Comparisons Drug Information.* St. Louis, MO: Facts and Comparisons. 1998 Apr: 305r.

Tian FS, Zhang HR, Li WD, Qiao P, Duan HB, Jia CX. Study on acupuncture treatment of diabetic neurogenic bladder. *Zhongguo Zhen Jiu.* 2007 Jul;27(7):485-7.

Tierra L. *The Herbs of Life.* Freedom, CA: Crossing Press, 1992.

Tierra M. *The Way of Herbs.* New York: Pocket Books, 1990.

Timofeev I, Steriade M. Low-frequency rhythms in the thalamus of intact-cortex and decorticated cats. *J Neurophysiol.* 1996 Dec;76(6):4152-68.

Ting W, Schultz K, Cac NN, Peterson M, Walling HW. Tanning bed exposure increases the risk of malignant melanoma. Int J Dermatol. 2007 Dec;46(12):1253-7.

Tisserand R. *The Art of Aromatherapy.* New York: Inner Traditions, 1979.

Tiwari M. *Ayurveda: A Life of Balance.* Rochester, VT: Healing Arts, 1995.

Todd GR, Acerini CL, Ross-Russell R, Zahra S, Warner JT, McCance D. Survey of adrenal crisis associated with inhaled corticosteroids in the United Kingdom. *Arch Dis Child.* 2002 Dec;87(6):457-61.

Tompkins, P, Bird C. *The Secret Life of Plants.* New York: Harper & Row, 1973.

Toomer G. "Ptolemy". *The Dictionary of Scientific Biography.* New York: Gale Cengage, 1970.

Triglia A, La Malfa G, Musumeci F, Leonardi C, Scordino A. Delayed luminsecence as an indicator of tomato fruit quality. *J Food Sci.* 1998;63:512-515.

Trivedi B. Magnetic Map" Found to Guide Animal Migration. *Natl Geogr Today.* 2001 Oct 12.

Tsinkalovsky O, Smaaland R, Rosenlund B, Sothern RB, Hirt A, Steine S, Badiee A, Abrahamsen JF, Eiken HG, Laerum OD. Circadian variations in clock gene expression of human bone marrow CD34+ cells. *J Biol Rhythms.* 2007 Apr;22(2):140-50.

Tsong T. Deciphering the language of cells. *Trends in Biochem Sci.* 1989;14: 89-92.

Tsuei JJ, Lam Jr. F, Zhao Z. Studies in Bioenergetic Correlations-Bioenergetic Regulatory Measurement Instruments and Devices. *Am J Acupunct.* 1988;16:345-9.

Tsuei JJ, Lehman CW, Lam F, Jr, Zhu D. A food allergy study utilizing the EAV acupuncture technique. *Am J Acupunct.* 1984;12:105-16.

Tubek S. Role of trace elements in primary arterial hypertension: is mineral water style or prophylaxis? *Biol Trace Elem Res.* 2006 Winter;114(1-3):1-5.

Tucker J. *Life Before Life: A Scientific Investigation of Children's Memories of Previous Lives.* New York: St. Martin's Press, 2005.

Tweed K. Study: Conceiving in Summer Lowers Baby's Future Test Scores. *Fox News.* 2007 May 9, 2007. (Study done by: Winchester P. 2007. Pediatric Academic Societies annual meeting.)

Udermann H, Fischer G. Studies on the influence of positive or negative small ions on the catechol amine content in the brain of the mouse following shorttime or prolonged exposure. *Zentralbl Bakteriol Mikrobiol Hyg.* 1982 Apr;176(1):72-8.

Ulett G. Electroacupuncture: mechanisms and clinical application. *Biological Psychiatry.* 1998;44(2):129-138.

Ullman D. Controlled clinical trials evaluating the homeopathic treatment of people with human immunodeficiency virus or acquired immune deficiency syndrome. *J Altern Complement Med.* 2003 Feb;9(1):133-41.

Ullman D. *Discovering Homeopathy.* Berkeley, CA: North Atlantic, 1991.

Unger RH. Leptin physiology: a second look. *Regul Pept.* 2000 Aug 25;92(1-3):87-95.

Vallance A. Can biological activity be maintained at ultra-high dilution? An overview of homeopathy, evidence, and Bayesian philosophy. *J Altern Complement Med.* 1998 Spring;4(1):49-76.

Van Cauter E, Leproult R, Plat L. Age-related changes in slow wave sleep and REM sleep and relationship with growth hormone and cortisol levels in healthy men. *JAMA.* 2000 Aug 16;284(7):861-8.

van den Berg H, Dagnelie P, van Staveren W. Vitamin B12 and seaweed. *Lancet.* 1988;1:242-3.

van den Eeden SK, Koepsell TD, Longstreth WT, van Belle G, Daling JR, McKnight B. Aspartame ingestion and headache: a randomized crossover trial. *Neurology.* 1994;44:1787-93.

Van Wijk R, Wiegant FAC. *Cultured mammalian cells in homeopathy research: the similia principle in self-recovery.* Utrecht: University Utrecht Publ, 1994.

Vandenbroucke JP. Should you eat meat, or are you confounded by methodological debate? *BMJ.* 1994 Jun 25;308(6945):1671.

Vaquero JM, Gallego MC. Sunspot numbers can detect pandemic influenza A: the use of different sunspot numbers. *Med Hypotheses.* 2007;68(5):1189-90.

Vargha-Khadem F, Polkey CE. A review of cognitive outcome after hemidecortication in humans. *Adv Exp Med Biol.* 1992;325:137-51.

Vauthier JM, Lluch A, Lecomte E, Artur Y, Herbeth B. Family resemblance in energy and macronutrient intakes: the Stanislas Family Study. *Int J Epidemiol.* 1996 Oct;25(5):1030-7.

Vescelius E. *Music and Health.* New York: Goodyear Book Shop, 1918.

Vickers A. Botanical medicines for the treatment of cancer: rationale, overview of current data, and methodological considerations for phase I and II trials. *Cancer Invest.* 2002;20(7-8):1069-79.

Vickers AJ, Kuo J, Cassileth BR. Unconventional anticancer agents: a systematic review of clinical trials. *J Clin Oncol.* 2006 Jan 1;24(1):136-40.

Vidgren HM, Agren JJ, Schwab U, Rissanen T, Hanninen O, Uusitupa MI. Incorporation of n-3 fatty acids into plasma lipid fractions, and erythrocyte membranes and platelets during dietary supplementation with fish, fish oil, and docosahexaenoic acid-rich oil among healthy young men. *Lipids.* 1997 Jul;32(7):697-705.

Vierling-Claassen D, Siekmeier P, Stufflebeam S, Kopell N. Modeling GABA alterations in schizophrenia: a link between impaired inhibition and altered gamma and beta range auditory entrainment. *J Neurophysiol.* 2008 May;99(5):2656-71.

Vigny P, Duquesne M. *On the fluorescence properties of nucleotides and polynucleotides at room temperature.* In. Birks J (ed.). Excited states of biological molecules. London-NY: J Wiley, 1976:167-177.

Volkmann H, Dannberg G, Kuhnert H, Heinke M. Therapeutic value of trans-esophageal electrostimulation in tachycardic arrhythmias. *Z Kardiol.* 1991 Jun;80(6):382-8.

Voll R. The phenomenon of medicine testing in elecroacupuncture according to Voll. *Am J Acupunct.* 1980;8:97-104.

Voll R. Twenty years of electroacupuncture diagnosis in Germany: a progressive report. *Am J Acupunct.* 1975;3:7-17.

von Schantz M, Archer SN. *Clocks, genes and sleep. J R Soc Med.* 2003 Oct;96(10):486-9.

Vyasadeva S. *Srimad Bhagavatam.* Approx rec 4000 BCE.

Wachiuli M, Koyama M, Utsuyama M, Bittman BB, Kitagawa M, Hirokawa K. Recreational music-making modulates natural killer cell activity, cytokines, and mood states in corporate employees. *Med Sci Monit.* 2007 Feb;13(2):CR57-70.

Wade N. From Ants to Ethics: A Biologist Dreams of Unity of Knowledge. Scientist at Work, Edward O. Wilson. *New York Times.* 1998 May 12.

Walker AF, Marakis G, Morris AP, Robinson PA. Promising hypotensive effect of hawthorn extract: a randomized double-blind pilot study of mild, essential hypertension. *Phytother Res.* 2002 Feb;16(1):48-54.

Walker M. *The Power of Color.* Gujarat, India: Jain Publ., 2002.

Wang R, Jiang C, Lei Z, Yin K. The role of different therapeutic courses in treating 47 cases of rheumatoid arthritis with acupuncture. *J Tradit Chin Med.* 2007 Jun;27(2):103-5.

Wang XY, Shi X, He L. Effect of electroacupuncture on gastrointestinal dynamics in acute pancreatitis patients and its mechanism. *Zhen Ci Yan Jiu.* 2007;32(3):199-202.

Waser M, *et al.* PARSIFAL Study team. Inverse association of farm milk consumption with asthma and allergy in rural and suburban populations across Europe. *Clin Exp Allergy.* 2007 May;37(5):661-70.

Watnick S. Pregnancy and contraceptive counseling of women with chronic kidney disease and kidney transplants. *Adv Chronic Kidney Dis.* 2007 Apr;14(2):126-31.

Watson L. *Beyond Supernature.* New York: Bantam, 1987.

Watson L. *Supernature.* New York: Bantam, 1973.

Wauters M, Considine RV, Van Gaal LF. Human leptin: from an adipocyte hormone to an endocrine mediator. *Eur J Endocrinol.* 2000 Sep;143(3):293-311.

Wayne R. *Chemistry of the Atmospheres.* Oxford Press, 1991.

WB Saunders; 1982, Fishman HC. Notalgia paresthetica. *J Am Acad Dermatol.* 1986;15:1304-1305

Weatherley-Jones E, Thompson E, Thomas K. The placebo-controlled trial as a test of complementary and alternative medicine: observations from research experience of individualised homeopathic treatment. *Homeopathy.* 2004 Oct;93(4):186-9.

Weaver J, Astumian R. The response of living cells to very weak electric fields: the thermal noise limit. *Science.* 1990;247: 459-462.

Wee K, Rogers T, Altan BS, Hackney SA, Hamm C. Engineering and medical applications of diatoms. *J Nanosci Nanotechnol.* 2005 Jan;5(1):88-91.

Weikl A, Assmus KD, Neukum-Schmidt A, Schmitz J, Zapfe G, Noh HS, Siegrist J. Crataegus Special Extract WS 1442. Assessment of objective effectiveness in patients with heart failure (NYHA II). *Fortschr Med.* 1996 Aug 30;114(24):291-6.

Weinberger P, Measures M. The effect of two audible sound frequencies on the germination and growth of a spring and winter wheat. *Can. J. Bot.* 1968;46(9):1151-1158.
Weiner MA. *Secrets of Fijian Medicine.* Berkeley, CA: Univ. of Calif., 1969.
Weinert D, Waterhouse J. The circadian rhythm of core temperature: effects of physical activity and aging. *Physiol Behav.* 2007 Feb 28;90(2-3):246-56.
Weiss B. *Many Lives, Many Masters.* New York: Simon & Schuster, 1988.
Weiss RF. *Herbal Medicine.* Gothenburg, Sweden: Beaconsfield, 1988.
Weller A, Weller L. Menstrual synchrony between mothers and daughters and between roommates. *Physiol Behav.* 1993 May;53(5):943-9.
Weller L, Weller A, Roizman S. Human menstrual synchrony in families and among close friends: examining the importance of mutual exposure. *J Comp Psychol.* 1999 Sep;113(3):261-8.
Welsh D, Yoo SH, Liu A, Takahashi J, Kay S. Bioluminescence Imaging of Individual Fibroblasts Reveals Persistent, Independently Phased Circadian Rhythms of Clock Gene Expression. *Current Biology.* 2004;14:2289-2295.
Werbach M. *Nutritional Influences on Illness.* Tarzana, CA: Third Line Press, 1996.
West P. *Surf Your Biowaves.* London: Quantum, 1999.
West R. Risk of death in meat and non-meat eaters. *BMJ.* 1994 Oct 8;309(6959):955.
Westman M, Eden D. Effects of a respite from work on burnout: vacation relief and fade-out. *J Appl Psychol.* 1997 Aug;82(4):516-27.
Wetterberg L. Light and biological rhythms. *J Intern Med.* 1994 Jan;235(1):5-19.
Wheeler FJ. *The Bach Remedies Repertory.* New Canaan, CN: Keats, 1997.
White AR, Rampes H, Ernst E. Acupuncture for smoking cessation. *Cochrane Database Syst Rev.* 2002;(2):CD000009.
White J, Krippner S (eds). *Future Science: Life Energies & the Physics of Paranormal Phenomena.* Garden City: Anchor, 1977.
White S. *The Unity of the Self.* Cambridge: MIT Press, 1991.
Whiten, A. and E. M. Widdowson (eds.). *Foraging Strategies and Natural Diet of Monkeys, Apes and Humans.* Oxford: Clarendon Press, 1991.
Whitfield KE, King G, Moller S, Edwards CL, Nelson T, Vandenbergh D. Concordance rates for smoking among African-American twins. *J Natl Med Assoc.* 2007 Mar;99(3):213-7.
Whittaker E. *History of the Theories of Aether and Electricity.* New York: Nelson LTD, 1953.
Whitton J. *Life Between Life.* New York: Warner, 1986.
WHO. *Guidelines for Drinking-water Quality.* 2nd ed, vol. 2. Geneva: World Health Organization, 1996.
WHO. How trace elements in water contribute to health. *WHO Chronicle.* 1978;32: 382-385.
Wilkinson SM, Love SB, Westcombe AM, Gambles MA, Burgess CC, Cargill A, Young T, Maher EJ, Ramirez AJ. Effectiveness of aromatherapy massage in the management of anxiety and depression in patients with cancer: a multicenter randomized controlled trial. *J Clin Oncol.* 2007 Feb 10;25(5):532-9.
Williams A. Electron microscopic changes associated with water absorption in the jejunum. *Gut.* 1963;4:1-7.
Williams G. *Natural Selection: Domains, levels, and challenges.* Oxford: Oxford Univ Press, 1992.
Wilson L. *Nutritional Balancing and Hair Mineral Analysis.* Prescott, AZ: LD Wilson, 1998.
Winchester AM. *Biology and its Relation to Mankind.* New York: Van Nostrand Reinhold, 1969.
Winfree AT. *The Timing of Biological Clocks.* New York: Scientific American, 1987.
Winstead DK, Schwartz BD, Bertrand WE. Biorhythms: fact or superstition? *Am J Psychiatry.* 1981 Sep;138(9):1188-92.
Wittenberg JS. *The Rebellious Body.* New York: Insight, 1996.
Wixted JT. A Theory About Why We Forget What We Once Knew. *CurrDir Psychol Sci.* 2005;14(1):6-9.
Wolf, M. Beyond the Point Particle - *A Wave Structure for the Electron. Galilean Electrodynamics.* 1995 Oct;6(5): 83-91.
Wolverton BC. *How to Grow Fresh Air: 50 House Plants that Purify Your Home or Office.* New York: Penguin, 1997.
Wood M. *The Book of Herbal Wisdom.* Berkeley, CA: North Atlantic, 1997.
Woolger R. *Other Lives, Other Selves.* New York: Bantam, 1988.
World Cancer Research Fund, American Institute for Cancer Research. *Food, Nutrition and the Prevention of Cancer: A Global Perspective.* 1997: 509.
Worwood VA. *The Complete Book of Essential Oils & Aromatherapy.* San Rafael, CA: New World, 1991.
Wright ML. Melatonin, diel rhythms, and metamorphosis in anuran amphibians. *Gen Comp Endocrinol.* 2002 May;126(3):251-4.
Wyart C, Webster WW, Chen JH, Wilson SR, McClary A, Khan RM, Sobel N. Smelling a single component of male sweat alters levels of cortisol in women. *J Neurosci.* 2007 Feb 7;27(6):1261-5.
Yadav H, Jain S, Sinha PR. Antidiabetic effect of probiotic dahl containing Lactobacillus acidophilus and Lactobacillus casei in high fructose fed rats. *Nutrition.* 2007 Jan;23(1):62-8.

Yadav VS, Mishra KP, Singh DP, Mehrotra S, Singh VK. Immunomodulatory effects of curcumin. *Immunopharmacol Immunotoxicol.* 2005;27(3):485-97.

Yamaoka Y. Solid cell nest (SCN) of the human thyroid gland. *Acta Pathol Jpn.* 1973 Aug;23(3):493-506.

Yan YF, Wei YY, Chen YH, Chen MM. Effect of acupuncture on rehabilitation training of child's autism. *Zhongguo Zhen Jiu.* 2007 Jul;27(7):503-5.

Yang HQ, Xie SS, Hu XL, Chen L, Li H. Appearance of human meridian-like structure and acupoints and its time correlation by infrared thermal imaging. *Am J Chin Med.* 2007;35(2):231-40.

Yeager S. *The Doctor's Book of Food Remedies.* Emmaus, PA: Rodale Press, 1998.

Yeung JW. A hypothesis: Sunspot cycles may detect pandemic influenza A in 1700-2000 A.D. *Med Hypotheses.* 2006;67(5):1016-22.

Yokoi S, Ikeya M, Yagi T, Nagai K. Mouse circadian rhythm before the Kobe earthquake in 1995. *Bioelectromagnetics.* 2003 May;24(4):289-91.

Yoshioka M, Doucet E, Drapeau V, Dionne I, Tremblay A. Combined effects of red pepper and caffeine consumption on 24 h energy balance in subjects given free access to foods. *Br J Nutr.* 2001 Feb;85(2):203-11.

Yu XM, Zhu GM, Chen YL, Fang M, Chen YN. Systematic assessment of acupuncture for treatment of herpes zoster in domestic clinical studies. *Zhongguo Zhen Jiu.* 2007 Jul;27(7):536-40.

Yuan SY, Lun X, Liu DS, Qin Z, Chen WT. Acupoint-injection of BCG polysaccharide nuclear acid for treatment of condyloma acuminatum and its immunoregulatory action on the patient. *Zhongguo Zhen Jiu.* 2007 Jun;27(6):407-11.

Zaets VN, Karpov PA, Smertenko PS, Blium IaB. Molecular mechanisms of the repair of UV-induced DNA damages in plants. *Tsitol Genet.* 2006 Sep-Oct;40(5):40-68. Review.

Zamora JL. Chemical and microbiologic characteristics and toxicity of povidone-iodine solutions. *Am J Surg.* 1986 Mar;151(3):400-6.

Zarate G, Gonzalez S, Chaia AP. *Assessing survival of dairy propionibacteria in gastrointestinal conditions and adherence to intestinal epithelia.* Centro de Referencia para Lactobacilos-CONICET. Tucuman, Argentina: Humana Press. 2004.

Zhang C, Popp, F., Bischof, M.(eds.). *Electromagnetic standing waves as background of acupuncture system. Current Development in Biophysics - the Stage from an Ugly Duckling to a Beautiful Swan.* Hangzhou: Hangzhou University Press, 1996.

Zimecki M. The lunar cycle: effects on human and animal behavior and physiology. *Postepy Hig Med Dosw.* 2006;60:1-7.

Zizza, C. The nutrient content of the Italian food supply 1961-1992. *European Journal of Clinical Nutrition.* 1997;51: 259-265.

Zou Z, Li F, Buck L. Odor maps in the olfactory cortex. *Proc Natl Acad of Sci.* 2005;102(May 24):7724-7729.

Index

-compliance